ADVANCES IN LIBRARY ADMINISTRATION AND ORGANIZATION

ADVANCES IN LIBRARY ADMINISTRATION AND ORGANIZATION

Series Editors: Edward D. Garten and
Delmus E. Williams

Recent Volumes:

Volume 1:   Edited by W. Carl Jackson,
                 Bernard Kreissman and Gerard B. McCabe

Volumes 2–12:   Edited by Bernard Kreissman and
                 Gerard B. McCabe

Volumes 13–19:   Edited by Edward D. Garten and
                 Delmus E. Williams

ADVANCES IN LIBRARY ADMINISTRATION
AND ORGANIZATION   VOLUME 20

ADVANCES IN LIBRARY ADMINISTRATION AND ORGANIZATION

EDITED BY

EDWARD D. GARTEN

*Dean of Libraries and Information Services, University of
Dayton, OH, USA*

DELMUS E. WILLIAMS

Dean of University Libraries, University of Akron, OH, USA

2003

JAI
An imprint of Elsevier Science

Amsterdam – Boston – London – New York – Oxford – Paris
San Diego – San Francisco – Singapore – Sydney – Tokyo

ELSEVIER SCIENCE Ltd
The Boulevard, Langford Lane
Kidlington, Oxford OX5 1GB, UK

First edition 2003

Library of Congress Cataloging in Publication Data
A catalogue record from the British Library has been applied for.

ISBN: 0-7623-1010-3
ISSN: 0732-0671 (Series)

⊗ The paper used in this publication meets the requirements of ANSI/NISO Z39.48-1992 (Permanence of Paper).
Printed in The Netherlands.

CONTENTS

vi

INTRODUCTION

Why is it that I hate to admit having more than a little of the "Chicken Little Syndrome" in my approach to management? And why, seeing my secretary place a few new "please call" messages on my desk, more often than not, do I privately agree with satirist Dorothy Parker's candid comment – "What fresh hell is this?" Upon considerable reflection, I'm left with some compelling evidence that, more often than not, when an experienced administrator thinks the sky is falling, the sky may, indeed, be falling. Management is not easy these days. The problems are complex. The answers, when they come, are less prone to satisfy. Such observations are only reinforced by articles like the one that appeared in a mid-August 2002 issue of The Chronicle of Higher Education noting that the average age of the American Library Association's members was 49 and that 68% of library directors planned to retire in 14 years or less. Fewer professionals appear to be positioning themselves for library administration. Perhaps this is not surprising.

Many in our profession are asking whether we will have the number of administratively inclined librarians necessary to step into future library management positions. Often we cite a wealth of anecdotal evidence (gained in the hallways when library directors gather), evidence that suggests that more than a few librarians are bringing different (read: not easily understood) attitudes to the job today. Such individuals, we sometimes suggest among ourselves, are, to our dismay, disinclined to take on the longer hours management roles require. Many even tell us that they simply don't care to deal with the personnel problems that often seem to dominate the contemporary library landscape. It would appear that still others have considerable distaste for the management of either flat or declining budgets. Where is the value to be gained in being an administrator, they ask?

ALA-accredited library school enrollments remain relatively flat with only minor enrollment fluctuations year to year. Fewer applicants for both entry level professional and entry point administrative positions appear to be making themselves available if the preponderance of shallow recruitment pools are to be believed. It is suggested that more of what available library school graduates exist are accepting alternative (and often more lucrative) information management positions, avoiding traditional libraries altogether. Perhaps at least part of the sky is falling. Perhaps we will see more academic libraries run by non-librarians and, perhaps, especially in universities, we will see more libraries subsumed by or incorporated into new organizational models and led by individuals who have not progressed through typical library advancement paths.

Why are many among our library staff so resistant to change? Indeed, why is change viewed as so hard for so many to accept? Why do more and more library administrators feel caught in the middle and frequently relegated to the sidelines in an increasingly more complex and challenging information environment? We could ask a dozen equally difficult questions. The literature in the field continues to address these questions and this volume offers eleven fresh perspectives to practitioners trying to make more sense of the change that daily must be confronted. First off, Gail Bader, William Graves and Jim Nyce offer an ethnographic study of the library as a "real world metaphor." Their contribution examines an important new set of metaphors now employed to reorganize work (or "new work" as they define it). They ask about what keeps library staff from embracing this new work as both an organizational and operational principle. They raise fundamental questions regarding the constructive and empowering possibilities of new forms of change in the workplace, changes that necessarily assume a clear break with the organizational models that have historically defined the library.

Next, José-Marie Griffiths continues her exploration of the role of the chief information officer (CIO) in today's university. A former CIO at the University of Michigan, Griffiths knows well the difficulties this administrative function has encountered over its relatively brief life. She raises the fascinating question of whether universities may have "too many chiefs" given the proliferation of "chief officers for this and chief officers for that." She offers no easy answers to a difficult question, but suggests that all campus executive team administrators must ultimately recommit themselves to a sense of shared responsibility for all areas of the organization, and especially for information technology.

Next up, readers will find an essay by Mary Jane Rootes that explores information ethics from several philosophical perspectives. Given the tragic events of the past year and the subsequent questions surrounding access to information raised by those outside of the profession, Rootes' compelling logic and framework for dialogue will be welcomed. Among the questions she surfaces are ones like this: If withholding information is necessary to secure generic rights – or for that matter any of the moral agents – is it morally correct to do so? Her concern here is to help us discern the moral imperative that should be followed in order to best serve the mission of librarianship.

Recent volumes in this series have offered practical accounts of several leading edge approaches to the support of distance delivered education. New ways of information support are emerging, particularly from the "new genre," entrepreneurial, virtual universities. At the same time, new approaches to the virtual library are emerging in many state university systems. My own recent consultative work with such places as Jones International University, Northcentral University, Walden University, and the North Dakota State University System Online, among others, suggests to me that library managers continue to ask good questions of – and provide strong solutions to – the online learning environment. The next two pieces in this volume present two excellent models of practice. Donna Meyer speaks to the step-by-step approach that her exciting, emerging virtual and doctoral-granting university has taken toward the creation of a broadly conceived virtual library. Harvey Gover, one of the leading lights behind the promulgation of the current ACRL Guidelines for Distance Learning Library Services offers a comprehensive and detailed discussion behind the development and evolution of Washington State University's model for library support of learners working at a distance. As Meyer and Gover both suggest, virtual libraries will continue to grow and change, and globalization of library services will continue to expand to support students' information needs.

Information as an asset is yet another topic that garners healthy debate within our profession. Charles Oppenheim, Joan Stenson and Richard M. S. Wilson from the United Kingdom next offer an intriguing paper that explores many of the issues surrounding the identification of attributes of information and the recognition of these attributes by senior administrators. In the end, they argue that the challenge for library and information professionals is to identify clearly those attributes that can assist managers recognize significant information to improve business performance.

Moving along, John Budd offers a view of the current state of graduate library school management courses. He examines the library management syllabi from a number of graduate library education programs and notes the variability in those course syllabi. Budd contends that, given the ubiquity of management in all organization, there is an urgency in the need to begin conversation about what should constitute solid, practical library management education.

Why do people enter our profession, much less desire administration (which is part and parcel of nearly every librarian's job description today) as an end? The answers are complex, but Bambi Burgard offers considerable insight into those elements that advance choice of profession, especially among women. Burgard argues that the challenge for the library administrator, in the end, becomes one of assisting new professionals who come up against the gap between their career expectations and the reality of the field.

Rush Miller and Sherrie Schmidt, both well experienced library administrators, address the need for more data regarding electronic resources and services. How do we collect such data; how do we make sense of that data? Doubtless, more academic libraries are engaged in cost analysis initiatives or at the minimum are tentatively attempting to analyze their costs in order to present better data when applying for funds or allocating resources. The authors detail the preliminary results from the Association of Research Libraries' New Measures Initiative, an important effort for library administrators who are beginning to manage hybrid libraries that are in transition from a primary focus on print to a primary focus on digital information resources and services.

Roswitha Poll then offers an intriguing summary of a project, sponsored by the German Research Council, wherein a comprehensive, integrated quality management system was developed for academic libraries. Using the Balanced Scorecard, she posits the central premise of the Balanced Scorecard approach: the exploration of different (and sometimes overlapping) quality aspects in separate fashion, while at the same time keeping all of them in full view. We believe this to be an important contribution to an emerging management trend. We conclude the volume with John Harer's Delphi-based study of measures of quality that can be used in applying Continuous Quality Improvement. Harer's work strongly suggests that libraries need to gauge the needs and expectations of their patrons in planning for quality services. Such projects as ARL's LibQUAL+ initiative and other quality assurance measures now being employed by libraries are testaments to the fact that we are seeing an increasing demand that we determine how well we are doing that can only bode well for our future.

With this volume, Del Williams and I bring to a score an annual series that has achieved a minor milestone in library science publishing history despite its editorially-acknowledged (and sometimes privately celebrated eclecticism). We heartedly thank JAI and Elsevier Science for their confidence in the value of this series and offer our sincere appreciation to the nearly 200 contributors who have been published in these pages since 1982.

Edward D. Garten
Co-Editor

CHOICE, RESPONSIBILITY AND WORK: RHETORIC IN A UNIVERSITY LIBRARY REORGANIZATION

Gail E. Bader, William Graves III and James M. Nyce

However men may analyze their experiences within any domain, they inevitably know and understand them best by referring them to other domains for elucidation. It is in that metaphoric cross-referencing of domains, perhaps, that culture is integrated, providing us with the sensation of wholeness. And perhaps the best index of cultural integration or disintegration, or of genuineness or spuriousness in culture for that matter, is the degree to which men can feel the aptness of each other's metaphors (Fernandez, 1986, p. 25).

INTRODUCTION

Fernandez knew, as did Kenneth Burke to whom Fernandez owed so much, that the fundamental human problem of maintaining what he elsewhere called the "inchoate sense of wholeness" was critically linked to the never-ending dilemma of "the degree to which men can feel the aptness of each other's metaphors." And since the publication of "Persuasions and Performances" nearly 30 years ago, a great deal of anthropological, sociological and historical work on "power and resistance," "hegemony," and "cultural reproduction and change" can be usefully framed as particular responses to a number of fundamental questions implicit in Fernandez' quote – When, and under what types of conditions, does any particular "metaphor" or "trope" serve to promote cooperation and social integration? When, and under what types of conditions, does it serve to promote conflict and social

Advances in Library Administration and Organization
Advances in Library Administration and Organization, Volume 20, 1–16
© 2003 Published by Elsevier Science Ltd.
ISSN: 0732-0671/PII: S0732067102200012

disintegration? When and how is the "aptness" of any given "metaphor" or "trope" lost? We believe these to be among the most central, enduring questions in the Human Sciences.

This paper will begin to examine an important new set of tropes that are being employed to re-organize work in a research library once again. These new tropes argue for and rationalize the re-organization of middle-class, professional work in ways that can be seen, depending on one's perspective, to liberate the individual's potential for creative work in a bureaucratic organization and to give free rein to individual initiative or to de-skill professional work practices, routinize such practices, or even to eliminate jobs completely.

We have just begun this study and much important ground remains to be covered, so in this paper we will focus quite specifically and, admittedly narrowly, on the institutional rhetoric of the "change agent," an individual whose official job it is to guide the changes occurring in the re-organization of work at this research library. What follows, then, represents our initial analyses of a number of open-ended, in-depth interviews with several key administrators against the background of our independent readings of an extensive set of recent "strategic planning" documents the library has provided us with. This is a critical starting point for our entire on-going study, for the rhetoric of the "change agent" clearly represents the present authoritative voice of strategic planning in this institution.

OUR FIRST ETHNOGRAPHIC STUDY: THE LIBRARY AS COMPUTER METAPHOR

The 1980s was a decade in which the imagination and attention of the U.S. middle-class was virtually consumed by utopian visions and dystopian nightmares of a "computer revolution" or, as some chose to call it, "an information technology revolution." In 1987 when we first studied change in the Brown University Library system, the Library was attempting to create and implement a multi-functional computer system (JOSIAH) that was supposed to seamlessly integrate all information, all staff, all units, all work and all library users (Graves & Bader, 1987). The envisioned all-encompassing technical functionality of the "computer" then became, as it did in a great number of different institutional settings throughout America in the 1980s, the "apt" rhetorical figure for planning, discussing and debating future definitions of information, library management, professional functions and staff work. "The library as computer," the Library of the 21st century, we heard again and again, would be a radically different type of institution because of "computerization."

During our research in the Library in the mid-1980s, perceptions and feelings of inexorable, accelerating "change" were voiced at all levels of the institution. Indeed, the fundamental "dilemma" was how the library was to deal with "change" – accelerating change in information technologies, change in the publishing industries, change in academic fields of knowledge, change in the library profession, change in library users' needs and interests, and change in the world at large. And when we did our first study, the metaphor of the LIBRARY AS COMPUTER seemed to provide necessary, fruitful and "apt" ways of responding to the perceived and felt "dilemmas" of rapid "change" at all levels of the organization. It did so by strategically calling attention to the need to focus on key aspects of the internal organization of the library itself.

However, as we carefully documented in that first study, the metaphor of the LIBRARY AS COMPUTER eventually became a contested trope within the library system. But what came to be contested was not the metaphor itself, but the degree to which the metaphor was perceived as "apt." And this took the form of debates concerning the appropriate enactment of that metaphor in redefining the organization and nature of routine work practices within the library. In essence, the fundamental, implicit question informing these debates was – *Is this specific metaphor "apt" because it predicates centralization and the technocratic rationalization of library work or because it predicates decentralization and increasing autonomy throughout the work place?* We have covered that history and those issues more thoroughly in previous publications (Graves, 1995, 2000; Graves & Bader, 1987), so we will not discuss them here. We only wish to underscore the key point that this institutional metaphor served quite powerfully to frame and channel institutional debates over the enactment of the metaphor itself in changing the library and the nature of work within the library.

OUR CURRENT RESTUDY: THE LIBRARY AS REAL WORLD METAPHOR

Thirteen years later we returned to the Brown University Library. We found that the formal institutional structure and the definition of work had changed very little since our last study. Now, however, we found the library in the midst of a new, even more ambitious wave of planning for reorganization and change. However, the dominant, compelling "computer" tropes about which we had heard so much had lost a great deal of their previous "aptness." Indeed, in our first key interviews with the Library's computer-systems staff, our questions about the role of "computerization" were turned away decisively, almost impatiently – "JOSIAH (the centralized library computer-system) is *just* a tool now." Once the major institutional metaphor for dealing with all fundamental questions of continuity and change, JOSIAH was now "JUST a tool," a taken-for-granted feature of the organization of information and work within the library. Apparently, the "computer revolution" was over.

If anything, thirteen years later the traditional perceptions of and feelings about "change" have become even more acute. The new planning for major reorganization of the library system is ever more driven by what university librarians and staff see now as "extraordinary" changes occurring in their environment, their professional community, their institutions and their client base. For librarians, while financial, political and demographic changes are an understood part of this, the most important issue seems to be perceptions of the increasing rate at which change is occurring (Shaughnessy, 1996).

Nevertheless, the speed with which change is occurring is still often talked about in reference to technology. Its perceived *pervasiveness* as a medium for information transfer in all sectors of society and its perceived *ubiquity* as a generalized work tool are felt to be blurring formal distinctions and divisions within library work itself. In response to these general perceptions of the rate of inexorable change and its link to the pervasiveness and ubiquity of new technologies, university libraries have begun to shift their focus away from their local holdings, storage and the organization of information to issues of "global access" and the provision of electronic and online forms of information and services to library patrons.

However, managing this shift from "local storage" to "global access" is now understood as requiring university libraries "to do more" than just address their own institutional "needs." Now the focus should be on customers and clients and their "satisfaction," but this, it is believed, will require a fundamental rethinking of library organization. From this will emerge a client-centered restructuring of what a university library is, how library staff positions are defined and organized, and how staff work is to be accomplished within the library.

The once dominant metaphor LIBRARY AS COMPUTER has lost its perceived "aptness" in these new considerations. As the shift from a focus on local storage to a focus on global access has come to dominate deliberations about how to deal with the "accelerating pace of change," a new set of tropes has recently emerged to replace the older LIBRARY AS COMPUTER metaphor. The new organizing metaphor is the LIBRARY AS REAL WORLD and in radical contrast to the previous LIBRARY AS COMPUTER metaphor, this new metaphor strategically calls attention to the perceived need to remove all internal divisions and external walls that separate the institution of the library from the "real world" of the *vividly imagined* free-ranging, unfettered, independent library patron.

Just as the LIBRARY AS COMPUTER metaphor should be understood as a particular institutional refraction of the broader middle-class enchantment with the "computer revolution" in the 1980s, we think the LIBRARY AS REAL WORLD metaphor should be understood as a particular institutional refraction of the contemporary widespread appeal of the dominant corporate rhetoric of "reengineering" or "reinventing" the corporation, "flattening hierarchy," "team-building," "participatory management," and a host of other closely related *corporate solutions* to the perceived dilemmas of change.

But what we find most striking and most significant about this shift from the metaphor of LIBRARY AS COMPUTER to the LIBRARY AS REAL WORLD is the extent to which the authoritative institutional rhetoric we outline below incorporates strong ideological claims about normative connections among notions of "choice," "responsibility" and "self" in the "real world" of contemporary American life. And it is these types of claims, we fully anticipate, that will become the new "contested terrain" over the degree to which the LIBRARY AS REAL WORLD metaphor will be perceived as "apt" for dealing with the perceived dilemmas of current accelerating change.

THE "OLD" LIBRARY AND THE "NEW" LIBRARY

The Brown University Library's reorganization at present is more talked about than enacted. It is a "strategic plan" for reorganization. Given this, what follows is an attempt to excavate the authoritative institutional rhetoric that defines how reorganization is currently understood, what it should be and what it should achieve.

In the remaining sections of this paper, we examine the rhetoric of the Library's designated "change agent" in order to understand what, exactly, will remove all internal divisions and external walls that separate the institution of the library from the "real world" of the *vividly imagined* free-ranging, unfettered, independent library patron. In particular, we will look at how notions of work, authority and institution are being redefined in the library's current reorganization efforts. To do this, we will focus on how the individual (here called Joanne) tasked by the University Librarian to help bring the library into the 21st century talks about work, the workplace and authority in both the "old" and the "new" library.

THE LIBRARY AS "PROTECTED ARENA"

The rhetorical contrast between the "real world" and the contemporary workplace is critically important to understanding the Brown University reorganization plan. According to Joanne, the problem with the way the workplace is currently organized is that it is "a protected arena" in marked contrast to the "real world."

In the "real world," she argues, adults are held accountable for their actions and decisions. For example, if an individual fails to pay his/her taxes, that individual, and no one else, is responsible. Her aim for the staff, as she phrases it, is for "everybody [to] act like an adult."

Reorganization is necessary, first and foremost, because the workplace is a "protected arena." And within this "protected arena," Joanne claims, staff are not able to act like adults because, as the workplace is currently organized, there is always someone "higher up" who can assume ultimate authority for a decision. At the same time, it is the formal division of labor within this "protected arena" that allows individuals to escape the consequences of their own actions by shifting responsibility to other individuals. In Joanne's eyes, it is this institutionally mandated lack of responsibility for one's own decisions that, in effect, reduces library staff to children. And children, of course, are not legally responsible for their own decisions.

This lack of responsibility in the workplace is contrasted with the responsibility she claims is demanded by the "real world." In life outside of work, adults are held by middle class Americans to be responsible for their own actions and decisions. As Joanne said to us, "I have to pay my bills myself, work should be like real life. Where do I go to [when I can't pay my own bills]." It is this lack of responsibility for our actions that makes workers into children. It is also this lack of responsibility that marks the work currently being done in the research library as "old work."

Joanne constantly refers to the current work in the Library as the "old work." And, from the perspective of strategic plans for reorganization, "old work" entails a number of undesirable characteristics. First, "old work" is work that is defined for one by someone else. Managers, unions, the canons of professionalism, and even individual patrons currently define for the staff member the work that is to be done. Thus, externally imposed objectives and goals define and shape the nature of the work staff members routinely accomplish.

In this "protected arena," waiting for someone else to define objectives or subordinating one's actions to externally defined goals essentially removes choice and the consequences of choice for individual staff members. This "waiting," in fact, is the hallmark of the "old work." Whether we consider the case of staff members waiting for patrons to come to them with problems, or waiting for directives from superiors, or accepting without question union or professional definitions of "the job," "old work" means work defined for one by others.

"NEW WORK" AND THE LIBRARY AS "REAL WORLD"

The workplace, Joanne claims, should be like the real world. As she says, "The principles of real life should be the principles of the workplace." There is no one outside of work who mediates our decisions. There is no "boss" or "higher up" to take the responsibility for an adult who makes a poor choice. If you fail to make the "right" choices, you pay the consequences. There, the middle class seems to believe, is no one else to "check" your choices or to ultimately take responsibility for your life choices. Joanne insists that the workplace should reflect these same conditions precisely because the conditions of the "real world" are real, commonsensical and "natural." Unmediated decisions, unconstrained by external structures and impositions, are what we, as individuals, should aspire to in the workplace. And this is because, in the real world, with its lack of mediators, individuals are defined and evaluated in terms of how they enact choice, exercise autonomy, and accept responsibility. Furthermore, because these conditions "bring out" creative and adult behavior in individuals in the "real world," such conditions should also inform the workplace.

The "old work" of the library organization must be replaced by the "new work," according to Joanne. The staff member should not simply "respond" to patron's needs, superior's directives or institutional structures. The staff member should be proactive and take the initiative. Thus, for example, the appropriate model of "new work" for staff members in Public Services would be that of a counselor, an interviewer, or a salesperson, not a passive information source at a help desk.

In the "old work," library staff responded to patrons' requests for assistance in using the resources of the library. But, in the "new work," library staff will take the lead in determining what patrons actually need. Thus, in contrast to the "old work," the "new work" does not recognize the boundaries and constraints legitimized by contractual, ideological or formal organizational definitions of work. "New work" will require that individual staff members take the initiative in redefining their own positions and choosing their own tasks.

"New work," then, will also require that individual staff members actually take the initiative in redefining institutional order. "Hierarchy does not serve us well when we want to initiate responsibility," argued Joanne. In fact, she continues, the formal organization of work in the library actually restrains staff from realizing their potential as active, creative individuals. According to Joanne, "You need structure, but it doesn't have to be hierarchy. [It can be based], not on position, but on competence, knowledge, skills, and so forth."

This rhetoric can be seen at work in the library's detailed strategic plans for reorganization. The plans call for replacing traditional elements of departmental structure and authority with very generally defined "task-forces" that have such general functions as "access and delivery," "scholarly resources" and "organizational support," for example. In keeping with the desirable characteristics and definitions of the "new work," individual staff members will choose, on the basis of their self-defined interests and claimed competencies, the "task-forces" they wish to belong to. In this way, traditional formal bureaucratic organization will be dramatically reduced, if not done away with completely, by the individual's own initiative, choice and acceptance of responsibility.

This rhetoric also underwrites major changes in the way the Library will form major administrative committees and special ad hoc task forces. In the "old library" under the strictures of the "old work," individual staff members were assigned to such committees on the basis of professional credentials, position in the hierarchy and departmental representation. In the "new library" with the advent of the "new work," such committees will be based, not on organizational criteria, but on the individual interests and competencies of specific staff members. Individual staff members will volunteer for committees, rather than be assigned to these by supervisors or department heads.

WHAT KEEPS THE LIBRARY STAFF FROM EMBRACING THE "NEW WORK?"

Why is it nearly impossible to do "new work" in today's library organization? According to the change agent, staff are currently constrained in two ways: they are constrained by traditional ideologies of work and by the role middle management plays in the organization. We will begin by looking at the ways Joanne views ideologies as constraining library staff from realizing their potential.

Staff's (over)identification with professional library work is one thing Joanne would like to change. Professionals have a fairly clear view of what constitutes the nature of their work. Professional work is defined through years of schooling and a focus on the "creative" aspects of their work, creative work that requires the independent judgment of a knowledgeable expert. In particular, they have a fairly clear set of understandings about what constitutes clerical or routine work in contrast to professional or knowledge-based work.

While professional work would seem, by definition, to fit into the category of "new work," it does not for the change agent. Professionalism, as Joanne frames it, is an artificial ideology that pre-defines the kind of work staff is supposed to do. This is an arbitrary, externally imposed boundary, Joanne argues, and it removes the ability to define work from the individual. In so doing, it keeps staff from realizing their full potential as adults. Not surprisingly, in fact, Joanne's own career exemplifies this. Even though she does not have a professional library degree, Joanne has moved up the hierarchy through positions in a number of library departments. At present, she is very near the top of the institutional hierarchy. She reports directly to the University Librarian.

For Joanne, unions pose the same problems as professionalism. Unions limit their members from realizing their full potential by defining the nature and kind of work they can do according to contractual agreements and categories. Unions bundle certain tasks into "jobs," allocate jobs, define workplace conditions and organize workplace relationships. In so doing, unions limit individual choice and potential by removing staff's ability to shape their own work.

The problem with both professionalism and unionism is that they are imposed ideological statements about work and its relation to self. More to the point, they do not reflect the "real world, i.e. life" outside the workplace. Like hierarchy then, these conventional structures arbitrarily constrain the individual and his or her potential in the workplace. But these ideologies are not the only things that currently limit staff's ability to perform the "new work." Staff is also constrained by the organization of work and work relations that have created middle management.

Middle management is a key obstacle to staff's ability to undertake the "new work." With the introduction of new technologies, middle management has lost their role as mediators between upper management and staff. Middle management, by the very nature of their jobs as "approvers" and "communicators" between staff and upper management, prevent staff from acting like creative self-actualizing adults. In their role as "authorities" who can legitimize action, they rob staff of their ability to make decisions and to act on their own initiative. "The problem is that hierarchy lets someone else decide [what you have to do]." After all, if one is only doing what one was allowed to do, staff is reduced to following orders. Their ability to act on their own is limited.

Middle management, as seen by Joanne, represents much of what is wrong with today's workplace. As mediators, middle managers interfere with staff's (natural) ability to act, make choices, accept responsibility for their choices and act autonomously. Middle management reduces staff autonomy. They constrain, stand in the way of, and interfere with natural choice and action on the part of the individual. In short, staff are trapped in an organization that allows them only to follow orders and directives.

THE CHANGE AGENT'S VISION OF MIDDLE-CLASS WORK

How should the workplace be organized, according to the change agent? The most desirable situation is to make the workplace as much like the "real world" as possible. In the real world we find no unnatural organizational structures or ideologies that rob individuals of their ability to make choices. In the real world individuals are free agents. They make their own choices and forge their own destinies. In short, library staff should be like Americans in their "real life," their non-work world.

Without the unnatural structures and ideologies of the workplace, library staff can be creative and realize their full potential because there is no one to tell them what they should or should not do. Given this, their actions both are products of and reflect an authentic self. This must be the shape of the new work and the new library.

To enable the "new work" we must get rid of the old organization. Rather than attempting to negotiate hierarchy and structure, Joanne believes that we should abandon structure. Joanne sees structure, not as just superordinate and imposed, but as "unnatural." It keeps us from realizing our potential as creative, responsible individuals. By "dissolving" hierarchy and structure, institutions will both valorize and emerge from the unmediated, individual actions and choices. Most importantly, the very key to "dissolving" hierarchy and structure is empowering individuals to take the initiative, define their own choices and accept the consequences of those choices.

These are the conditions that will bring about the "new work." Work and real life currently have little in common, according to Joanne, but they should have everything in common. Library staff must be persuaded to do at work what they naturally do in real life. If the staff members will accept the commonality between the real world and work and rid themselves of limiting ideologies, hierarchy and structure will be seen as irrelevant, mere impediments to self-actualization, and will ultimately wither away.

THE CHALLENGE OF THE NEW METAPHOR
LIBRARY AS REAL WORLD

What we find remarkable about this new metaphor is that it practically negates the previous LIBRARY AS COMPUTER metaphor. That older institutional metaphor established the framework for debates about the appropriate and proper relationships between routine work practices and the traditional formal organizational structures and divisions that defined the library. On the one hand, this older metaphor was used to argue the primacy and precedence of rational, formal organizational structures over irrational, unruly, irregular routine work practices that needed to be rationally ordered. On the other hand, by bringing the disjunctures between formal organizational structures and irrational, unruly, irregular work practices into sharper focus, this same metaphor also enabled staff members to reclaim those same "irrational, unruly and irregular" work practices as embodying the "real" and enduring systematic logic of the organization of work within the library, a logic which should drive, not be driven by, fundamental organizational change (Graves, 1995).

However, the new LIBRARY AS REAL WORLD metaphor radically reframes the debates about organizational change by bringing the individual into sharp focus while simultaneously pushing the traditional formal organizational structures and divisions far into the background. Within the framework of the LIBRARY AS COMPUTER metaphor, the formal characteristics of the organization itself were submitted to intense scrutiny. Now, within the framework of the LIBRARY AS REAL WORLD, the characteristics of the person will be submitted to the same intense scrutiny.

As the Library proceeds with its planned reorganization, what is bound to be contested within the framework of this new metaphor will be the perceived nature of the connections among choice, action, and the notion of the self at work in the library setting. However, in the rhetoric of the change agent and in the general strategic plans for reorganization, we see that the fundamental solution to the perceived need for reorganization rests on a very clear set of assumptions about the nature and significance of the connections among choice, action and the self.

The rhetoric of this reorganization effort makes an explicit link between "right" choice, "legitimate" action, and an "adult" notion of self. What bridges and links them is a direct, unmediated appeal to "individual responsibility." In this way, the rhetoric of the change agent gives us a remarkably clear and simple picture of how choice, action and self can so often "go together" in just such a common-sense, taken-for-granted way in American culture. Furthermore, the persuasiveness of this particular rhetoric of the connection of choice-action-self is that it has the power to make hierarchy "go away" by redefining it in such a way that it literally disappears into the background and, finally, totally out of view.

It is worth noting, of course, that whatever else these reorganization efforts achieve, hierarchy and structure do not "go away." And this, of course, is bound to create specific problems for the "change agent" and the plans for reorganization. Nevertheless, for middle class Americans, what these efforts at reorganization offer is an opportunity to rewrite what hierarchy and structure mean in the workplace – about the only place where Americans today "believe" there is structure that is, to some limited extent, necessary.

What these reorganization efforts (and the rhetoric that accompanies them) do is move these terms away from a strictly sociological reading in which power, class and structure overlap. The result is that, for the middle class, these issues are literally taken off the table. The end result is that hierarchy and structure are being rewritten in the most compelling and convincing of American terms – in reference to the autonomous, voluntaristic self.

POSTSCRIPT: QUESTIONS FROM THE
LIBRARY FLOOR

We are witnessing a radical redefinition of conceptions of library organization throughout the United States. The Brown University Library System is hardly unique in this respect. As the dominant metaphor of THE LIBRARY AS COMPUTER, so characteristic of the 1980s and 1990s, yields to the 21st century metaphor of THE LIBRARY AS REAL WORLD, fundamental questions about the relationship between new technologies and the organization of library work have been overshadowed by a host of new questions about the relationship between user needs and the skills, and the knowledge and creativity required of each library staff member.

As we have attempted to show in this paper, the traditional functional and structural principles of "collections maintenance" are clearly perceived as the primary obstacles to forging a new dynamic, fluid relationship between the require-ments of addressing user needs and the demands of coordinating the human resources of the library. And it is assumed that a more suitable set of organizational principles will emerge through time from a new strategic focus on user needs, rather than management of the collections. In time, it is assumed, traditional hierarchies, formal channels of communication and reporting, authority and responsibility based on the distinction between "professional" and "support" staff and functional divisions all will be recast radically as individual staff members voluntarily transform their work routines to better serve the needs of library users. Thus, the fundamental purpose of the strategic plan has been to establish the appropriate conditions to set this "transformation" into motion. In turn, this would empower staff to assume "stewardship of the library."

In point of fact, this revolutionary strategic plan follows rather closely the logic and basic principles of well-known and popular corporate models for reorganization, including "total quality management," "policy management," "process management" and "just-in-time management," among others. All of these corporate models call for reorganization based on detailed, continuous assessment of changing client and customer needs, team-building, "just-in-time" organizational responsiveness, and a fundamental commitment to maintaining a flexible, goal-oriented organizational framework based on continuous assessment and development of individual skills, knowledge and core competencies.

A question all this raises is – *how have non-administrative professional and support staff responded to this new strategic vision?* In the months following our examination and analysis of the strategic plan itself, we have interviewed a number of non-administrative staff in the Technical Services and Public Services divisions of the library in an attempt to understand general staff perceptions of both recent changes and plans for future changes. Many of our interviewees have worked in this library for more than 15 years, and several of them first introduced us to the problems and prospects of technology and change in the library in the mid-1980s.

These research activities will continue. Thus, in what follows, we make no claims to a comprehensive assessment of staff perceptions of the strategic planning process. We also do not presume to make policy recommendations to the library administrators who have developed and managed this "process" and who understand the long-term goals of the library far better than we do. Instead, here we choose the much more limited goal of providing a preliminary sketch of some of the basic issues and concerns about reorganization being expressed and, in some cases debated, on the floor of the library today. In this way, we hope to highlight some of the more difficult problems embedded in the logic of the strategic planning process itself.

One of the most commonly expressed concerns is the definition and operationalization of the notion of "user needs" itself. This, of course, is a traditional problem that has generated a significant amount of empirical library research over the years. That it continues to be a very difficult problem was clearly revealed in an interview with one Department Head. In the course of that interview, she described her attempts to follow-up on survey data provided to the staff by the Library's standing "User-Needs Team." The data clearly documented basic faculty and student dissatisfaction with the quality of holdings in one specific area of the collections –

> I felt I really had to go myself to the faculty and grad students and ask them to explain WHY they were 'dissatisfied' with the collections.

To her surprise, she was unable to get the faculty and grad students to be more specific and she drew the following conclusion from her meeting with them –

> Oh, you know it really shows how difficult it is dealing with 'user-needs.' That's why the patrons need librarians. All too often they are really not terribly clear about exactly what those needs are.

This is neither a new problem nor an unfamiliar one to library staff. However, the traditional organization of the library subordinated this problem to the routine needs of managing the collections. To put it simply, "user needs" were traditionally defined and operationalized in terms of the routine, ongoing "needs" of the collections.

The new strategic plan, however, seeks to invert the priorities. As the Library's Change Agent clearly articulated this in one interview –

> We need to be starting with the needs of the end-user and then working backwards, rather than what we now do, which is to start with materials and work forward to the end-user.

However, this is a daunting challenge for most library staff, who are, in effect, being asked to envision new ways of defining, identifying and serving end-user needs, freed now from the traditional considerations attendant upon management of the collections. In fact, a number of "process workshops" have been held to stimulate library staff to "brainstorm" about just these issues and so lay the foundations for the emergence of new work teams, interest groups and collaboratives.

Our interviews, however, have so far indicated a basic sense among rank-and-file library staff that the ultimate responsibility for operationalizing new notions of "end-user needs" and forming work collaboratives to meet those needs should rest with the top administrators of the library, not with the staff. More than one of our interviewees expressed the following sentiments –

> There has been too much emphasis put on making sure the reorganization is perfect before actually implementing it. I disagree completely. I do not understand why they don't just do it – just form the work groups. The problem here is that there has been so much talk, so much discussion, so much planning, that I feel the staff are suspicious and wary. I think they feel that there is a hidden agenda. I think they believe that the REAL PLAN is hidden and that they are being maneuvered into accepting something that in the long-run is NOT going to be in their interests.

It is important to note that this particular staff member does *not* believe that there is a "hidden agenda" waiting to ambush the staff. In point of fact, we find no clear evidence to suggest any "hidden agenda." Furthermore, extrapolating from our interview data, it seems apparent that only a small number of staff actually suspect a "hidden agenda."

Nevertheless, two things are clearly being contested on the floor. The first is the perceived vagueness and absence of any operational definition of "end-user needs," upon which the reorganization itself is widely understood to depend. The second concerns more general notions of "accountability" and "responsibility" at the very heart of the foundational principles of the strategic plan for reorganization.

As we have discussed at length in this paper, the "new work" of the new library is based on the assumption that individual staff members should take the initiative in defining their own positions and in choosing their own routine tasks. In the Change Agent's view, it is the "old" organizational structure and "corporate culture" of the library that imposes severe constraints on the abilities of individual staff members to take these initiatives.

The logical problem, as we have noted, is that hierarchy and structure do not just disappear. More importantly, from the perspective of most library staff, hierarchy and structure do much more than constrain or limit "change." They also constitute enabling mechanisms for rendering "change" intelligible, manageable and acceptable. Thus, the difficulty with the Change Agent's view of hierarchy and structure in relationship to individual initiative is that it ignores the equally important enabling functions of hierarchy and structure.

Stark reminders of this classic sociological principle are reflected in a number of our interviews with individual staff members. After clearly acknowledging the need for new changes in the library, one Department Head reflected on her own perceptions of the consequences of "change" as defined by the strategic plan –

> We're all trying to change. I am the Department Head, so I could certainly say that being Department Head has clearly defined responsibilities and I don't NEED or WANT to be involved in any initiatives or projects that are not clearly part of my Department. *But that is the old way of thinking.* So I myself do a lot of different things and am involved in a lot of different initiatives that really go beyond the traditional definition of Department Head . . . But, you know, I have mixed feelings. Sometimes I feel that I am involved in too much. I feel fragmented. Sometimes I feel like I'm becoming a jack-of-all-trades and probably not good at any of them. Maybe I'm not as good a Department Head as I should be.

After further ambivalent reflections on the new mandate for "change," she added the following –

> I really do understand why so many staff just don't want to get involved in taking new initiatives and getting involved in library-wide interest groups. Some just want to do the jobs they were hired to do and go home. Some just don't want to get involved in anything they feel goes beyond their expertise, interests or jobs. Some just feel that they want to concentrate on their jobs and become better at those jobs. I really do understand how many feel about this. It's difficult.

This Department Head's candid and open reflections on "change" underscore two important points, echoed in a number of our other interviews. First, she fully acknowledges the need for change in the organizational structure and in the traditional "corporate culture" of the library. In all of our past and present work in the library, in fact, we have very rarely found any direct resistance to or outright rejection of change. In point of fact, library staff have always insisted that change in the library is constant, yet manageably incremental and fairly smooth. Overall, we have consistently found that library staff welcome change and fiercely resent all suggestions to the contrary.

Second, the very real sense of "mixed feelings," "being fragmented," and the fear that "Maybe I'm not as good a Department Head as I should be" follows not from the experience of change itself, but, we would argue, from dealing with visions of change that have become radically disconnected from the critical counterbalancing mechanisms of continuity in the institutional history. This raises yet another key difficulty in the philosophy of the strategic plan – the library cannot be divested of its own history and structure any more than it can be divested of its permanent and growing collections.

The type of "anomie" so clearly expressed by this Department Head in this instance does not, of course, characterize the experience of all staff in the library.

Perhaps, in fact, it characterizes only a few. Nonetheless, such a case does raise fundamental questions about new strategies for change that assume a radical break.

REFERENCES

Fernandez, J. (1986). Persuasions and performances: Of the beast in every body and the metaphors of everyman. In: *Persuasions and Performances: The Play of Tropes in Culture*. Indiana University Press.

Graves, W. III, & Bader, G. E. (1987). *The library as information system: Aspects of continuity and change in the staff's world. IRIS Technical Report Series, Nr. 87–7*. Brown University.

Graves, W. III. (2000). Instrumentalism and the social consequences of technological choice. In: G. L. Carter (Ed.), *Empirical Approaches to Sociology* (3rd ed.). Allyn & Bacon.

Graves, W. III. (1995). Ideologies of computerization. In: M. Shields (Ed.), *The Social Construction of Academic Work and Technology*. Erlbaum Press.

Shaughnessy, T. W. (1996). Lessons from restructuring the library. *Journal of Academic Librarianship, 22*, 251–256.

THE EVOLVING ROLE OF CHIEF INFORMATION OFFICERS IN HIGHER EDUCATION[☆]

José-Marie Griffiths

INTRODUCTION

During the 1980s, as organizational uses of information technology (IT) increased in both number of users and amount of use, and as more technology options presented themselves, organizations began to appoint senior personnel as "technology czars." For executives outside the IT industry, particularly those focused on other aspects of running an enterprise (various business units, finance, human resources, etc.), the IT world seemed to be chaotic, out of control and full of terminological confusion. IT budgets and expenditures were growing rapidly and demands for service continued to increase both in scale and scope. Meanwhile organizational IT units seemed unresponsive, and curiously resistant to change. Central IT units in universities seemed stuck in the mainframe culture of home-grown, customized system development and controlled access at a time when distributed client-server computing offered the promise of low cost, local control and agility. As a result, many local IT support units evolved throughout academic institutions, placing even greater demand on scarce institutional resources and fuelling the potentially explosive tension between central administrative and local authority.

☆This article is based on "Role of the CIO in Universities." In: M. Drake (Ed.), Encyclopedia of Library and Information Science. New York: Marcel Dekker, Inc., 2001. Copyright of this original entry is owned exclusively by Marcel Dekker, Inc. url: http://www.dekker.com/index.jsp.

Advances in Library Administration and Organization
Advances in Library Administration and Organization, Volume 20, 17–36
© 2003 Published by Elsevier Science Ltd.
ISSN: 0732-0671/PII: S0732067102200024

The evolving strategic nature of IT decisions, the growing and unresolved tension between central and distributed IT, and the seemingly endless demand for additional resources necessitated the development of the "technology czar" role. Academic institutions differed in their view of the designated "IT person." Some institutions saw the role as focused exclusively on IT, others began to view information and supporting technologies as a strategic asset and created positions with broader responsibilities such as libraries, institutional research and strategic planning. Some appointed a Vice President, Vice Chancellor or a Vice Provost; others began to use the actual title of Chief Information Officer (CIO); yet others use various Director titles. But all of these positions had in common the notion of a single point of responsibility for information technology (sometimes information *and* technology) for the institution.

CHIEF INFORMATION OFFICERS – THE ROLE EVOLVES

The first designated "technology czars" were appointed to resolve a variety of IT problems. Woodsworth (1988) identified four reasons for establishing such positions in higher education: fiscal control; fears that decentralized purchasing of IT would lead to chaos and incompatibility; a sense of need for coordination and leverage; and the desire of executives and senior administrators to consolidate reporting lines. In an excellent overview of the first ten years of evolution of the CIO role, Penrod, Dolence and Douglas (1990) report that two factors were frequently cited in the literature as rationales for establishing a CIO function: dissatisfaction with current information systems management, performance, productivity or investments; and acknowledgement by the CEO that information is a strategic resource significant enough to warrant executive-level attention. They also state that the earliest CIO functions in higher education tended to reflect the strategic focus rather than the operational one.

Early CIO appointments tended to be accompanied by a restructuring of central administration IT units (typically, administrative computing or MIS, academic computing, and telecommunications (data and/or voice)) into a single central unit. If the CIO's responsibility extended beyond IT per se, the IT unit and other organizations tended to remain separate units reporting to the same CIO. Unfortunately during these reorganizations, the question of the relationship between central and local IT units tended to be pushed aside as CIOs focused on the differing cultures of administrative and academic computing, the evolution of campus networks, the growing use of personal computers, the need to upgrade or replace legacy systems, and the opportunities presented by large enterprise-wide administrative systems, to name but a few issues.

A VARIETY OF CIO MODELS EMERGE

The need for and definition of the CIO function in higher education depends on the way institutions and, perhaps more accurately, the executive leadership of institutions, view the role of IT in the institution. Fleit (1988) categorized institutions according to three IT perspectives that led to differing views of the CIO role. The first group of institutions has a strategic view of IT as key to their long-term success. These institutions tended to be early adopters in creating CIO positions reporting to the institutional CEO (President, Chancellor or Provost). The dominant roles of the CIO in these institutions relate to strategy and architecture, the sphere of influence is within and beyond the institution, and key responsibilities are leadership and the search for new opportunities. The second group of institutions has an operational view of IT. While acknowledging that IT is important, it plays a supporting role in improving institutional efficiency and effectiveness. These institutions have directors of computing organization(s) who typically report to a Vice President or Assistant/Associate Vice President. The dominant role they play is as the custodian of machines and data, their sphere of influence is within the computing unit, and their key responsibility is operational efficiency. The third group, thought to be the largest at the time, was confused by the role of IT in the strategic development of the institution. These institutions have senior IT officers who report to a Vice President or Vice Chancellor. The dominant role they play is to solve all technology-related problems, typically without other senior administrator involvement. Their sphere of influence is within defined technology areas, and their key responsibilities are the coordination and integration of diverse areas.

Three surveys of academic CIOs conducted between 1986 and 2001 reveal some interesting patterns and trends. While these surveys were not based on formal statistical samples and tend to have small sample sizes, the results nevertheless convey a general idea of the position and role of the CIO in academe. Woodsworth (1988) surveyed 28 CIOs in research universities; Penrod et al. (1990) 58 CIOs identified from CAUSE and EDUCOM national conference attendance lists and referrals, and Cain (2001) 150 CIOs through an informal survey. They found that CIOs report to various executives in academic institutions as shown in Table 1. There seems to

Table 1.　Proportion of CIOs Reporting to Various Executives.

Reports to:	Woodsworth (1986–1987) $n = 28$	Penrod et al. (1989) $n = 58$	Cain (2001) $n = 150$
President	29%	40%	30%
CAO/President	36%	19%	41%
CFO	25%	36%	21%

Table 2. Proportion of CIOs with Responsibility for Various Units.

Responsibility	Woodsworth (1986–1987) $n = 28$	Penrod et al. (1989) $n = 58$	Cain (2001) $n = 150$
Academic Computing	89%	86%	97%
Administrative Computing	71%	90%	96%
Telecommunications	79%	data 97%, voice 69%	79%
Library	14%	16%	20%

be a similar proportion of CIOs reporting to a President, Academic Vice President or Provost, and Chief Financial Officer. Differences in the proportions most likely reflect the different samples. However, it does appear that by 1989, CIOs tended to report to the President or CFO much more than to the Chief Academic Officer, and by 2001 they tended to report to the President or Chief Academic Officer. This trend may reflect the increased concern of the late 1980s and early to mid-1990s with telecommunications; legacy system replacement, Y2K and ERP implementations; and the resurgence of interest in distributed learning of the mid to late 1990s.

The range of responsibilities of CIOs also varied from institution to institution. The typical range of organizational units for which CIOs had administrative responsibility included academic and administrative computing, and telecom-munications. Some CIOs had responsibility for other units, most frequently institutional libraries, but also media resources units, institutional research, insti-tutional planning, etc. Table 2 shows the proportion of CIOs with responsibility for the four unit types most frequently identified. The trends show a steady increase to almost 100% of CIOs responsible for both academic and administrative computing. The proportion of CIOs responsible for telecommunications seems to be fairly steady at just under 80%. However, the 1989 data show that most CIOs were responsible for data communications, while just over two-thirds were also responsible for voice communications. The proportion of CIOs with responsibility for libraries grew very slightly to about 20%. The idea of bringing disparate IT units and libraries/media centers under the umbrella of a CIO emerged in the early 1980s (Hardesty, 1998). Interest in consolidations rose for a few years but seemed to have waned by 1989 (Moholt, 1989). A resurgence of interest occurred in the mid-1990s, particularly among smaller colleges. Some of these organizational mergers were successful and continue today, while others were considered disasters.

Thus, while the early views of CIO roles seemed to suggest that institutions were recognizing the nature of information as a strategic asset, the evidence suggests that this has not been a key trend. It could be that as more institutions struggled with IT issues and created CIO positions, the relationship between information and information technology tended to focus almost exclusively on administrative information. Indeed, most IT investments in academe, until recently, have been in support of administrative rather than learning or research functions.

One of the observed developments in the maturing of the CIO role is the changing nature of the key functions of the CIO. Woodsworth (1988) in 1986–1987, found that the key functions identified by CIOs themselves were: major hardware and software purchases, contracts for initial major purchases, formulation of policies, and formulation of long-range goals. By 1989, Penrod et al. (1990) determined that CIOs perceived their four most important functions were leadership and management (cited by 81%), planning (71%), communications (62%), vision (35%), managing the IS budget (35%), coordination (23%), technical expertise (15%), consensus building (14%) and problem solving (8%). Clearly, the major focus of the CIOs in the late 1980s seems to have shifted from the technological issues to broader leadership and management issues. It is interesting to note that Passino and Severance (1988) found that corporate CIOs had experienced a similar shift over the same time period.

Penrod and his colleagues also asked CIOs to identify the four activities on which they spent the most time. Activities most frequently mentioned were human resources management (cited by 80%), planning/strategizing (61%), vendor relations (59%), meetings (59%), and budgeting (41%). Penrod et al. concluded that the CIOs' perceptions of their functions and the activities they actually engage in are closely aligned.

Penrod et al.'s survey also asked CIOs to rank, in order of accuracy, a list of statements describing the role that their senior administrations expected them to play. The rankings from top to bottom were: provide leadership on technological issues, coordinate and integrate technology initiatives, develop a strategic planning process for information resources, formulate information technology policy, make the important technology decisions, "fix" information resource problems, relieve [top executives] from worrying about technological issues, and authorize information technology purchases by user departments.

As a further validation of CIO and administrator perceptions of key functions and roles, Penrod et al. asked CIOs to indicate the top four characteristics of a successful CIO. They indicated communications and interpersonal skills (cited by 74%), good general management skills (60%), technical competence and knowledge (53%), vision for information technology (42%), negotiating and consensus building (38%), global institutional view (26%), leadership (19%), planner (13%), and perseverance and energy (11%).

Penrod et al. concluded that the CIO perceptions of senior administrator expectations, their own roles within the institution, their allocation of time, and characteristics for success were consistent with each other. Differences in CIO

Table 3.   Characteristics of Successful CIOs, (Penrod et al.).

Function/Characteristic	CIOs indicating importance	CIOs indicating characteristic for success
Leadership	81%	19%
Management	81%	60%
Planning	71%	13%
Communication/Liaison	62%	74%
Vision	35%	42%
Managing IS Budget	35%	
Coordination	23%	37% (negotiate and build consensus)
Technical Expertise	15%	53%

models were identified: between CIOs who report to the President or Chancellor and those who report elsewhere; and between CIOs whose responsibilities included academic and administrative computing and telecommunications and those with a broader scope of responsibility.

However, a closer "Monday morning" review of the Penrod et al.'s results show a number of seeming inconsistencies, particularly between the CIO perceptions of key functions and characteristics deemed necessary for success. Table 3 displays the results side-by-side. On the surface, at least, the greatest inconsistencies seem to be with leadership, planning, managing budgets and technical expertise. Leadership, cited by 81% of the CIOs as a key function and ranked as the top senior-level expectation, was considered a top success characteristic by fewer than 20%. It could be that leadership was considered in a narrow way – referring especially to leadership on technology issues alone. Vision is considered a critical component of leadership and was identified as a success characteristic by 42%, even though only 35% considered it a key function of the CIO. The importance of planning shows similar inconsistency, viewed as a key function by 71% yet as a success characteristic by only 13%. Managing budgets was not specifically mentioned as a success characteristic and may well have been included in the general management category, so there may not have been an inconsistency there. Finally, technical expertise was identified as a success characteristic by 53%, yet as an important function by only 15%.

It is also worth noting some key differences between CIOs responsible only for IT and those with broader responsibilities. Those with broader responsibilities tended to see communications as a key function (67%) more than those with IT-only responsibilities (50%). This probably reflects their need to communicate across a more diverse population. Interestingly, both groups of CIOs identified "lack of understanding" as institutional weaknesses, IT-only CIOs more than the others (53% to 49%). Finally, IT-only CIOs were more likely to consider vision or technical expertise as key functions (44% and 25%, respectively) than CIOs with broader responsibilities (27% and 7%, respectively). This may reflect that in the latter situation, institutional leaders had already defined or bought-in to the vision of information and supporting technologies as a strategic resource.

The survey results, in retrospect, indicate that the CIO role was predominantly focused on IT; that institutional climate, presidential and executive preferences, and individual characteristics shaped the specific CIO role within an institution; and that CIOs, with rare exception, were perceived as IT leaders, not as institutional leaders.

More recently, based on the move to very large-scale ERP implementations, scaled up interest in instructional technologies, or the perceived lack of success of the CIO role within the institution, some institutions moved to separate or (re-separate) academic from administrative computing and split the CIO role across two or more IT managers. In the corporate sector, in an even more unusual move, Capital One Financial Corporation recently "split the CIO role between an IT expert and a business professional" (Trombly, 2000). Perhaps these developments indicate a further maturing of the CIO role into more of a distributed responsibility. I will return to this issue at the end of this article. Nevertheless, today, the existence of an institutional CIO is very common, although the role itself has evolved well beyond the management of central IT resources.

Looking back over the years since the CIO role first came into existence, several key trends affecting the perception and use of IT in universities can be identified. First, IT is no longer a specialized resource for use by an elite few. IT today touches everyone in the academy one way or another. Second, most users of IT are no longer willing or able to spend much of their time learning about current and emerging IT application and operation. They simply want to use the new tools; thus, demands for user technical support are growing and, increasingly, the technical support staff needs to know and understand what the user is trying to accomplish through the application and use of IT.

Recently conducted surveys at the University of Michigan (Griffiths, 1999, 2000) confirm these trends. Over the period 1996–2001, faculty and student use of IT changed dramatically. First, the user population expanded to almost 100% of faculty and students, most staff, and even came to include prospective students and alumni. Second, the amount of time spent using IT expanded. Third, the perception of both the importance of IT to the work being performed and individual success grew. Fourth, the IT skill levels attained by faculty, students and staff improved, and this improvement was accompanied by increasing anxiety about the adequacy of their IT skills and learning opportunities. Fifth, the locations at which people use IT are increasing. Sixth, people are not just using IT as an individual activity, but are beginning to engage in collaborative communities of many kinds. And seventh, faculty and students, in particular, are expanding their use of IT beyond traditional research and scholarship to creating new ways to do things as well as new things to do.

All of these changes have caused the leadership of academic institutions to seek help in the IT arena by appointing a CIO to be responsible for IT and its role in the enterprise. Given the changes in IT and IT use by faculty, students and staff, it is not surprising that today's CIO role is different from the original role, at least in terms of focus. The change is best articulated by a shift from IT management to IT leadership.

FROM IT MANAGEMENT TO IT LEADERSHIP

The nature of leadership and management, their similarities and distinctions, have been topics of debate over the years. Kotter (1990), for example, views leadership and management as "separate and distinct but complementary systems of action, each with its own function and characteristic activities ... management about coping with complexity, leadership about coping with change." He sees the necessity of both for success in "today's business environment." Zaleznik (1977), on the other hand, considers managers and leaders as two very different types of people. He sees the manager focus as ensuring that an organization's business gets done; while leaders seek out or create potential opportunities and rewards. Managers excel at diffusing conflicts; leaders engage in intense and often chaotic interactions. Zaleznik expresses concern that larger organizations, in particular, favor a management rather than a leadership culture; thereby over-emphasizing people who rely on and strive to maintain orderly, stable work patterns, collective forms of decision-making and risk avoidance.

Gardner (1993), who has been writing about leadership for over 35 years, asks why there is a continual call for better leadership. In addition to citing what he describes as conventional and shallow views on leadership, he also points to the fact that attention to leadership alone is both sterile and inappropriate. Instead he places leadership within a context of the "accomplishment of group purpose" and considers some of the issues that underlie the ongoing call for effective leadership. The issues he focuses on are motivation, values, social cohesion and renewal. Bennis (1991), another long-time author on the subject of leadership, exposes and describes a worsening of "the unconscious conspiracy" against effective leadership. In particular, he makes suggestions on how to counter the turmoil, inertia and routine that work against the best-laid plans.

IT leadership faces the same challenges as leadership in other parts of an enterprise. The larger and more complex an organization and the more distributed its culture, the more the role of the leadership is direction setting and coordination, rather than direction setting and operation. Leaders and managers, in the IT arena or elsewhere, do have similar roles (otherwise the debate and confusion over the nature of each would not have raged for so long), but they differ significantly in terms of their frame of reference. The IT manager's frame is the unit, process, service or system to be managed, its user community and its competition (actual or potential). The IT leader's frame is the entirety of the enterprise – the institution, its current and prospective communities, its resource base, its competitors, external influences, etc. This distinction in frame of reference can make it difficult for some IT managers in colleges and universities to step into IT leadership positions without considerable exposure to and understanding of the culture, vision, goals and success criteria espoused by academics. Recently, Cartwright (2002) indicated that CIOs, along with other executive leaders needed to demonstrate "proven leadership skills, strong management skills, and a solid grasp of the difference between the two."

FIVE CRITICAL LEADERSHIP ROLES OF A CIO

In today's fast-paced, global, competitive environment, the IT leader needs to be careful to focus time and effort on those areas that are most important to the success of the institution. It is all too easy to engage in extended discussion of the details of an ongoing project, or to delve into the inner workings of the latest hi-tech device. Indeed, for many technology savvy CIOs, such discussions can provide a welcome relief from the more business-oriented, strategic issues they must address. The real focus of the CIO of any organization should be the enterprise of the organization. All CIO activities should be performed from that broader perspective. What is the organization's mission/business and how can IT play a role in furthering that mission/business? Can IT be used as a catalyst to transform the organization in positive directions? Are there traditional supporting roles for IT that are no longer needed or viable? These are the kinds of issues the CIO should consider.

In higher education these issues relate to whether and how IT can help an institution in its educational mission. Can IT be used in the teaching/learning process and, if so, how and when? Are there aspects of IT application and use that can fundamentally change the way students learn? How would that affect how we teach – and even what we teach? How can the societal implications of the IT revolution be incorporated into today's curricula? What is IT's role in discovery and research? Certainly, IT can now be used to process and analyze volumes of data that it would otherwise be impossible to handle in a lifetime. Furthermore, IT can today support complex models, simulations, visual and virtual forms of presentation that encourage comprehension and challenge old understandings. And today's IT can change the perception and nature of interpersonal relationships, such that the age-old lines between teacher and student can blend into a more symbiotic relationship with interchangeable roles as teacher and student embark on a journey of mutual discovery and learning.

Today's CIO roles are just beginning to mature to the point where the day-to-day operation of IT itself is not, and probably should not be, the primary role of the CIO. Rather, the CIO should be responsible and accountable to the institution for its investments in IT and the value that IT adds to the institution's business or mission. My years as a CIO in higher education have led me to identify five critical and essential leadership roles for the university CIO of today.

Role 1: Strategic IT Direction Setting

The CIO has a critical role to play in determining how IT can help further the interests of the institution. In so doing, the CIO must be in a position to know and fully understand the mission and business of the institution and the prevailing vision, direction, goals and success indicators/metrics of its current leadership. The CIO must, therefore, have a place at the leadership table to engage in discussion of institutional strategy. To be accepted as a member of the executive team, the CIO must be a "full-spectrum contributor to the development and management of business strategies and directions rather than a niche player in the limited band of IT" (Zastrocky & Schlier, 2000). As the institutional vision, directions, goals, and success indicators are developed and implemented, it is the role of the CIO to consider and bring forward ways in which IT could help or hinder the fulfillment of the vision. This requires a knowledge of whether existing and emerging IT could be applied; whether new IT specifications are required, and who could develop and provide them; where IT would offer and deliver the greatest help; whether the existing institutional environment (both the cultural and IT environment) could support the proposed vision or whether other issues would need to be addressed first (to improve the likelihood of success); and so on. In effect, the CIO needs to bring forward a clear vision for the development, implementation, and use of IT by the institution in the context of the institution's vision. The IT vision should be clear in relating its contribution to the overall institutional vision and should include metrics relevant to the various communities served by the institution.

An example of this level of decision-making is the decision of whether to require all students to have their own computer, or whether to require all faculty to create course web sites. The CIO should be involved in understanding what the institution expects to accomplish through such decisions – it could be to propel the institution to a state perceived by prospective students and employers of its graduates as offering an educational experience relevant to today's society in terms of e-business trends, e-consumerism, etc. Of course, requiring computers or web sites alone will not necessarily achieve this goal, but, coupled with a move to incorporate e-activity in curricula, in campus service delivery, and so on, this requirement could help evolve a more technologically savvy community, engaged, not only in using the technology, but also in discussing the implications that using the technology brings to the individual, the community and to society at large.

The other key aspect of the CIO's involvement in strategic direction setting is in educating other institutional decision-makers about the underlying support and infrastructure needs that accompany a move in a particular direction. Will the support be available to students and faculty as they ramp up their use of technology? Is the existing technological infrastructure sufficient to fulfill expectations for service delivery?

Role 2: IT Priority Setting

Since it is highly unlikely that an institution can afford to bring forward all of its ideas to fruition, the CIO along with other leaders at the institution must engage in setting priorities. Within the framework of institutional priorities, the CIO is responsible for setting priorities for IT that will support the broader priorities. The process for IT priority setting must be based on knowledge and understanding of the existing institutional environment, particularly of IT and other resource availability; of the range of possible IT directions, and the development, implementation, operational and economic implications of each; of the institutional capacity for change; and of the institutional culture for identifying and defining priorities. The output of the priority-setting role should be a strategic IT plan for the institution.

Role 3: IT Standards Development and Implementation

The importance of IT standards to an institution cannot be overemphasized. With the proliferation of IT options and IT-based resources and services, standards are essential to ensuring interoperability and access. There are tradeoffs in selecting standards, particularly in selecting open versus proprietary standards. Consequently, a decision on which areas of IT should adopt and adhere to standards is as important as the decision as to which specific standard to adopt.

On the other hand, the adoption of particular standards can result in barriers or constraints to some users and can result in greater or lesser cost to the institution. These implications need to be explored, articulated and communicated to institutional leaders by the CIO.

Role 4: IT Policy Development and Oversight

As IT has extended its reach into our lives, and as IT uses and abuses have increased dramatically over recent years, the need for development and enforcement of policies and procedures has increased. Policies and procedures related to IT should be aimed at encouraging the kinds of uses and outcomes intended by the institution as much as, if not even more so than, discouraging abuses. In particular, policies can help define expectations and norms for conditions of IT access, use, rights, privacy, security, etc. They can also help to manage the allocation of limited resources.

The CIO can anticipate the need for IT policy, based on understanding how the IT application/service can be used/abused. It is also important to understand what is needed to implement and monitor policy, in terms of resource needs. Procedures for monitoring compliance and addressing non-compliance should be established at the time of policy development. Policies and procedures should be reviewed for relevance periodically and revised as necessary.

Role 5: Institutional Return-On-Investment (ROI) in IT and Other Metrics Development

In many organizations today, there is no institutional view of the totality of IT budgets and expenditures. IT has become so pervasive that it can be hidden (deliberately or unintentionally) in many different accounts and financial reports. This situation can result in sub-optimization of IT investment and returns on that investment. For example, economies can be derived from aggregating demand, sharing infrastructure and services, adopting common standards, etc. However, the potential benefits that could be derived from careful consideration of aggregation and leveraging of common needs and interests are not fully realizable unless an institution-wide approach is taken. The CIO must have both the responsibility and the authority to generate this institutional perspective. The CIO is also the leader who is expected to have a broad knowledge of the IT needs and uses across the entire institution. The CIO can, therefore, connect individuals from one part of the organization to others with similar or complementary needs and interests.

Another key contribution the CIO can make to an institution is in the development of relevant metrics. Such metrics need to be defined in terms to which the various constituencies of the institution can relate. Such metrics should be published on a regular basis so that the entire community of the institution can track progress and provide feedback on potential changes in need or emphasis. At the University of Michigan, the development and publishing of such metrics provided information useful to various planners and decision-makers (Griffiths, 1999, 2000).

The five roles outlined above constitute for me the definition of a CIO exercising institutional leadership in IT. While I view all five roles as essential, it does not mean that CIOs do not perform other roles; they often do. However, if all five roles are performed, a sixth, derived, role emerges.

Derived Role: Representing Institutional IT Interests to Internal and External Communities

The CIO is well positioned to be the focal point for IT information and communication, both within and outside the institution. By performing the other critical CIO roles, the CIO will gather a wealth of knowledge of IT matters throughout the institution, as well as representing the institutional position vis-à-vis IT. As such, the CIO can function as a clearinghouse for IT information that makes referrals; coordinates institutional IT surveys, responds to external surveys; benchmarks against other peer institutions; and acts as the IT spokesperson for the institution.

FACTORS RELATED TO THE SUCCESS OF A CIO

Institutions of higher education vary a great deal from one to another. In considering the evolving, and often misunderstood role of CIOs, it is not easy to identify factors that will contribute to the success or failure of CIOs as a whole. However, the experiences shared among CIOs have led me to observe several factors or issues that can affect the potential success of a CIO, particularly if they are not recognized or addressed overtly.

Responsibility With Authority

Most institutions give their CIOs the responsibility for all major IT decisions and consequences. But not all of them give the CIO the authority to "get the job done." The CIO must have the authority (directly or indirectly through the visible support of the CEO) to require the engagement of others in IT-related deliberations, standards and policy implementation, etc., to ensure success. This is especially the case in institutions that operate in a decentralized mode.

The implications of this need for responsibility with authority are that CIOs must have executive or senior level positions in the institutions. They do not need to have direct responsibility for day-to-day operational IT management, but they should have the responsibility to coordinate across IT organizations and activities throughout the institution. They must also have a coordination relationship and authority with those to whom the managers of IT organizations report. As an example, if an institution has a central IT organization and several school or college IT organizations, the CIO should have authority to coordinate across the managers of all the IT organizations, and across the deans/directors of the schools or colleges on IT-related matters. This dual level coordination authority is important. While few would argue the coordination across managers of IT organizations, the need for coordinating the IT efforts of the schools or colleges and their deans is not always recognized. This lack of recognition tends to derive from the perception that the CIO role is to take care of the IT organization rather than to take care of the institution through the application of IT. This latter view requires interaction with all major areas of an institution's "business." Even the coordination of the IT managers will be sub-optimized if the coordinator has no direct knowledge of what each entity supported by each IT manager is trying to accomplish.

Centralized Versus Decentralized Organization

The more centralized an institution is, the greater likelihood of success for the CIO. A relatively centralized organization is accustomed to central authority and control and tends to acknowledge them. The culture of such institutions is conducive to central coordination and decision-making.

In decentralized institutions, the degree of decentralization can have a significant effect on the sustained effort required to balance the role of the central versus the distributed authorities. In such institutions, the open discussion of where coordination can be mutually beneficial (across the decentralized units as well as between the decentralized and the central units) is helpful. Rather than trying to tackle all the possible areas of coordination, the CIOs might be more successful by taking on one or two areas and demonstrating successes, thereby making the case for further coordination. Discussions can then proceed on the extent to which functions should be centrally and/or locally managed, funded, etc.

Technical Versus Non-Technical Skills

Traditionally, the CIO position has been considered a technical role. However, more recently, organizations have come to recognize that, while the CIO needs to have some technical knowledge and understanding, the CIO must also possess more traditional leadership traits, and these traits may be equally, if not more, important than technical skills. These include the ability to communicate with both technical and non-technical audiences, strategic planning, budgeting, and resources management. A recent discussion among CIOs on the need for a CIO to be qualified in technical areas tended towards the consensus that "business skills and people skills" are essential for a successful CIO, but that deep technical skills are not (Computerworld Executive Suite, 2001). Similarly, in identifying the top 10 requirements of the CIO position, Polansky (2001) only mentioned technical skills in the context of "expertise in aligning and leveraging technology for the advantage of the enterprise" and that skills related to specific facets of technology such as ERP, web services, etc., are often preferred qualification rather than required ones.

A similar question is often asked of me, namely, should the CIO of a large organization be the manager of a central IT unit? I used to think that it was beneficial to have a large resource base behind you to give some "weight or clout" to IT decisions and actions. However, over the last few years, I've become convinced that the day-to-day operational needs of any sizeable IT organization can impose considerable distraction from strategic-level issues and concerns (as Bennis, 1991 argued). The CIO needs to be able to envision and enable change without being associated directly with only one part of the IT community within an institution. The CIO should have the same relationship with all IT units (again, here's where a more centralized organization may be easier to work with).

Executive Ownership of IT Issues

Executive ownership of IT issues varies considerably from institution to institution. In the early days of IT use within academic institutions, it was easy for executives to abdicate responsibility to the "technology czars." But as IT has now evolved almost to the point of ubiquity, academic executive leadership must acknowledge and accept ownership and responsibility for IT in the same way as they do for the financial and human resources of the institution. This implies an executive-level appointment for the CIO (an issue I will address again, later.)

The well publicized "Y2K or Millennium Bug" presented an illustrative case for most organizations of executive abdication of responsibility for the issue until within a year or so of a critical deadline. Many institutional leaders saw the problem solely as an IT problem. But, in fact, it was the catalyst that revealed significant institutional shortcomings in inventory control, disaster preparedness, institutional interdependencies and communications channels, re-investment in systems, awareness of the extent of embedded controls, lack of clarity in institutional priorities, etc. Apart from a few leading institutions, most academic executives only became engaged in the flurry of activity during the year 1999. Unfortunately, having seen no major disasters befall any institution, many of those executives have retreated from the IT arena, believing they were dragged into making substantial efforts based on "much fuss over nothing."

Organizations with executive leadership that remains disengaged from IT, even if they appoint a CIO, are at risk. Earl and Feeny (2000) recently defined seven Chief Executive Officer (CEO) archetypes, based on CEO attitudes towards IT (9). Ranging from the least to most ready for the Information Age, they are:

Hypocrite Espouses the strategic importance of IT.
           Negates this belief through personal actions.
 Waverer   Reluctantly accepts the strategic importance of IT.
           But not ready to get involved in IT matters.
 Atheist   Convinced IT is of little value.
           Publicly espouses this belief.
  Zealot   Convinced IT is strategically important.
           Believes he or she is an authority on IT practice.
Agnostic   Concedes IT may be strategically important.
           Requires repeated convincing.
 Monarch   Accepts that IT is strategically important.
           Appoints best CIO possible, then steps back.
 Believer Believes IT enables strategic advantage.
           Demonstrates belief in own daily behavior.

The role-model CEOs for the Information Age are defined as "IT believers rather than IT-literate CEOs." CEOs who demonstrate their fitness for the Information Age see IT as "a first-order factor of strategy making, not second-order." In other words, they recognize that IT can both create new business opportunities and threats, and they ensure that these opportunities and threats are placed high on their strategic agendas.

Earl and Feeny cite today's conventional wisdom that the CIO should report to the CEO. They indicate that this could work well if the CEO were a believer, and that believer CEOs invariably work closely with their CIO; but that it might be less fruitful if the CEO fell into one of the other categories. Nevertheless, they insist that a good relationship between CIO and CEO is key to "ensuring that IT is regarded and exploited as an asset."

KEY ATTRIBUTES OF A CIO

During the EDUCAUSE 2000 Annual Conference, EDUCAUSE President, Brian Hawkins, stated that a CIO needs three primary skills: communications, alliance building, and collaboration. Reporting on a panel presentation at the conference, a group of academic CIOs with over 100 aggregate years of experience in managing IT organizations, offer advice to help new CIOs apply their skills in Hawkins' three areas (Bucher et al., 2001). They recommend starting by establishing friendly relationships, meeting with constituents, and getting to know staff. To prepare for success they recommend learning about the institutional culture, learning about budgets, building a relationship with their bosses, setting and managing expectations. And, for setting a new agenda they recommend identifying outstanding problems and difficult issues, and evaluating one's role as a change agent on campus. The group identifies five key skill areas for CIOs: flexibility in dealing with a new environment, pragmatism in approaching all problems, and excellence in managing various relationships, budgets, and expectations.

Oblinger (2000) recently confirmed that academic institutions are calling for new leadership from CIOs; that the position often originated from a data processing manager base and was, therefore, often viewed as an IT manager rather than a leader. She indicates that some universities abandoned CIO positions in favor of separating (in fact, often re-separating) academic and administrative computing, but that new demands, a need for diverse skills, and opportunities for synergy are causing many to reconsider hiring a CIO. She goes on to define five primary characteristics of today's emerging CIOs: strategist, bridge builder, implementer, communicator, and change agent.

In teaching leadership and organizational design, I have evolved a model of leadership that combines elements of many models, but that I have found useful as a CIO. The model is depicted in Fig. 1. The model identifies four major characteristics of IT leaders. They must be visionary (and not simply able to envision the IT future, but be able to understand the vision on a much broader future for the institution, its communities, and the role of IT in that future). They must have and behave with the utmost integrity (trust is one of the single most important attributes for leaders today). They must have a sufficient amount of common sense to be able to bring their vision to fruition. Finally, they must have the courage to make difficult decisions and argue for what they believe to be right.

IT leaders also need to understand and work within the culture of their institutions. They must know and understand their communities (actual and potential, user and provider), be able to be collaborative, building and nurturing win-win partnerships with both internal and external entities, and be able to communicate effectively with vastly differing groups with both converging and diverging interests.

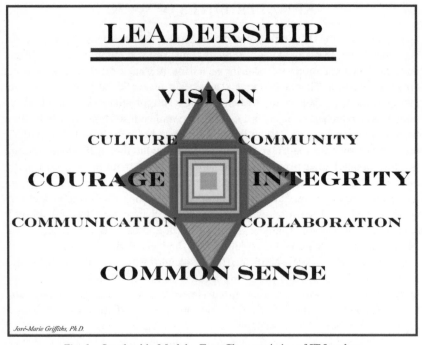

Fig. 1.   Leadership Model – Four Characteristics of IT Leaders.

TOO MANY CHIEFS?

While I believe that IT issues must be addressed at an executive level within an institution, I am also aware that executive-level positions have proliferated of late. Today, in addition to the traditional CEO, Chief Academic Officer, Chief Financial or Business Officer, Chief Operating Officer, there are increasing calls for the Chief Information Officer, Chief Investment Officer, Chief Diversity Officer, Chief Privacy Officer, Chief Communications Officer, Chief Technology Officer, Chief Research Officer, Chief Accounting Officer, Chief Marketing Officer, Chief Knowledge Officer and even Chief People Officer (Dunham, 2001; Morgan, 2001). As a result, the questions facing any organization are when is an area important enough to warrant a distinct executive-level (Chief or VP) position, and how many such positions can the organization support? On the other hand, should an area that is so important that it pervades the entire organization (i.e. it is everybody's responsibility) negate the need for a position that focuses specially on that issue? How can organizations reconcile their need for executive ownership and responsibility for an area with community ownership and operational responsibility for that area?

Not that I have all the answers, but in considering the dilemma of today's CEOs in creating executive teams, I believe that "Information Age CEOs" need to think how best to pay attention to critical areas, both as they begin to emerge and require special attention, and over the longer term, as they diffuse throughout the culture of an organization. Such attention to the role of executives and senior administrators with respect to critical issue areas could help avoid the difficulties the CIO role has had over its lifetime to this point. Finally, executive team members, while having specific areas of responsibility, should also recognize and accept that, ultimately, they have a shared responsibility for all areas of an organization, IT included.

REFERENCES

Bennis, W. (1991). *Why leaders can't lead: The unconscious conspiracy continues.* San Francisco: Jossey-Bass Publishers.

Bucher, J., Horgan, B., Moberg, T., Paterson, R., & Todd, H. D. (2001). The realities of a new senior-level IT position. *EDUCAUSE Quarterly, 24*(2), 34–38.

Cain, M. (2001). http://www.educause.edu/asp/doclib/abstract.asp?ID=CSD1600

Cartwright, C. A. (2002). Today's CIO: Leader, manager, and member of the "executive orchestra." *EDUCAUSE Review* (January/February), 6–7.

Computerworld Executive Suite (2001). Does a CIO need to be technical? Closed discussion group (May).

Dunham, K. J. (2001). Law firms, in a competitive bid, appoint chief marketing officers. *The Wall Street Journal, Career Journal* (May 15), B14.

Earl, M., & Feeny, D. (2000). How to be a CEO for the information age. *Sloan Management Review* (Winter), 11–23.

Gardner, J. W. (1993). *On leadership.* New York: The Free Press.

Griffiths, J.-M. (1999). *Technology enhancing tradition.* Ann Arbor: University of Michigan.

Griffiths, J.-M. (2000). *University of Michigan faculty information uses and needs: A Report on the 1999 survey.* Ann Arbor: University of Michigan.

Hardesty, L. (1998). Computer center-library relations at smaller institutions: A look from both sides. *CAUSE/EFFECT, 21*(1), 35–41.

Kotter, J. P. (1990). What leaders really do. *Harvard Business Review* (May-June), Reprint 90309.

Moholt, P. (1989). What happened to the merger debate? *Libraries & Computer Centers: Issues of Mutual Concern* (May), 1.

Morgan, M. (2001). Traditional companies play with titles. *Ann Arbor News, Business Section* (June 3), E1.

Oblinger, D. (2000). Higher Ed's new CIO activities lead to new responsibilities. *Multiversity* (Fall), 17–21.

Passino, J. H., & Severance, D. G. (1988). The changing role of the chief information officer. *Planning Review, 16*(September/October), 38–42.

Penrod, J. I., Dolence, M. G., & Douglas, J. D. (1990). *The chief information officer in Higher Education.* Boulder: CAUSE.

Polansky, M. (2001). The top 10 requirements of the CIO position. Posted March 22. http://www.cio.com/research/executive/questions/220320011402

Trombly, M. (2000). Capital one fills CIO slot with business, tech execs. *Computerworld* (February 28).

Woodsworth, A. (1988). Libraries and the chief information officer: Implications and trends. *Library Hi Tech*, 6(1), 37–44.

Zaleznik, A. (1977). Managers: Are they different? *Harvard Business Review* (May-June), Reprint 92211.

Zastrocky, M. R., & Schlier, F. (2000). The higher education CIO in the 21st century. *EDUCAUSE Quarterly*, 1, 53 & 59.

INFORMATION ETHICS,
A PHILOSOPHICAL APPROACH

Mary Jane Rootes

Information ethics is a growing concern in library science. Part of this concern centers around how much assistance a librarian is obligated to give when the information sought potentially can be used to harm one's self or others. Some argue that, if it is suggested that the information will be used in a harmful way, the librarian should be able to show discretion; there should not be unlimited access to information. Others argue that a limitation on access to information presents the greatest threat to those whom the library serves. Each position makes a valid point, but I must question how these positions are reached. Upon what kind of moral argument are these positions based? It is my goal in this paper to do the following: identify the underlying moral principle that libraries in the United States must serve; define moral agency, and thereby the moral agents served by the moral principle; and argue for the best way that such a principle be served.

The central mission of the libraries in the United States is to facilitate the acquisition of information by its users. It is through the use of the library that ideas are both developed and disseminated. The objectives of a library vary according to the constituency served, but the mission remains the same, to promote an informed society. The purpose of this paper is to discern the moral imperative that should be followed in order to best serve this mission.

An informed society is achieved, in part, through the access to information. Thomas Jefferson recognized the role that information plays in preserving a free society. According to Jefferson, freedom is achieved when the people are governed by their own informed consent (Alfino & Pierce, 1997, p. 93). Jefferson writes, "If

Advances in Library Administration and Organization
Advances in Library Administration and Organization, Volume 20, 37–66
Copyright © 2003 by Elsevier Science Ltd.
ISSN: 0732-0671/PII: S0732067102200036

a nation expects to be ignorant and free, in a state of civilization, it expects what never was and never will be" (Bartlett & Kaplan, 1991, p. 344). This marked the birth of the principle that libraries in the United States of America are founded on the premise that a consenting society requires an informed society. Libraries, ideally, serve democracy through the promotion of a consenting society, but does this imply that libraries should be governed by this democratic principle? Is there an underlying principle that is even more fundamental to their function?

Dialogue is important in promoting an informed society. British philosopher John Stuart Mill in *On Liberty* writes: "There is the greatest difference between presuming an opinion to be true because each opportunity for its refutation has not disproved it, and assuming its truth for the purpose of not permitting refutation" (Mill, 1985, p. 79). Mill argues, in part, that truth is found, not through acceptance, but through debate. Democracy governs according to consent. Consent is reached through debate. The public library is an institution that promotes informed consent, a vital part of a democratic society. While from this one rightfully may conclude that the library is an important part of a democratic society, it does not follow that the library is a democratic institution. But if it is not democracy, what ideals should govern libraries in the United States?

To answer this question I must ask, what ideals support democracy? It is not enough to say that democracy relies on consensus, and consensus is achieved only through an informed public. It is necessary to consider how the public is informed. The public is informed through access to information. The question is, what should govern or moderate this access to information? To determine this I will look at the counterpart to information access, censorship.

The nemesis of information access is censorship. Censorship can be practiced in different ways. Censorship, in the proper sense, occurs when a government's action is used to prevent the distribution of information to the public; this is an active form of censorship (Andre, 1983, p. 25). There is also the passive form censorship – not promoting the conveyance of information. This is the action most commonly referred to when the term censorship is used in the action of a reference librarian. This is due to the role assigned to reference service, which is to take an active role in providing the library clientele with the information sought (Shaw, 1926, p. 27). "In a sense, librarians made the dilemma possible by offering to mediate the patron's request in the first place." (Alfino & Pierce, 1997, p. 7). Censorship has a history in libraries in the United States. Judith Krug, of the Intellectual Freedom Committee, of the American Library Association, recognizes the checkered past of libraries in the United States in regard to information access.

In 1877, it was written that it was the librarian's duty "to see that a good book be sought where a poor one had been preferred" (Harris, 1976, p. 286). Fictional work was made available in the public library in order that its "confectionary of literature would ensure an interest of the lower tastes, only to be led to a 'higher level of reading' " (Harris, 1976, p. 286). During World War II there were increasing levels of censorship throughout Europe. It is due, in part to this, that libraries in the United States became concerned with censorship. It was at this time that the American Library Association codified a Bill of Rights to protect library users from censorship.

The concept of intellectual freedom in United States libraries traces back to 1939, when the American Library Association drafted its Library Bill of Rights. There are three articles in the first version of the ALA's Bill of Rights. The first article assures that the selection of materials be based on the interest and values of the community served. The second article guarantees the representation of different points of view, stressing that all possible sides of an issue should be represented – that the library cannot represent a particular partisan position. The third article defines the library as "an institution for democratic living," guaranteeing equal access of meeting rooms to the public (ALA, 1996, pp. 5–6).

The Intellectual Freedom Movement itself is recognized as beginning in the 1960s. John F. Kennedy defended intellectual freedom when he said, "If this nation is to be wise as well as strong, if we are to achieve our destiny, then we need more new ideas for more wise men reading more good books in more public libraries. These libraries should be open to all – except the censor... Let us welcome controversial books and controversial authors. For the Bill of Rights is the guardian of our security as well as our library" (American Library Association, Office for Intellectual Freedom, 1996, p. 259).

The Intellectual Freedom Movement brought recognition to the pluralistic society served by libraries in the United States. In 1980, Article VI of the Library Bill of Rights, the article ensuring equal access to meeting rooms on the principle of democratic living was changed because the term *democratic living* reflects a partisan position. Democracy, in its strict sense, means majority rule, but the library is not designed for the majority, but for everyone (ALA, 1996, p. 15). The American Library Association's Bill of Rights serves as the library profession's interpretation of the First Amendment of the Constitution. These First Amendment rights are not based on a democratic principle, but on liberty. Historian Mary Ritter Beard writes, "The Constitution [does] not contain the word or any word lending countenance to [democracy], except possibly the mention of 'We, the people' in the preamble" (Bartlett & Kaplan, 1991, p. 618).

Through intellectual freedom, the library plays an important role in supporting a democratic society. Intellectual freedom in libraries today, as expressed in the Library Bill of Rights, is not based on democracy, but on the foundation of our democratic government – liberty, as expressed in the Constitution. But it is not enough to say that intellectual freedom should be based on the principle of liberty, this type of liberty must be defined. In *Two Concepts of Liberty*, Isaiah Berlin delineates two distinct, though related concepts of liberty: a liberal concept of liberty and a rationalistic concept of liberty. Berlin refers to these as negative and positive liberty, respectively. Negative liberty is concerned with the extent to which government impedes on one's freedom; it is the "freedom from." Negative liberty provides at least a minimum amount freedom, "which on no account may be violated; for if it is overstepped, the individual will find himself in an area too narrow for even that minimum development of his natural faculties which alone make it possible to pursue and even to conceive the various ends which men hold good or right or sacred" (Berlin, 1998, p. 196). Positive liberty addresses one's need to be his/her own master; it is the "freedom to." It is a rationalistic concept of liberty because it requires that the ends sought be rational.

In order to determine how libraries can best achieve liberty, and thus intellectual freedom, I will first define the basic elements of liberty. Liberty is defined as the quality or state of being free. (Merriam Webster's Collegiate Dictionary, 10th ed., s.v. "liberty"). Freedom is "the absence of necessity, coercion or constraint in choice or action;" (*Merriam Webster's Collegiate Dictionary*, 10th ed., s.v. "freedom") it is to act autonomously. Autonomy is central to liberty. An autonomous agent is one who acts free of imposed constraints. Positive liberty ensures freedom from one's own passions, internal forces; it is the freedom to seek a particular end. Negative liberty ensures freedom from external forces; it is the "freedom from." Which form of liberty should libraries serve?

Today, the Intellectual Freedom Movement tries to advocate liberty in the negative sense by not promoting any position outside of unlimited access to information. Such a position advocates the security of the rights of the individual, regardless of what it could mean to the general welfare. But the foundation of liberty, and thus intellectual freedom, is not limited to individual liberty. In negative liberty, common welfare does not come at the expense of individual liberty.

Information ethics is an issue central to intellectual freedom. Throughout my paper I will use the terms "ethics" and "morality" interchangeably. The definition of morality/ethics as it is used in this paper is: "[the] requirements for action that are addressed at least in part to every actual or prospective agent, and that are concerned with furthering the interests, especially the most important interests, of persons or recipients other than or in addition to the agent or the speaker" (Gewirth, 1979, p. 1).

Martha Montague Smith refers to the discipline of information ethics as info-ethics. Smith defines info-ethics as "[an] ethical reflection on information, information professionals, information technologies, or related phenomena, such as libraries and librarians" (Montague-Smith, 1996, p. 2). The field of information ethics is recognized as beginning in 1988, but information ethics is not a new moral issue in libraries.

This paper is built on an argument between two librarians; each with a different view of just what intellectual freedom implies. One of these librarians, Robert Dowd, argues that information access is a fundamental part of intellectual freedom, and that such access should not be hampered. Robert Hauptman, on the other hand, argues that unlimited access to information is not equivalent to intellectual freedom but is equivalent to abjuring any moral responsibility on the part of the information provider (Hauptman, 1976, p. 627).

Robert Hauptman did his seminal work in information ethics in 1976. In his study, Hauptman posed as a person of questionable character who was seeking information for the construction of an explosive with the potency required to blow up a house. In answering this information request, Hauptman argues, the librarian is faced with the choice between a responsibility to society and a responsibility to his or her role as librarian, a disseminator of information (Hauptman, 1998, p. 127). Hauptman's work expanded the moral question beyond the librarian's responsibility to the patron to that of the librarian's responsibility to the society as a whole. Hauptman argues that the librarian act out of concern for the welfare of those affected by the action "secured" through dispensation of information. I will show that these two roles are not mutually exclusive. Rather, the common good and individual liberty are interdependent when promoting negative liberty.

In 1989 Robert Dowd did a similar study of the moral implications in a reference transaction. Dowd found dissimilar results in his study; Dowd found the librarians to be morally judgmental. Dowd went further to say that the librarian's duty is to the security of the individual patron's rights: ". . . I applaud the efforts of those librarians whose professional responsibility truly lies with each patron requesting help" (Dowd, 1989, p. 492). Dowd argues that intellectual freedom implies an "unfettered" access to information. As I stated earlier, in negative liberty, the common good and individual liberty are not mutually exclusive. Intellectual freedom must take into consideration the well being of both the individual and the common welfare. Negative liberty is actualized when each agent is allowed to seek her own good in her own way (individual liberty), provided it does not put the welfare of others in danger (common welfare). In "Review of Library Literature," I will show how, ironically, both Hauptman and Dowd are arguing for aspects of negative liberty, but that they each fall short of achieving such freedom. And for this reason, neither can be used to support intellectual freedom.

I will then turn to two moral philosophers, Immanuel Kant and Benjamin Constant, as they confront a moral conflict similar to that of Dowd and Hauptman. Kant and Constant, like Dowd and Hauptman, are concerned with freedom and autonomy and how these concepts relate to individual liberty and the common good. While reviewing Kant and Constant, I hope to bring out both the strengths and weaknesses of their respective theories.

The strength of each of their arguments is found in the distributive property of morality. The distributive property of morality is demonstrated in how the moral rule is distributed or executed; how both moral agents and moral cases are treated. A categorical rule/principle is one that is always applied in the same way in all cases. This categorical nature is the distributive property of such a principle. Both Kant and Dowd argue for a categorical nature to morality. It is a strength because little deliberation is required by either theory when determining the morally correct action. The strength is in the consistency of the principle – it is categorical. The weakness of the arguments presented by both Kant and Dowd is in the justification of such a principle – should it be categorical? Kant argues that reason itself is justification for morality and its categorical nature. Dowd's argument is based on the premise that the mission of libraries is to provide an unfettered access to information (Hauptman, 1998, p. 294).

The questions raised by the respective positions of Dowd and Kant are: can morality be reduced to reason alone and can the mission of libraries be reduced to providing an unfettered access to information? I will attempt to answer these questions by presenting the counterviews given by Hauptman and Constant. The strength in the arguments presented by Hauptman and Constant is also in the distributive property of the respective moral theory; each of them base the moral imperative on a principle of simple consistency. The principle of simple consistency treats similar cases similarly; it takes into consideration the context of moral situations. The weakness in each of the arguments is that neither Hauptman nor Constant provide a method for determining how to formulate the morally correct action for these similar cases.

I will then argue that moral philosopher Alan Gewirth has resolved the limitations of Kant and Dowd and those of Constant and Hauptman, while preserving the strengths of each of their arguments. Gewirth does this with his moral theory, the Principle of Generic Consistency. Gewirth argues for the categorical nature of morality, but adds that "although one moral requirement may be overridden by another, it may not be overridden by any non-moral requirement, nor can its normative bindingness be escaped by shifting one's inclinations, opinions or ideals" (Gewirth, 1979, p. 1). Gewirth argues that reason is necessary for morality, but that morality consists of both reason and action (Gewirth, 1979, p. 21). Gewirth goes on to say that morality is necessary in a social context (Gewirth, 1979, p. 129).

To conclude this paper, I will demonstrate how the Principle of Generic Consistency can resolve the dilemma raised by librarians Hauptman and Dowd. I will begin by reviewing their positions, recognizing both the strengths and weaknesses of each of their arguments and then apply the Principle of Generic Consistency to these scenarios to show how Gewirth would address these moral conflicts. Gewirth's moral theory would appeal to the consistency principle found in the arguments presented by Hauptman and Constant, while preserving the categorical nature of morality, as exhibited by both Kant and Dowd. Such a resolution supports neither unlimited access to information nor strong censorship; it supports intellectual freedom.

REVIEW OF LIBRARY LITERATURE

Robert Hauptman first raised awareness about the ethical issues of reference service in 1976. Hauptman, a library school student at the time, did a study on the culpability, or lack thereof, in reference service provided by librarians. In his study, Hauptman posed as a library patron seeking potentially dangerous information. The behavior examined was how librarians respond to the request for material on how to build a bomb that would be powerful enough to blow up a house. Hauptman tried to present himself as a person of questionable character. He used six public and seven academic libraries in this study. Hauptman first made sure that he was speaking to the reference librarian. He then requested information for the construction of a small explosive, requesting specifically the chemical properties of cordite. He then asked for information on the potency of such an explosive, whether or not it could blow up a suburban house (Hauptman, *Wilson Library Bulletin*, 1976, p. 626).

Hauptman was surprised to find that not one of the librarians hesitated to answer his question on ethical grounds. It could be argued that these librarians chose *to* help for ethical reasons, but Hauptman argues that the "majority of these librarians gave the question, within an ethical context, little thought." (Hauptman & Stichler, p. 292). Hauptman's study raised two questions: is reference service morally neutral, and does unlimited access to information imply moral neutrality? Hauptman argues that reference service is not morally neutral and that unlimited access to information implies moral neutrality. "But the danger of confusing censorship with ethical responsibility is too obvious to require further elucidation. To abjure an ethical commitment in favor of *anything* is to abjure one's individual responsibility" (Hauptman, *Wilson Library Bulletin*, 1976, p. 627). Hauptman's argument is that unlimited access to information abjures ethical responsibility.

Hauptman argues that librarians are professionals, and

professionals view the freedom to function independently, the exercise of discretion, and the formulation of independent judgments in client relations based upon their own standards and ethical views as essential to professional performance (Hauptman & Stichler, p. 292).

Hauptman argues that autonomy is essential to professionalism. But does this autonomy come at the expense of the autonomy of the library patron? The question goes further than just whether access to information should come at the expense of the common good; it posits whether the autonomy of the librarian and the autonomy of the library clientele are mutually exclusive. It implies that they are, but are they?

Hauptman recognizes that in its Code of Ethics, the American Library Association recognizes professional librarians as "independent thinkers functioning in a societal context," but argues that this is counter to the claim made by ALA advocates (Hauptman & Stichler, p. 292). Advocates of *Libraries: An American Value*, drafted by the 21st Century Intellectual Freedom Statement Committee, a division of the American Library Association, argue for unlimited access to information. Unlimited access to information insists that the freedom of the library clientele should not be impeded for any reason. Hauptman argues that this abjures moral responsibility (Hauptman, 1976, p. 627).

The American Library Association's stance implies a form of liberty in the negative sense, the least restrictive liberty. It is obvious that Hauptman's position does not align with that of the American Library Association; he argues that that there are times when it is morally justified to limit the access to information. But can it be said that Hauptman is preserving liberty in the positive sense?

Liberty in the positive sense, as defined by Berlin in *Two Concepts of Liberty*, is a form of liberty that entails the freedom to pursue a particular end. This particular end is the state of liberty achieved when the agent acts autonomously, free of the persuasion of one's passions. Hauptman suggests that the librarian act in a way that will prevent the patron from using information in a way that will be detrimental to the common welfare. Hauptman is trying to deter an action, rather than promote a particular behavior. He does not suggest that a particular end be sought by the patron, only those acts that infringe on the liberty of others should be deterred. Therefore, he is not suggesting the promotion of liberty in the positive sense.

Hauptman's argument suggests that all agents have the duty to not intentionally harm others. John Stuart Mill, described by Berlin in *Two Concepts of Liberty* as an advocate for liberty in the negative sense, argues that liberty must be restricted when the exercise thereof hinders the freedom of another agent (Berlin, 1998, p. 199). Isn't this what Hauptman is attempting to do?

To clarify Hauptman's position on liberty and its relationship to intellectual freedom, I will review a contrasting position taken by Robert Dowd. Dowd's experiment followed a format very similar to that of Hauptman. Dowd, like Hauptman, surveyed thirteen libraries – six public and seven academic. Contextually, the studies were similar. Hauptman's request for information on how to build a bomb was done in the mid-1970s, a time when terrorism was a topical issue. In his study, dating from the late 1980s, Dowd requested information on how to free-base cocaine. Dowd chose free-basing cocaine because at the time of the study this behavior was a hot topic – it was illegal and was considered to be anti-social and dangerous (Dowd, 1989, p. 485).

In Dowd's study there was little question of what would be done with the information sought and the legal implications thereof. Dowd reported that none of the librarians in the survey (public or academic) followed the usual protocol of a library request. The reference librarian is expected to ask questions to determine the specific information needs of the patron and to assist the patron in finding this information. This is referred to as the reference interview. The librarians in this study did provide minimal to good service in finding information for Dowd, but none of them tried to refine the question or show him how to find information on his own (Dowd, 1989, p. 490).

Dowd went into this survey expecting to find righteous librarians, or morally indifferent librarians. Dowd did not view the behavior of these librarians as morally indifferent, but as morally judgmental (Dowd, 1989, p. 491). Because these librarians did not follow the library protocol of the reference interview, Dowd felt that they were not respecting his autonomy. He concluded that reference service should not discriminate on the basis of the nature of the query or the character of the person requesting the information; such judgment violates the autonomy of the agent requesting the information (Dowd, 1989, p. 491). In his argument, Dowd argues that there should be no restriction on the information service provided to the library clientele. Dowd is arguing for the "freedom from," an aspect of negative liberty.

Negative liberty is realized when each agent is allowed to seek her own good in her own way (individual liberty), provided it does not put the welfare of others in danger (common welfare). Dowd argues that each library patron be allowed, through access to information, to seek her own good in her own way. Dowd argues for the autonomy of the library clientele. Out of respect for such autonomy, Dowd argues that reference service should be free of any moral judgment (Dowd, 1989, p. 491). But could this individual liberty – the right to seek one's own good in one's own way – put the welfare of others in danger?

Both Hauptman and Dowd argue for the spirit of negative liberty. Dowd argues for the library patron's right to seek her own good in her own way, and that there should be unlimited access to information, regardless of what the request of such information may imply. Hauptman argues that the library patron has the right to seek her own good in her own way, but there are instances in which the librarian has a moral duty to impede such access. These instances would include circumstances in which the well being of others is at stake, e.g. an attempt to find the chemical properties necessary to blow up a house. Individual liberty and the common good are both necessary for negative liberty. So, can the positions of Hauptman and Dowd be reconciled?

Isaiah Berlin in *Two Concepts of Liberty* refers to John Locke and John Stuart Mill as proponents of liberty in the negative sense. According to Berlin, Locke and Mill agree, "The only freedom which deserves the name, is that of pursuing our own good in our own way" (Berlin, 1998, p. 199). Berlin goes on to explain why such philosophers believe that this is the only kind of freedom that deserves to be called freedom. Berlin quotes Mill,

unless the individual is left to live as he wishes in 'the part [of his conduct] which merely concerns himself,' civilization cannot advance; the truth will not, for lack of a free market in ideas, come to light; there will be no scope for spontaneity, originality, genius for mental energy, for moral courage. Society will be crushed by the weight of 'collective mediocrity' (Berlin, 1998, p. 199).

Both are necessary, but which is more important to negative liberty, individual liberty or the common good? Neither is more important than the other. Negative liberty is distinct in the freedom that it ensures to the individual, but this does not mean that individual welfare precludes the common welfare, or vice-versa. Mill argues, "The only freedom which deserves the name, is that of pursuing our own good in our own way" but notes that this freedom cannot be exercised when it directly brings harm to others. "The principle is that the sole end for which mankind is warranted, individually or collectively, in interfering with the liberty of action of any of their number is self-protection" (Mill, 1985, p. 68). Mill argues for individual liberty, but not at the expense of the welfare of others.

According to Mill, negative liberty ensures not only a person's liberty but a similar liberty for others as well. But individual liberty and the common good are not always congruent. Mill gives one primary circumstance under which an individual's liberty can be restrained: when the exercise of such a liberty would cause harm to others (Mill, 1985, p. 68). But does limiting the accessibility of information prevent harm to others? A better question when attempting to apply Mill's position to the current debate is does unlimited access to information bring harm to others, or would the limitation of this accessibility bring an even greater harm? Supporting access to information does not indicate an approval of how that information may be used. One may protect access to information simply out of concern for the dangers of suppressing information.

Mill would not advocate Hauptman's restriction of access to information. But would Mill's stance on the free expression of ideas support Dowd's argument? Dowd argues for individual liberty on that grounds that, "the patrons [Dowd and Hauptman] requesting information on these two admittedly controversial topics neither intended to blow up a house nor use cocaine. What better argument in favor of wholesale information dissemination could there be?" (Dowd, 1989, p. 491). Mill's argument in regard to the freedom of ideas is not that the suppression of free ideas is not warranted because we cannot know the consequences/correctness of such expression, as Dowd argues, but because we do know the consequences of the suppression of ideas, regardless of whether these ideas are right or wrong, and these consequences are detrimental to a free society (Mill, 1985, p. 82). Mill would not support the grounds for Dowd's argument that the greatest argument for the free exchange of ideas is that we cannot know the result of such dissemination.

The moral positions of both Robert Hauptman and Robert Dowd raise important concerns for the reference librarian, but they each address only part of library service's promotion of negative liberty through intellectual freedom, the common good and individual liberty, respectively. They each argue for negative liberty, but in so doing imply that the liberty of one must come at the expense of the other. In this section, I have tried to deconstruct the theories of Hauptman and Dowd in order to examine their respective moral implications. In so doing, I argued that, though both Hauptman and Dowd make arguments advocating negative liberty, that neither position is able to preserve such liberty.

In "A Philosophical Approach," I initially will review the work of two 18th century philosophers, Immanuel Kant and Benjamin Constant. Kant and Constant address a very similar argument regarding the right to truth. They debate the limitations on such a right, taking positions similar to Dowd and Hauptman, respectively. Kant argues for the categorical nature of morality. Constant argues that in his preservation of moral truths, Kant disregards the rights of the moral agents that are affected by such an action. In this section, I will attempt to analyze the argument made by Kant and that made by Constant. I will identify the strengths and weaknesses of each of their arguments and apply them to the argument presented by Dowd and Hauptman, respectively.

In the second part of this section, I will present another moral position advocating the rights of the moral agent and the rights of the recipients of such an action – Alan Gewirth's argument for the Principle of Generic Consistency. I will review how he defines moral agency and moral action. I will explore how Gewirth addresses both duty and rights, while preserving the categorical nature of morality. In so doing, I hope to show that Gewirth's moral theory is able to preserve the strengths of Kant's Categorical Imperative without neglecting the theory of rights exemplified by Benjamin Constant. I will then extrapolate this to the arguments presented by Hauptman and Dowd. I will then apply the Principle of Generic Consistency to the moral arguments presented by Hauptman and Dowd.

A PHILOSOPHICAL APPROACH

The quandary presented by Hauptman and Dowd is not new to moral philosophy. In this section I will review a similar argument between two 18th-century moral philosophers, Immanuel Kant and Benjamin Constant. In their moral argument, Kant and Constant agree that the truth-telling principle is an important moral imperative, but they disagree on the relationship duty has to rights. Hauptman and Dowd would agree that information access is a duty upheld by the reference librarian, but they disagree on how this duty applies to rights. It is my hope that Kant and Constant as moral philosophers will bring light to the fundamental differences between the positions of Hauptman and Dowd. I will begin this discussion by reviewing the moral theory of Kant.

Immanuel Kant's moral theory centers upon morality as duty, and the categorical nature of morality. An imperative is an obligatory act or duty (Webster, s.v. 'imperative'). According to Kant, there are three forms of imperatives: the technical imperative, belonging to art; the pragmatic imperative, belonging to welfare; and the moral imperative [Categorical Imperative], belonging to free conduct (Kant, pp. 26–27). Kant's moral theory is unique in two ways; the law governing the moral imperative is categorical, and this imperative is derived from strictly formal principles.

In *Grounding for the Metaphysics of Morals: On a Supposed Right to Lie Because of Philanthropic Concerns*, Kant begins by clarifying good will: "There is no possibility of thinking of anything at all in the world, or even out of it, which can be regarded as good without qualification, except a good will" (Kant, p. 7). Kant goes on to refer to duty as that which emerges from good will. An action is moral if the agent is acting out of duty, not simply in accordance with duty. The action must be done out of principle, not simply in accordance with a principle.

Kant does not try to formulate rules for ethical action, but provides a test for the rules of conduct – a principle on the basis of which to determine whether or not an action is moral, the Categorical Imperative. The three formulations of the Categorical Imperative are:

(1) one must always act in a way that can be willed, at the same time, that it may become a universal law;
(2) one must always treat the rational agent as an end, and never as a means to an end, without at the same time as an end;
(3) act in conformity with the idea of the will of every rational being as a will which lays down universal laws of action (Hastings, 1928, p. 252).

The first formulation of the Categorical Imperative applies directly to action; it prescribes the moral action. The second formulation addresses how moral agents should be treated in such an action. The third formulation applies to moral agency and the qualifications thereof. Next, I will review the limitations in the Categorical Imperative.

First, I shall address the categorical nature of action in Kant's moral theory. A criticism of Kant's Categorical Imperative is its inability to consider the context or consequences of an action to determine the moral weight of such an action. It is the categorical nature of action prescribed by the Categorical Imperative that precludes, for example, the action of telling a lie, even under dire circumstances, in attempt to prevent a greater injustice. Kant argues that "telling a lie can never be justified by the evil that it is intended to prevent. An action done from duty has its moral worth, not in the purpose that is to be attained by it, but in the maxim according to which the action is determined" (Kant, 1928, pp. 12–13).

Kant's Categorical Imperative is based on purely formal principles. Kant argues that morality is based on logical grounds, that context plays no role in the moral situation. How one should act in regard to the welfare of others is addressed in the pragmatic imperative, not the moral imperative. Here, Kant differs from moral philosophers, such as Alan Gewirth, who argue that morality is primarily concerned with how one's actions affect others. Kant views moral truths as existing independent of the agents and the affects on others, while Gewirth argues, "Morality, however, is primarily concerned with interpersonal actions; that is, with actions that affect persons other than their agents" (Gewirth, 1979, p. 129).

While Kant argues that moral truths are independent of moral agents, he does take the treatment of moral agents into consideration when determining a moral action. The second formulation of the Categorical Imperative – treat the rational agent as an end, and never as a means to an end, solely – dictates how moral agents should be treated. It is important to note that Kant equates rational agency with moral agency, and equates rational agency with that which accepts the moral truth of the Categorical Imperative. The moral agent is duty-bound to reason and those of rational agency, and is not obligated to those outside of rational agency, as Kant defines it.

The moral agent's obligation to reason is apparent in the third formulation of the Categorical Imperative – act in conformity with the idea of the will of every rational being as a will which lays down universal laws of action. The truth of the third formulation of the Categorical Imperative rests on the premise that morality can be derived through reason alone. In which case, the formulation makes an analytic claim. An analytic statement is a statement whose truth or falsehood can be derived through the analysis of the statement (Magee, 1998, p. 228). Analytic statements are analytic because they do not reveal anything to the agent. If it does not reveal anything to the agent, it is superfluous.

French political theorist Benjamin Constant, a contemporary of Kant, explicitly challenged the truth in the Categorical Imperative. Constant argued that moral imperatives cannot be derived through reason alone and exist independent of the moral agent. Constant wrote a rebuttal to Kant's Categorical Imperative entitled "On Political Reactions." Constant had a different approach to interpreting duty. According to Constant, duty cannot be addressed without also considering rights; where there is duty, there must also exist the right to what that duty entails. An example of a moral duty where Kant and Constant find disagreement is in the duty of truth telling.

Constant uses the scenario of a moral agent being questioned by a potential attacker as to the whereabouts of a potential murder victim: is the moral agent obligated to tell the perpetrator whether or not the person is hiding in his house? Constant states, "no one has the right to a truth that harms others" (Kant, p. 65). It is Constant's view that if the moral agent were to divulge that the potential victim is in his house, then this agent should be held morally responsible for the murder.

Constant argues that it is necessary to take into consideration more than just the maxim served when determining the moral character of an action. This is because,

> In every case where a principle that has been proved to be true appears to be inapplicable, the reason for this lies in the fact that we do not know the middle principle that contains the means to its application (Kant, p. 65).

Constant goes on to argue that what may be morally sound, generally, is not always true in particular cases. Constant does not question the moral importance of the maxims produced by Kant's theory. He only questions whether these maxims apply in all cases.

What is this middle principle to which Constant refers? The middle principle is the individual's contribution to the formation of the moral imperative to be followed; it is consent to this moral principle. Constant writes "no man can be bound by any laws other than those to whose formation he has contributed" (Kant, p. 65). According to Constant, the moral agent must contribute to the formation of the law, in this case the moral law, either in her own person or through representation, if she is to be under such a law. In the case of truth telling, the moral agent cannot be bound to tell the truth if it is in conflict with a moral duty she deems more urgent.

How does this argument relate to the debate between Robert Hauptman and Robert Dowd? The most obvious parallel between these two debates is that in each case, Kant versus Constant and Dowd versus Hauptman, the authors debate whether the obligation of truthfulness is in conflict with other moral precepts. Kant and Dowd each argue that there is no real conflict, that truth is always mandated. Constant and Hauptman each disagree.

Let's take a closer look at the parallel between Kant and Dowd. In their respective cases, Kant and Dowd argue that the conflict in moral obligation does not really exist. Though for different reasons, Kant and Dowd each urge that the agent should not take into consideration the extenuating circumstances of the case at hand but should act only according to the primary obligation. According to Kant, the agent is ultimately responsible to the Categorical Imperative and that such moral responsibility requires telling the truth (Kant, p. 65). According to Dowd, the moral responsibility of the reference librarian is always to the individual library patron, and such responsibility requires unlimited access to information (Dowd, 1989, p. 491).

Does Kant's Moral Theory Shed Any Light on the Limitations in Dowd's Argument?

Kant argues for the Categorical Imperative, and Dowd argues for unlimited access to information. Kant and Dowd are both arguing on categorical grounds; they are each making an absolute claim. The advantage to an absolute moral rule is that it is not conditional – it offers clear and unconditional guidance. The disadvantage of an absolute moral rule is that it denies that moral rules can conflict. I maintain that the rule of truth-telling/information access is not the only moral rule to which the moral agent is bound. The moral agent acts within a social context; there are competing obligations – obligations which do not all hold the same moral value. The librarian acts within this broad, societal context. The general welfare is promoted through the access to information. But are there not times when the general welfare comes in conflict, and must supersede unlimited access to information? The fundamental question is, is it possible to argue for the categorical nature of morality while recognizing that there are instances in which moral rules conflict?

Constant and Hauptman each recognize that moral rules may conflict. In such instances, they each argue that the moral agent acting must play a role in the legislation of the moral imperative to be followed. Constant argues that no one should be required to follow a rule or law if she did not contribute to its legislation (Kant, p. 65). Similarly, Hauptman argues that the professional nature of librarianship requires that the reference librarian be able to act independently, be able to show discretion based upon her own standards (Hauptman & Stichler, p. 291).

Do Constant and Hauptman contest the categorical nature of morality? Not necessarily. Both Constant and Hauptman argue on deontological grounds; they each argue from a moral principle based on duty. But to say that one moral obligation may conflict with another is not to say that moral obligation is contingent: "Thus, although one moral requirement may be overridden by another, it may not be overridden by any non-moral requirement, nor can its normative bindingness be escaped by shifting one's inclinations, opinions or ideals" (Gewirth, 1979, p. 1). That one moral duty takes precedence over another does not imply that the former is categorical and the latter is contingent. Is this what Constant and Hauptman are saying? This is not clear. Let's look more closely at the objections raised by Constant and Hauptman.

Constant and Hauptman each argue for two very important points: morality necessarily exists in a social context, and the moral agent must consent to the moral action. Neither the position of Hauptman nor that of Constant denies the categorical nature of morality, but neither provides a further definition of what constitutes consent or what this social context implies. The chief failure of the respective arguments is that neither Constant nor Hauptman provides an unbiased method for determining when the action in question will bring harm to others and this should be overridden by an even greater moral commitment. They each leave such judgment to the moral agent's discretion. The arguments raised by Constant and Hauptman do not rule out the categorical nature of morality, nor do they rule out a hypothetical nature.

Is it possible to resolve the dispute between Kant and Constant and that between Dowd and Hauptman? Is it possible to preserve the categorical nature of morality, as exhibited in the arguments made by Kant and Dowd, while placing it within a social context where moral rules do conflict? This moral theory would be justified on its own terms; it would be logically consistent (Kant). It must be categorical (Kant and Dowd). This moral theory must address both moral obligation and the rights that such obligation entails (Constant). Such a moral theory must secure the autonomy of the moral agent (Hauptman and Constant). It must be both logically justified, and accepted within the framework of the moral agent. In so doing, such a principle would be self-legislated; the moral agent would be able to concede to the morality of such an action, while recognizing the necessarily categorical nature of the moral imperative. To do this, this principle must provide guidance on how to resolve moral conflicts, conflicts between the common good and individual liberty. How can such a principle be achieved?

The most obvious difficulty is in finding a moral theory that is rationally justified *and* requires that the moral agency be an agency of volition as well. Could that which is rationally justified and categorical in nature require that the moral agent both accept and act in accord with such a principle? This moral theory must promote negative liberty, the freedom from; it must secure the moral agent's self-directed autonomy. This self-directed autonomy must not threaten the autonomy of other moral agents. To do this, the rights of all persons affected by moral actions must be taken into consideration; the respective rights must be a factor in the moral equation. To clarify, the ideal moral principle to be followed must be categorical in nature; it must ensure autonomous agency; and it must promote the rights of all moral agents. In meeting these requirements, such a moral theory will promote liberty in the negative sense, thus promoting intellectual freedom.

Through the Principle of Generic Consistency, moral philosopher Alan Gewirth ensures the categorical nature of morality through formal necessity. The categorical nature of Gewirth's theory is found in the principle, "Act in accord with the generic rights of your recipients as well as of yourself" (Gewirth, 1979, p. 135). This principle makes it formally necessary that the rational agent uphold the moral law; an agent cannot violate the principle without self-contradiction. I will begin with what makes Gewirth's theory of formal necessity distinct from other theories of formal necessity.

The Principle of Generic Consistency, like other formally necessary principles, requires impartiality, mutuality and reciprocity. This requires consistency in the application of such principles. Gewirth refers to moral theories that appeal to logical consistency, like the Principle of Generic Consistency, as consistency principles. Gewirth compares the Principle of Generic Consistency with two other consistency principles: simple consistency and appetitive-reciprocity consistency. The simple consistency principle argues that the same principle should be applied in similar cases: that if it is held that a moral rule is correct, it should be applied impartially to all similar cases. The appetitive reciprocity principle is a version of the Golden Rule – that one should act toward others with the same rules she would want applied to herself (Gewirth, 1979, p. 162). Each of these rules appeals to the consistency principle; each appeals to the law of distribution; the moral imperative is distributed equally to its moral agents.

The key to the problem encountered with both the simple consistency and appetitive-reciprocity consistency principles is in the hypothetical statement – if it is held that a moral rule is correct, it should be applied impartially to all similar cases. Neither of these principles provides a method to determine if the moral rule is correct. The simple consistency principle requires that similar cases be treated similarly, but provides no method to determine what fair treatment is. The appetitive-reciprocity principle bases the correctness of a moral rule on the moral agent's preference of treatment – to act toward others according to the same rules one applies to one's self. Here there is a method to determine how agents should be treated, but there is no method to determine the correctness of the rules the moral agent applies to herself.

Each of these principles, simple consistency and appetitive reciprocal consistency, requires that a similarity in conditions calls for a similarity in action. This requires consistency in the way in which a moral rule is applied; a violation of the principle commits the agent to holding that though the principle should be applied to all similar cases that fall under it, it needn't be applied to some of the cases that fall under it. In so doing, the agent contradicts herself (Gewirth, 1979, p. 163). Is this sufficient for a fair/just moral imperative? Political philosopher John Rawls argues that, treating similar cases similarly is necessary for substantive justice [morality], but it is not a sufficient guarantee thereof.

> There is no contradiction in supposing that a slave or caste society, or one sanctioning the most arbitrary forms of discrimination, is evenly and consistently administered, although this may be unlikely. Formal justice, or justice as regularity, excludes significant kinds of injustices (Rawls, 1971, p. 59).

It is necessary that the moral theory be administered fairly, but the content of this moral theory must be fair as well.

Formal necessity appeals to the considerations of reason. But Gewirth's moral theory requires more than simply formal necessity; it requires material necessity. Material necessity is the substantive criterion for the application of a moral principle; it consists of the necessary condition of action (Gewirth, 1979, p. 164). Gewirth argues that a viable moral theory is reached through the "analysis of certain considerations about both reason and action" (Gewirth, 1979, p. 21). Formal necessity appeals to reason, material necessity appeals to action. The crucial difference between the Principle of Generic Consistency and other consistency principles is that the Principle of Generic Consistency has not only a necessary form, it has a necessary content. This necessary content is material necessity.

In an attempt to define material necessity, I will delineate the necessary conditions for moral action. Gewirth argues that reason and action are the necessary conditions for moral action. Rational agency is necessary for moral agency. While rational agency is necessary to promote a particular structure of action, this structure of action that such agency must promote is that which is purposeful and voluntary (Gewirth, 1979, p. 158).

This coherent plan of life ensured by this particular structure of action must exhibit both volition and purposiveness. Gewirth refers to this volition and purposiveness as the generic features of action, the necessary features of action. Thus, volition and purposiveness are necessary for moral action. In order for an action to be voluntary the agent must "choose to act in accordance with its [moral principle] requirement rather than in other ways left open to him" (Gewirth, 1979, p. 138), which makes the action materially necessary (Gewirth, 1979, pp. 24–25). Moral action must be in accord with the Principle of Generic Consistency, and it must be voluntary. Is this not a contradiction? If the Principle of Generic Consistency dictates what a moral agent must do, how is the action voluntary? What, according to Gewirth, makes moral action voluntary?

First, does the Principle of Generic Consistency dictate moral action? Gewirth argues that, if the Principle of Generic Consistency were simply telling the moral agent that she ought to respect the rights of herself and other agents, and such an agent knows rights to mean that from which one ought to refrain from interfering, then the truth of such a statement is found in the meaning of the constituent terms. This would make the statement analytic. An analytic statement is a statement whose truth or falsehood can be derived through the analysis of the statement (Magee, 1998, p. 228). Analytic statements are analytic because they do not reveal anything to the agent. Gewirth recognizes that if a statement is analytically true, it cannot guide actions. A moral principle must guide actions. Gewirth argues that this would be the case for the Principle of Generic Consistency if it was simply an analytic statement, but it is not (Gewirth, 1979, p. 177).

The truth in the Principle of Generic Consistency is not simply analytic because its truth is found as the moral agent upholds it. The Principle of Generic Consistency is not simply about the "goodness/rightness of X;" it is about the goodness/rightness of X from the standpoint of the moral agent, and how this evaluation motivates action. Gewirth refers to this as dialectical necessity. To be dialectical, the moral theory must begin from the judgment, statements or assumptions made by the moral agent. "As dialectical, the method proceeds from within the standpoint of the agent, since it begins from standpoints or assumptions he makes" (Gewirth, 1979, p. 44). It is to say, for example, X is good from the standpoint of agent B. As a necessary method, dialectical necessity is based not simply on what some agent may think or believe, but on the premise that it is what every purposeful prospective agent would think or believe. "And the method is dialectically necessary insofar as this portrayal is restricted to what every purposive agent is logically or rationally justified in claiming from within this standpoint" (Gewirth, 1979, p. 160).

Because it is a generic feature of action, voluntary/autonomous activity is necessary for moral action. For an action to be voluntary this action must be under the agent's control; she must choose to act as she does. The agent chooses to act in such a way because it is what every purposive agent is logically or rationally justified in accepting. The action must be under the control and choice of the moral agent. Is this sufficient for moral action? No, moral action must also be purposeful (Gewirth, 1979, p. 27). In order for an action to be purposeful, the moral agent must act for some end or proximate outcome, and this must justify the action.

Purposiveness in action is achieved through rational agency, but rational agency is not sufficient for purposiveness in moral action. Purposiveness in action also requires autonomy or volition, of course, but the agent must also be motivated. Purposeful activity is directed toward the good as the moral agent defines it. The moral agent, according to Gewirth, "regards his purposes as good according to whatever criteria are involved in his action" (Gewirth, 1979, p. 51).

There are three kinds of goods to which this purposeful activity may be directed: basic goods, nonsubtractive goods, and additive goods. A basic good is that which serves as a necessary precondition for purposeful action. Freedom and well being are basic goods. A good is nonsubtractive when the loss of such a good would result in the diminution of the goods one has. Additive goods are those that increase the level of purpose fulfillment for the moral agent (Gewirth, 1979, pp. 56–57).

The goods sought through moral action are of two different views – the particularly occurrent view and the generically dispositional view. These views differ in how the good serves the function of the moral agent. The particularly occurrent view of the good is based on the particular end/purpose the moral agent is attempting to fulfill through her action. The particularly occurrent view of the good varies from agent to agent. Nonsubtractive and additive goods are evaluated according to this particularly occurrent view of the good. The right to these goods is referred to as a prudential right and is evaluated according to how this action enables the agent to achieve such a good through purposeful activity, while not hampering the basic goods – that which is necessary for purposeful activity – of other moral agents or of oneself.

The generically dispositional view of the good is based on that which is necessary for moral action, the conditions necessary for purposeful action (Gewirth, 1979, p. 58). It does not vary from agent to agent; it is constant. The basic good is that which is necessary for moral action (freedom and well-being). The basic good is concerned with the moral agent's capacity of action, and thereby agency, not the particular ends sought or achieved (Gewirth, 1979, pp. 58–59). The generic dispositional view of the good has an invariability that cannot be achieved by a particularly occurent view of the good. This is because the particular end sought by different moral agents will vary, but the requirements for moral agency remain constant (Gewirth, 1979, p. 59).

Freedom and well being are the necessary conditions for action that is both voluntary and purposeful activity, which is required for moral agency. Because freedom and well being are necessary to meet the conditions for moral agency, it is thereby a right of those with a capacity for moral agency – a rational coherent plan of life. Moral agency implies the right to freedom and well being. Gewirth argues,

> the justifying reason of generic rights as viewed by the agent is the fact that freedom and well-being are the most general and proximate necessary conditions of all of his purpose fulfilling actions, so that without his having these conditions his engaging in purposive action would be futile or impossible (Gewirth, 1979, p. 65).

Every agent must act within the generic rights (i.e. freedom and well-being) of her recipients as well as of herself. The agent needn't secure this freedom and well being, but cannot impede upon this freedom and well-being. This makes freedom and well being a negative right. If an agent rejects this negative right, through the Principle of Generic Consistency, she logically must reject the antecedent statement, that she has generic rights (freedom and well-being, the necessary conditions for moral agency), and thereby forfeits moral agency" (Gewirth, 1979, p. 135).

Purposiveness in action is achieved through rational agency – a coherent plan of life, but rational agency is not sufficient for purposiveness in moral action. Purposiveness also requires that the agent be motivated. Purposeful activity is directed toward the good as the moral agent defines it. The moral agent, according to Gewirth, "regards his purposes as good according to whatever criteria are involved in his action" (Gewirth, 1979, p. 51).

There are three kinds of goods to which this purposeful activity may be directed: basic goods, nonsubtractive goods, and additive goods. A basic good is that which serves as a necessary precondition for purposeful action. Freedom and well being are basic goods. A good is nonsubtractive when the loss of such a good would result in the diminution of the goods one has. Additive goods are those that increase the level of purpose fulfillment for the moral agent (Gewirth, 1979, pp. 56–57).

The goods sought through moral action are of two different views – the particularly occurrent view and the generically dispositional view. These views differ in how the good serves the function of the moral agent. The particularly occurrent view of the good is based on the particular end/purpose the moral agent is attempting to fulfill through her action. The particularly occurrent view of the good varies from agent to agent. Nonsubtractive and additive goods are evaluated according to this particularly occurrent view of the good. The right to these goods is referred to as a prudential right and is evaluated according to how this action enables the agent to achieve such a good through purposeful activity, while not hampering the generic rights, that which is necessary for purposeful activity, of other moral agents or of oneself.

The generically dispositional view of the good is based on that which is necessary for moral action, the conditions necessary for purposeful action (Gewirth, 1979, p. 58). It does not vary from agent to agent; it is constant. The basic good is concerned with the moral agent's capacity of action, and thereby agency, not the particular ends sought or achieved (Gewirth, 1979, pp. 58–59). The generic dispositional view of the good has an invariability that cannot be achieved by a particularly occurent view of the good. This is because the particular end sought by different moral agents will vary, but the requirements for moral agency remain constant (Gewirth, 1979, p. 59).

To review, the moral agent must know the action, its purpose, the proximate outcome and the recipients of such an action. This must serve as the motive of such an action (Gewirth, 1979, p. 31). This requires that moral agency be voluntary and purposeful. Such volition and purposefulness requires the freedom and well being necessary for voluntary action. The moral agent has the generic right to this freedom and well being because such freedom and well being are necessary for moral action. Any moral agent, by definition, has the right to moral action. The only case in which the agent would not have the right to this freedom and well-being would be one in which this agent denies these same generic rights to other agents with the qualifications of moral agency – the freedom and well-being necessary for autonomous purposeful activity.

Moral agency and moral action are key concepts in any moral theory. It is in his criteria for both moral agency and moral action that Gewirth is able to redress the limitations found in the moral principles put forth by Kant/Dowd and Constant/Hauptman. Next, I will show how Gewirth's Principle of Generic Consistency re-mediates the limitations of Kant's requirement for a strictly formal moral principle and how this applies to the argument put forth by Dowd.

Kant argues that morality must be based on reason alone. Because the Categorical Imperative is based on reason alone it is formally necessary. This limitation to formal necessity is problematic. It is problematic in how it derives the morally correct action; according to Kant's theory, the action itself must be universalized, and if such universalization results in inconsistency, the action is immoral. For example, the universalization of the act of lying destroys the concept of truth; it is for the preservation of the concept of truth that the moral agent must tell the truth.

Kant argues that the validity of the Categorical Imperative is found in reason itself. But how does Kant know that reason alone can dictate moral action? Kant's moral imperative is true if, and only if, rationality does indeed lay down the universal laws of action. If it does, then the third formulation of the Categorical Imperative is analytic. An analytic statement – by definition – does not reveal anything, it simply elucidates what is already evident. Gewirth argues that analytic statements cannot guide actions. A moral imperative must guide actions.

The key difference between Kant and Gewirth is what they each see to be the foundation of morality. Both Kant and Gewirth argue for formal necessity in the moral theory of action. But Gewirth argues that formal necessity is not sufficient for a moral principle. According to Kant, the foundation of morality is reason itself. Gewirth's argument does not rest on the premise that what must be logically accepted is morally right, as Kant's does. Gewirth argues that if the criterion of 'right' is taken to be simply rational or logical, such a 'premise' is not a normative moral one (Gewirth, 1979, p. 156). This is because reason alone cannot guide actions. Gewirth argues that formal necessity is not enough for a moral imperative, that a moral imperative must also have a material necessity. Material necessity is found in the generic rights ensured by the Principle of Generic Consistency. It is the generic rights that guide the actions of the moral agent and the necessity of logical consistency that prevents one with moral agency from denying such rights to one's self or other moral agents. The logical consistency in Gewirth's theory applies to the rights rather than the action.

It is in the application of rights that Gewirth differs from both Kant and Dowd. The consistency in Gewirth's principle of Generic Consistency is in the rights of the moral agent. Dowd, like Kant, looks for consistency in the rule, rather than in the rights. It is the material principle of rights that distinguishes Gewirth from both Kant and Dowd. Kant does not factor rights into the moral equation. Though Dowd does refer to the rights of the library clientele, he argues for an unqualified right – unlimited access to information. Gewirth argues that rights are qualified. Rights can be qualified as generic or prudential. While moral agency requires the generic rights, prudential rights are evaluated according to their consistency with generic rights.

The Principle of Generic Consistency redresses limitations presented by the categorical nature of both Dowd and Kant. This is because Gewirth's theory goes beyond formal necessity with the material necessity and application of generic rights, without losing the categorical nature of morality. The Principle of Generic Consistency does not limit rational agency to those seeking a particular end (i.e. that which is rational in the strict sense), as the Categorical Imperative does, but promotes generic rights, and thereby freedom and well-being to all purposive agents – agents with a coherent plan of life. Nor does it present an unqualified right, like Dowd.

Can the Principle of Generic Consistency resolve the limitations in Constant's argument? Hauptman/Constant and Gewirth agree, where there is moral duty there must exist a corresponding right to what that duty entails. To address these rights, Constant and Hauptman appeal to a simple consistency principle; to treat similar cases similarly. Gewirth would agree that similar cases should be treated similarly, but Gewirth goes further to determine what this similar treatment should be. Neither Constant nor Hauptman provide a method for determining just what rights and corresponding duties a moral agent must uphold; what lays the foundation for rights and corresponding moral duty? In the Principle of Generic Consistency, Gewirth provides the foundation of moral duty based on rights. This foundation is that which is necessary for voluntary and purposeful activity, the generic features of action. Gewirth refers to the rights that are necessary for voluntary and purposeful activity as generic rights. The generic rights consist of the freedom and well being that are necessary for purposeful activity.

Both Constant and Hauptman are concerned with preserving the moral agent's autonomy when determining a moral action. Constant argues that "no man can be bound by any laws other than those to whose formation he has contributed" (Kant, p. 65), and Hauptman argues that the librarian, as a professional, should have the "freedom to function independently" in her judgment of intellectual freedom (Hauptman & Stichler, p. 292). It is through dialectical necessity that this concern is resolved. Gewirth argues that the moral agent must "choose to act in accordance with its [moral principle] requirement rather than in other ways left open to him" (Gewirth, 1979, p. 158). This choice will be from the standpoint of the moral agent. The Principle of Generic Consistency is dialectical because it must begin from the judgment, statements or assumptions made by the moral agent. It is necessary because it is not based simply on what some agent may think or believe. Rather, it is based on a premise that every purposeful prospective agent would accept (Gewirth, 1979, p. 44).

In the case of a potential victim hiding in one's house in an attempt to evade the would-be murderer, would it be immoral to answer truthfully to the would-be murderer's request for information in regard to the location of his potential victim? Whether or not it would be immoral to disclose such information would be determined by whether such an action is a denial of the generic rights of any of the agents involved. Does the potential murderer have a generic or prudential right to this information? The disclosure of such information would be considered a prudential right because such information is not necessary to secure a basic good, a generic right. But regardless of whether such disclosure is a prudential right or a generic right, such an agent would forfeit such a right. The would-be murderer forfeits moral agency, and thereby generic and prudential rights, in the attempt to commit an act that would deny another moral agent of her generic rights.

So, telling a lie in the would-be murder case would not hamper the rights of the agent requesting such information. Because the potential victim would be deprived of freedom and well-being by the action of disclosing the truth, it would be morally required to not disclose the truth. Though Constant's argument is incomplete, I argue that Gewirth's Principle of Generic Consistency would support Constant's position; no one has the right to a truth that harms others, when harm is meant as the denial of moral agency.

So, how does Gewirth's moral theory relate to the moral debate within the field of information ethics in library service? The argument I am making is that the library must support intellectual freedom, and this intellectual freedom is achieved through negative liberty. Does the Principle of Generic Consistency promote negative liberty? Gewirth secures negative liberty through the Principle of Generic Consistency's relation to generic rights and the necessary conditions of action.

Negative liberty must secure both individual liberty and the common good, without one being at the expense of the other. The Principle of Generic Consistency does this by protecting the generic rights necessary for moral agency. Negative liberty cannot promote certain actions, like positive liberty, but it must prohibit that which infringes upon the liberty of others or of one's self. Gewirth's concept of moral agency does not require that one secure the necessary conditions of action – freedom and well-being – for other moral agents, only that they not impede on such conditions. Freedom and well being are negative rights, thus promoting negative liberty.

When presented with the moral scenarios presented by Hauptman and Dowd, how would the Principle of Generic Consistency evaluate the moral duty and rights of the librarian and the library clientele? In such an evaluation it would be necessary to take into consideration the following ethical questions: what constitutes moral agency; how do we determine the rights of the agents; what are the respective duties of the moral agents; how do we achieve the necessary balance of moral duty and moral rights. First, I will identify the generic rights in question.

A generic right is that which is necessary for autonomous, purposeful activity. Purposeful activity requires freedom and well-being, the generic features of action. Generic rights are generic to all agents affected by the action. In the case of the library, the moral agents would include: the library patron, the librarian(s), the community served by the library. Each of these agents has generic rights. According to the Principle of Generic Consistency, freedom and well-being are necessary for voluntary and purposeful activity. Voluntary and purposeful activity is required for moral agency. Therefore, freedom and well-being are generic rights. All moral agents, by virtue of being moral agents, have these generic rights. Because all moral agents have these generic rights, they each have the corresponding duty to respect such rights of other moral agents. They each must be taken into consideration when determining the morality of an action.

So, what are the rights of moral agents? As argued by Gewirth, because basic goods consist of those which are necessary for moral agency, the moral agent necessarily has a right to them. What are these basic goods? Basic goods consist of that which is necessary for moral agency; it is the freedom necessary for autonomous, purposeful activity. What makes activity autonomous and purposeful? Activity is autonomous and purposeful when it promotes a coherent plan of life. What makes an activity align with a coherent plan of life? A plan of life is coherent if it does not deny the generic rights of one's recipients or of one's self. Other moral agents do not have the duty to secure such rights, but only the duty to not impede upon such rights.

A generic right is an unqualified right; it does not vary by agency. Moral agency requires generic rights, but moral agency is not limited to generic rights. The other rights that exist in moral agency are prudential rights. Prudential rights are not unqualified. Prudential rights vary according to the goals and desires of particular agents. Moral agency secures the generic right to basic goods and the prudential right to non-subtractive goods (the particular goods necessary to sustain what the moral agent has, but not required for moral agency) and additive goods (the particular goods sought by the moral agent, but not required for moral agency). While prudential rights are not part of the necessary conditions for moral agency, prudential rights are necessary to motivate action.

Prudential rights, like generic rights, must be in accord with a coherent plan of life – these rights cannot run counter to the generic rights of one's recipients or of one's self. Generic rights must be in accord with a coherent plan of life in order to qualify as a generic right, and prudential rights must be in accord with a coherent plan of life in order for the agent to have such a right. The difference – if a "generic right" is not in accord with a coherent plan of life, it is not a generic right to begin with. Generic rights are unconditional and prudential rights are conditional. What is the right in question here? The right in question is intellectual freedom. It is general consensus that intellectual freedom is a necessary condition for agency in the library; the right to intellectual freedom is unconditional, it is a generic right. Intellectual freedom is a generic right because it is necessary for autonomous, purposeful activity. Activity is autonomous and purposeful when it promotes a coherent plan of life. This plan of life is coherent when the moral agent seeks non-subtractive and additive goods that do not violate the Principle of Generic Consistency.

Because intellectual freedom is a generic right, any denial of intellectual freedom is a denial of moral agency. Hauptman and Dowd agree that intellectual freedom is a necessary condition for the library to fulfill its mission. The disagreement is in just what this intellectual freedom implies. Dowd argues that the denial of access to information is the denial of the library patron's ability to act autonomously; it is the denial of agency. Hauptman argues that unlimited access to information is a denial of the librarian's generic rights, autonomous agency, and that complicity with this unlimited access to information can deny the rights of those affected by such an action of agency.

The question is, can unlimited access to information be equated with intellectual freedom? Is unlimited access to information necessary for autonomous, purposeful activity, as Dowd argues? Or, as Hauptman argues, can unlimited access to information hamper autonomous, purposeful activity, and thereby not be a generic right? There are cases in which unlimited access to information impedes autonomous, purposeful activity, e.g. the Kant-Constant scenario. Because there are cases in which unlimited access to information runs counter to a coherent plan of life – it is not in accord with either the generic rights of one's recipients or of one's self – it is not a generic right, it is a prudential right. Intellectual freedom is a generic right because it is necessary for voluntary and purposeful activity.

Unlimited access to information cannot be equated with intellectual freedom. The former is a prudential right, and the latter is a generic right.

Unlimited access to information is not equivalent to intellectual freedom, but was Dowd's intellectual freedom hampered? Gewirth argues that while generic rights are necessary for moral agency, they are not sufficient for moral action. The action within morality is purposeful activity. The moral agent, according to Gewirth, "regards his purposes as good according to whatever criteria are involved in his action" (Gewirth, 1979, p. 51). Purposeful activity is directed toward the good as the moral agent defines it. The good to which the action is directed is a prudential good. Basic goods consist of the necessary conditions for moral agency, but it is the prudential goods that motivate the agent to action. The goods sought are prudential goods, and the right to seek such a good is a prudential right. To determine whether the exercise of such a prudential right is in fact a right in a particular case, it must be determined whether or not the seeking of such good would hamper any of the basic goods in question – that which is necessary for autonomous, purposeful activity for all agents involved.

But does this mean that Dowd should not be given access to information on how to free-base cocaine? Not necessarily. Information on how to free-base cocaine is not a basic good; it is, at best, an additive good. Information on how to freebase cocaine is an additive good because such a good is not required for moral agency. This does not mean that Dowd does not have the right to this additive good, only that for it to be a right it cannot come in conflict with the generic rights of Dowd's recipients or of himself.

The question is, do the additive goods that Dowd seeks come in conflict with the basic good of himself or of others? The question is not whether such a good *should* be sought. Gewirth's argument for rationality does not require that the end sought by the moral agent be rational, it only requires a particular structure of action: purposeful activity that is in compliance with the Principle of Generic Consistency – it does not obstruct the generic rights of one's recipients or of one's self. What is this additive good? The additive good is *information* on how to free-base cocaine. Dowd's request for information on how to free-base cocaine does not present imminent danger to the generic rights of other moral agents or of his own person. Because Dowd's right to seek his own additive good in his own way does not deny other moral agents or Dowd himself of these generic rights, it is the duty of other moral agents, e.g. the reference librarian, to not interfere. I equate the denial of reference assistance with such interference.

Does this imply that the application of the Principle of Generic Consistency would run counter to the claim made by Hauptman? Not necessarily. The moral agents in Hauptman's scenario consist of: the person seeking information on an explosive powerful enough to blow up a suburban house. The generic rights of the librarian and others affected by such an action must be preserved. The generic rights of each of these moral agents must be preserved. These generic rights consist of that which is necessary for moral agency, e.g. freedom and well being. Would the withholding of information necessary to build a bomb powerful enough to blow up a house preserve such rights or deny such rights? Let's take a look.

Intellectual freedom, as stated earlier, is the basic good in question; intellectual freedom is necessary for moral agency. But a particular request for information qualifies as either a non-subtractive good or an additive good. Therefore, while intellectual freedom is a basic right, unlimited access to information is not. Would the patron requesting information on how to build a bomb to blow up a suburban house have the right to this information? Not necessarily. Because such a request seeks an additive good, rather than a basic good, a better question is, would the release of such information deny the generic rights of the person(s) acting or being affected by such an action?

If withholding such information is necessary to secure generic rights, basic goods, or any of the moral agents, it is morally correct to do so. Autonomous agency is a generic feature of action (Gewirth, 1979, p. 22). Hauptman's primary concern is with the autonomy of the reference librarian and the well being of those affected by such an action. First, would the withholding of such information be necessary to secure the autonomy of the reference librarian? A better question would be whether the reference librarian's autonomous agency is threatened by the release of such information?

Autonomous agency, as defined by Gewirth, is the generic feature of action found in the dialectical necessity of the method. The Principle of Generic Consistency is dialectical because it "proceeds from within the standpoint of the agent, since it begins from standpoints or assumptions he makes" (Gewirth, 1979, p. 44). The Principle of Generic Consistency is necessary because it is based on a premise that *every* purposeful prospective agent must accept. Hauptman's argument is that the librarian should be granted the authority to act according to her own judgment. Would the exercise of discretion that Hauptman argues for be based on a premise that every purposeful prospective agent must accept? Not necessarily. Dialectical necessity requires that the premise accepted be one that is both voluntary and one that every purposeful agent must accept. So, the information request does not deny the autonomous agency of the librarian.

Does such discretion inhibit the generic rights of purposeful agents? Does the dispensing of information on how to build a bomb powerful enough to blow up a suburban house threaten the generic rights of other moral agents? Basic goods ensure the generic rights of moral agents. In a case where one moral agent's additive goods come in conflict with the basic goods of his recipients or of his own person, the additive goods must come second to the basic goods. The basic goods in question are the goods of those who could be affected by the patron's quest for such additive goods, (i.e. the information on how to build a bomb powerful enough to blow up a suburban house). But is it clear that the generic rights of other moral agents are threatened? Hauptman presented himself in a manner to suggest such an intent. If it is clear to the librarian that it would present imminent danger to other moral agents, e.g. individuals or the community, it would be morally sound not to assist the person in the clarification of the material that would aid him in his endeavor because such an endeavor would deny the generic rights, e.g. freedom and well-being, of other moral agents. The key to this is the *imminence* of this danger, not simply the possibility of danger.

The request for information on how to build a bomb that would be powerful enough to blow up a suburban house is quite distinct from the request for information on how to freebase cocaine. They are each requests for information from reference librarians; terrorism and free-basing cocaine are both illegal acts. But these are the only similarities. The difference, as it relates to ethics, is in the action associated with each request. In the case of Dowd and the information on how to freebase cocaine, because this information does not present imminent danger, the right in question is Dowd's right to seek his own additive goods. And because these additive goods do not present imminent danger to the basic rights of other moral agents or his own person, it is Dowd's right to pursue his own good in his own way that should be respected. Because Hauptman's request suggests imminent danger, and thus the denial of basic rights of moral agents, the librarian should not be morally obligated to ensure that such information be found. While everyone should be given complete service in learning to use the tools of the library, it should not be required that the librarian assist a particular patron in finding this particular information if the manner of the request suggests imminent danger to the basic goods of any moral agent(s).

REFERENCES

Alfino, M., & Pierce, L. (1997). *Information ethics for librarians*. North Carolina: McFarland & Company, Inc.

American Library Association, Office of Intellectual Freedom (1996). *Intellectual freedom manual*. Chicago: American Library Association.

Andre, J. (1983). Censorship: Some distinctions. *International Journal of Applied Philosophy, 1*(Fall), 25–32.

Bartlett, J., & Kaplan, J. (Eds) (1991). *Bartlett's familiar quotations*. Boston, Toronto, London: Little, Brown and Company.

Berlin, I. (1998). Two concepts of liberty. Reprinted In: H. Hardy & R. Hausheer (Eds), *The Proper Study of Mankind*. New York: Farrar Straus and Giroux.

Dowd, R. (1989). I want to find out how to freebase cocaine or yet another unobtrusive test of reference performance. *Reference Librarian, 25–26,* 483–493.

Gewirth, A. (1979). *Reason and morality.* Chicago: University of Chicago Press.

Harris, M. (1976). Portrait in paradox: Commitment and ambivalence in American librarianship. *Libri, 26,* 281–301.

Hastings, J. (1928). *Encyclopedia of religion and ethics.* New York: Charles Scribner's Sons.

Hauptman, R. (1998). Professionalism or culpability? An experiment in ethics. In: R. Hauptman & R. Stichler (Eds), *Ethics, information, and technology: Readings.* Jefferson, NC: McFarland (original work published in 1976).

Hauptman, R. (1976). Professionalism or culpability? An experiment in ethics. *Wilson Library Bulletin, 5,* 626–627.

Kant, I. Grounding for the metaphysics of morals. In: J. Ellington (Trans.), *Grounding for the Metaphysics of Morals: With On a Supposed Right to Lie Because of Philanthropic Concerns* (3rd ed.). (Original work published in 1785).

Magee, B. (1998). *The story of thought: The essential guide to the history of western philosophy.* Great Britain, Dorey Kindersley Ltd., New York: Quality Paperback Book Club.

Montague-Smith, M. (1996). Information ethics: An hermeneutical analysis of an emerging area in applied ethics. Dissertation Abstracts International. Ph.D. dissertation, University of North Carolina, Chapel Hill.

Mill, J. (1985). *On liberty.* Introduction by G. Himmelfarb, New York: Penquin Books USA, Inc. (Original work published in 1859).

Rawls, J. (1971). *A theory of justice.* Cambridge, Massachusetts: Harvard University Press.

Shaw, R. K. (1926). *Samuel Sweet Green.* Chicago: American Library Association.

LEARNER-CENTERED LIBRARY SERVICE AT A DISTANCE

Donna K. Meyer

The red light is flashing on the phone console as I enter my office. The light's pulse means students are seeking answers and help from the Electronic Learning Resource Center (ELRC). As I take notes from the voice mailbox, my computer hums into life and the night's e-mail messages boldly appear, filling the inbox screen. A little green flower appears in the lower right-hand corner signifying that the virtual librarian awaits a chat with a student, a faculty mentor or a staff member. The eye of the video cam awakens and its green light means the camera is ready to record and display a videoconference. And so the day begins.

At Northcentral University (NCU) "We Put People First in Distance Learning," permeates each day. It is not only a motto, but also a way of working. Faculty mentors are assigned to work with students one-on-one, giving each student individual attention. Learner Affairs communicates with students to identify problems that might interfere with academic progress and to encourage success. The University's commitment to active self-learning guides the development of its academic programs so that adult students can earn a degree without having to interrupt their careers or home life. This educational delivery model allows students to develop and utilize lifelong learning skills through the application of course concepts and skills in current professional roles. Interactivity is based on a student's working environment, learner-to-learner interaction, and mentor to learner communication. This allows the student opportunities using an experiential model with feedback applicable to the evaluation of the student's objectives, and course concepts and program outcomes. A fundamental belief underlying this

Advances in Library Administration and Organization
Advances in Library Administration and Organization, Volume 20, 67–81
Copyright © 2003 by Elsevier Science Ltd.
ISSN: 0732-0671/PII: S0732067102200048

educational delivery model is that new knowledge is more effectively assimilated when the student has an experiential frame of reference.

As of June 2002, NCU offers undergraduate and graduate programs in Psychology and Business & Technology Management. Total distance student enrollment numbers around six hundred and fifteen students with a faculty of seventy-seven. Being at a distance, faculty mentors and students interact frequently via e-mail, telephone contact and other computer mediated conferencing tools. The individualized attention given to students supports and enhances their learning. In the ELRC, this idea drives each day's interactions. "Because students removed from their instructors and fellow students must work more independently than those in traditional settings, a strong sense of ownership is especially critical for distance learners" (Barsun, 2000, p. 20). But as Beagle reminds us, "Library service has traditionally been oriented toward the individual and not toward aggregate classroom groups" (1998) (Fig. 1).

Instead of a traditional library with shelves of books stored at a specific location, the University has developed a virtual library, called the Electronic Learning Resource Center (ELRC), that may be accessed by students, faculty mentors, and staff from anywhere in the world. The 1994 research into "digital libraries," funded by the U.S. government, provided for experimentation into the feasibility of providing materials digitally. But these projects did not take into

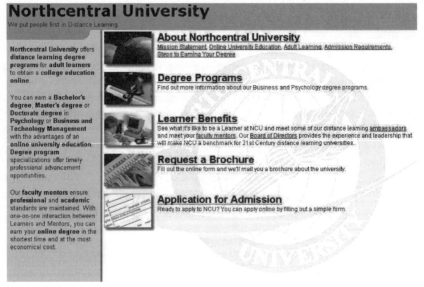

Fig. 1.

account the traditional services libraries offer. So, in the 1990s additional funds became available to broaden the research to include custodianship, sustainability, interoperability between collections, and relationships to a community of users (Besser, 2002).

The virtual library concept extends beyond database searches and obtaining journal articles or books utilizing document delivery and interlibrary loan. It encompasses preparing individuals to locate, use, and evaluate information resources. Students use the ELRC to access online databases, libraries in other university systems, public and private libraries, and Internet and research guides. Tutorials and courses are provided on how to conduct electronic research, improve study skills, and write in a particular format such as APA. The ELRC staff of reference librarians answer resource questions and provide one-on-one instruction in the use of the Internet, tips on database navigation, citation verification, and reference tools. The ELRC staff assists undergraduate and graduate students, as well as, faculty mentors and staff in their research activities. Assessing needs through surveys, NCU remains closely in tune with user needs. A sense of community rests on the exchange of ideas in discussion forums, a monthly newsletter, and daily interaction with individuals.

Today, a "best practices" virtual library . . .

- Provides content and imposes a structure to present that content to patrons.
- Offers search capabilities of databases and catalogs.
- Grants access to full-text documents.
- Provides tutorials for database use and information literacy.
- Links to course specific web sites reviewed and annotated by subject librarians.
- Links to general reference tools.
- Encourages interaction through e-reference options and discussion forums.
- Provides Interlibrary loan and document delivery.
- Presents 24-hour accessibility and reference service 7 days a week.
- Survey user needs and seeks input from all constituencies.

Lead by the Director of Information Resources (DIR), the ELRC staff's basic understanding of library processes provides the necessary foundation for the organization and operation of the ELRC. The DIR translates the vision of providing learner-centered library service into realistic goals, policies, and procedures and provides ongoing management of the web sites. The DIR keeps the administration and staff informed of changes and recommendations for future services and resources by organizing and presenting information on strategic plans, time lines and implementation of added resources and services. The Director negotiates with vendors to purchase access to resources. The distance learning environment requires web authoring skills, content evaluation skills, searching skills, negotiation skills, reference skills, communication skills, writing skills and teaching skills. By working with the Information Technology Department on such matters as site design, structure, and architecture, DIR stays informed of trends in web technologies, instructional technology and design.

Information overload bombards people everyday. Organizing the ELRC's content into categories and creating an interface to support those categories helps users find what they need. The staff evaluates resources for inclusion in the ELRC web site based on user needs, relevant content, and the curriculum.

A virtual library presents organized, pertinent information in an easily accessible online package. By creating consistent and functional navigation, graphics, page layout and categories, the user knows where to go and what to do. A virtual library encourages students and faculty to return. Sanchez (2000) outlines concepts to keep in mind:

- Take an editorial viewpoint.
- Regularly update content that's important to the customers.
- Touch your customer.
- Respond promptly.
- Give your customer a useful resource.
- Be a 'niche pad.'
- Create a community.
- Look at the long term.

Echoing many of Sanchez's ideas, Fichter (2000) states that a library can build support for itself and ensure continued funding by becoming a "sticky site." The regular updating of content builds confidence in your virtual library as a useful resource. Prompt response to reference questions and material requests help develop an educational community of students and faculty who rely on library resources. NCU's ELRC offers a monthly online newsletter that includes brief information on research strategies, writing skills, and web sites. A "Tip of the Week" adds fresh content on a weekly basis.

Resources on NCU's ELRC student web site include: OCLC First Search, full-text databases, indices, course-related Internet Guides, reference tools, journals, tutorials, request forms, dissertation resources, research tips, interlibrary loan and document delivery information. A separate site for faculty mentors provides resources for distance mentoring, mentor orientation, and faculty suggestions. Add-a-Resource allows all users to submit useful web sites for possible inclusion on the ELRC sites. Besser states, "Users don't want to learn several search syntaxes, they don't want to install a variety of viewing applications on their desk, and they want to make a single query that accesses a variety of different repositories. Users want to access an interoperable information world, where a set of separate repositories looks to them like a single information portal" (2002). NCU's selection of OCLC's First Search service offers a common interface to a variety of databases thereby simplifying searching.

Information literacy comprises an important aspect of a virtual library program. NCU's LS107 Information Research Methods, a required undergraduate course, provides an introduction to the scholarly research process with an emphasis on using both print and electronic information resources and services. LS610 Information Research Strategies, a required graduate course, provides a foundation in keyword searching, OPACs, database usage, evaluation of information, locating and using information, APA-style formatting and other research skills. This also provides graduate students prerequisite skills for dissertation work. LS510 Strategies for Distance Mentoring, for faculty mentors, offers an introduction to resources with an emphasis on using electronic information for syllabus improvement and/or development. NCU encourages students, faculty mentors, and staff to establish patterns of life-long learning. The skills fostered in these three courses provide a framework for developing these patterns. Currently, five librarians with M.L.S degrees and areas of specialization, plus the Director of Information Resources teach these courses.

Beyond the accessibility of information and resources on the ELRC web sites, the reference librarians answer resource questions, verify citations, locate materials, and provide interlibrary loans. Through a variety of communication tools, the ELRC staff encourages students, mentors, and staff to become independent, discerning, life-long information seekers. Tutorials, chats, videoconferences, e-mails, telephone contacts, and course offerings for students and mentors provide venues for teaching information strategies (Fig. 2).

From the patrons' point of view, evaluating distance learning library resources should involve answering the following questions:

- How do I access the resources?
- Does the university provide a real librarian behind the virtual reference desk? How do I contact the librarian? How quickly will my questions be answered?
- Are online databases available for my use? Do the databases include full-text journal articles?
- Does the library provide document delivery? Will articles be mailed, faxed, or emailed to me? Can I access the articles over the web with a provided web address?
- Does the library provide interlibrary loan services? Will I incur charges for interlibrary loans?
- Will online reserve readings be available on my course web page? How do I access the course web page and its resources?

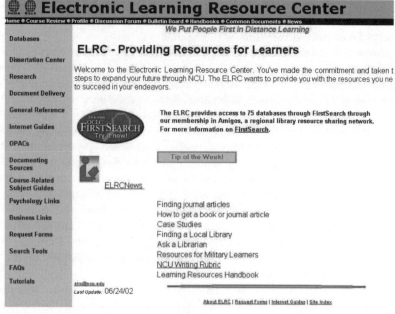

Fig. 2.

• Does the virtual library include Internet links, tutorials, and orientation
  modules?

The patron base at NCU includes adult students who share certain characteristics.
NCU students, with an average age of 44, strive to balance work, family, and
community involvement with educational goals. As mid-career professionals,
Campbell (1999) states that adult students exhibit responsibility for their learning
and a capacity for self-direction. The students bring life experience to NCU,
and project an internal motivation to learn. They demand learning situations
based on real-life problems with obvious application components. They demand
opportunities to set their own educational goals.

The Association of College and Research Libraries (ACRL) Guidelines for
Distance Learning Library Services establish the main philosophy governing the
ELRC:

> Access to adequate library services and resources is essential for the attainment of superior
> academic skills in post-secondary education, regardless of where students, faculty, and programs
> are located. Members of the distance learning community are entitled to library services and
> resources equivalent to those provided for students and faculty in traditional campus settings.

Survey responses indicate that students value the following services: database access, document delivery, and reference help. Students reported difficulties with searching efficiently on the Internet or in databases. The ELRC tackled these issues first by designing online tutorials, information literacy courses, e-reference through e-mail, instant messaging, web forms, telephone and videoconferencing. To provide meaningful and intuitive access, the ELRC continually seeks comments from the users to pinpoint their needs. Surveys, e-mails, phone calls all contribute to continuous needs' assessment. Post-Course Questionnaires gather information on how often a student used library resources for a particular course and how many books and journal articles were needed. The questionnaire inquires about how much money the student spent on photocopies, interlibrary loan, and fee-based document delivery. Students list specific library services used for the course and any local libraries used for resources. Survey results guide decisions on ELRC resources, services, and library agreements. The "Guidelines for Information Services" prepared by Reference and User Services Association (RUSA), provide a reality check for the services and resources provided by the ELRC. The guidelines also outline the key obligations surrounding accessibility, personnel, assessment, and ethics (RUSA, 2000). According to the guidelines, A library, because it possesses and organizes for use its community's concentration of information resources, must develop information services appropriate to its community and in keeping with the American Library Association's Library Bill of Rights. These services should take into account the information-seeking behaviors, the information needs, and the service expectations of the members of that community. Provision of information in the manner most useful to its clients is the ultimate test of all a library does (RUSA, 2000).

Organizing the virtual library at NCU involved acquiring access to resources and developing an interface for the ELRC. Adult students want clear menu structure, relevant examples, frequent entry and exit points, control over options and search functions (Campbell, 1999). To this end, the ELRC currently acquires database access through the regional consortia, Amigos, for OCLC services. Our students use one interface to access information and this simplifies orientation. First Search provides students, faculty mentors, and staff with access to WorldCat and subscriptions to a number of full-text and bibliographic databases. First Search provides reports on usage that may be used for evaluating selection decisions and the timing of moving from a per-search to subscription status on individual databases. The Institution's community reaches beyond the boundaries of the United States, offering global educational opportunities. The ELRC continually evaluates resources that will service the research needs of students regardless of locality. OCLC provides global access.

The staff discusses ways to improve and streamline document delivery, collection development issues, and effectiveness of the web site navigation; develops tutorials, and writes the online newsletter and daily tips. Through mass e-mails and individual responses to reference requests, the staff works to provide friendly and helpful assistance. The reference librarians recommend appropriate databases and strategies for forming search strings or the subject headings for catalog searches.

The Director of Information Resources designed and maintains three web sites. A public web site introduces potential students to the resources and services of the ELRC. The student website provides course-related subject guides, tutorials, First Search access, general reference links, a Dissertation Center, and research guides for the programs offered. The faculty mentor site offers course-related subject guides, resources for distance mentoring, First Search access, general reference links, and mentor orientation.

The web sites need to be evaluated frequently for navigation ease and link checking. The ELRC Research Guides annotate listings of academic print and non-print resources for the University's programs. Sixty-eight course-related Internet Guides provide links to over 450 Internet sites that support specific courses. Students, faculty mentors, or staff members may recommend web site addresses by submitting an "Add-a-Resource" request. After review by the ELRC staff, sites appear under all related topics. The University also offers course web sites that include areas for course discussion, and links to Internet sites and reserve readings. Access to reserve readings remains restricted to those currently enrolled to protect against copyright infringement. Faculty mentors that require extensive journal support for their courses' use XanEdu (http://www.xanedu.com) to provide course packs for students. The ELRC acquires interlibrary loans and document delivery through a variety of agreements with other libraries and document delivery vendors.

The importance of identifying members of the University community regardless of location requires remote authentication to protect library resources. Rather than identifying students and faculty mentors by IP address (identifies a machine) verification occurs through user selected ID and password. The University database of current students, faculty mentors and staff provides the necessary access control.

The Director of Information Resources keeps the administration and staff informed of changes and recommendations for future services and resources by organizing and presenting information on strategic plans, time lines and implementation of added resources and service. By serving on the Academic Affairs Committee, the Director stays alert to program changes, curriculum revisions and other academic issues. The committee meetings provide an avenue to disseminate information about the ELRC. The Director negotiates with vendors to purchase access to resources. A mass e-mail system housed on the University server allows sending announcements about services to selected groups: mentors (by department or all), students (by department or level), or staff.

STUDENT SUPPORT

When a new student enrolls in his/her first class, the ELRC emails a welcome letter outlining the services and resources available to NCU students. The welcome letter includes information on how to access the virtual library site and how to contact a reference librarian. A new student receives the link to the ELRC after establishing a user name and password. The ELRC produces a *Learning Resources Handbook*, available on the website or in hardcopy upon request. The manual outlines policies and procedures, and introduces resources available through the ELRC. The website provides research tips and how-to pages on database use, Internet searching, research guides, links to online catalogs, general reference tools, Dissertation Center, and FAQs. Additional online tutorials cover study skills and information for students new to the Internet. The Dissertation Center includes strategies on dissertation research, formatting guides, writing resources, dissertation tutorials, and links to other dissertation resources. Course-related subject guides provide links to resources of interest to those enrolled in a particular course. Mentors or students may suggest sites through "Add-a-Resource," an online form. Learner Affairs and the ELRC provide step-by-step orientation to the web site via telephone to students requesting assistance.

Ask-a-Librarian offers e-reference through e-mail, phone, fax, videoconference, instant messaging, and request forms. The reference staff responds to questions within twenty-four hours with feedback to students regarding resources to consult for information, answers to questions, and encouragement. 'Asynchronous anxiety' is a term used to describe the feeling of not being connected (Crouch & Montecino, 1997). The lack of feedback or a delay in feedback from fellow students and from the instructor [or reference librarian] is a definite cause of frustration (Barsun, 2000, p. 21; Burge, 1994).

The ELRC resource referral service verifies citations, locates resources, suggests document delivery services for specific material not available through the University, helps patrons locate general reference sources, and explores local library options. The ELRC acquires interlibrary loans and document delivery through a variety of agreements with other libraries and document delivery vendors. ELRC staff members use *The Internet-Plus Directory of Express Library Services* (Coffman, Kehoe & Wiedensohler, 1998) and databases available on the Internet to advise students on the location and services provided by libraries in the student's geographical area. When students need reference tools unavailable through interlibrary loan, the ELRC staff members locate the reference tool in a library near the student. The University assists students by reimbursing part of any access fees charged by a local library.

The funding for library services and resources originates from the tuition payments and is allocated as budget line items. The University provides toll-free numbers, servers, and other communication services. Library agreements through Amigos Library Services, Inc., our regional provider for OCLC services, provide a major part of the virtual library resource base. Users demand the benefits of digital resources, keyword search capabilities, up-to-date material, and access to information from their homes and offices over the Internet. The list is growing through the use of the local library consortia, Amigos, to help keep costs down. A long-term plan provides a framework for the library staff and administration to discuss and build on the present virtual library. The plan outlines the mission and purposes of the ELRC and future goals with specific timelines for acquiring additional resources.

"Many, if not most, graduate student online learners have traditionally been mid-career students. Because they've been out of school for some time, they not only lack up-to-date study and research skills; they lack confidence in their ability to master new ideas and technologies. Librarians are often intimidating to such students, so librarians working in the for-profit graduate institutions often must make a substantial effort to diffuse this fear before they can work effectively and supportively with these students" (Garten, 2001, p. 9). Learner Affairs "coaches" new students in a combination hands-on and voice conference, through the ELRC web site and works closely with the ELRC to assist new students in developing the skills and confidence needed to flourish in the online environment. The reference librarians spend time on the phone and in e-mails reassuring new students or students new to online databases, search engines, document formats, etc. "The level of technology resources and expertise varies radically from learner to learner, which makes it somewhat challenging for librarians ... to find the right level at which to position information and online guidance" (Garten, 2001, p. 9).

The University provides staff to maintain the online environment, train students, and mentors in computer skills, and provide assistance as needed. The IS department provides suggestions to students, faculty and staff concerning recommended hardware and software requirements. Software evaluations of products to enhance communication, learning and instruction, including correlations between such software; model lesson plans for the use of the software; informal and formal evaluations on the results of its use; and other instructional resources will be provided by the IS department.

MENTOR SUPPORT

LS510 Strategies for Distance Mentoring offers an introduction to resources with an emphasis on using electronic information for curriculum development and distance education. The course helps mentors recognize the importance of information literacy – the ability to locate, evaluate, and use information – to improve course design and online mentoring. The overall thrust of all user instruction is to encourage independent and effective information literacy skills. LS510 includes the following topics:

- Learning principles and the online environment.
- Copyright and plagiarism.
- Electronic Learning Resource Center.
- Searching (electronic, database); keywords; Boolean logic; strategies.
- Search engines, directories, and subject guides.
- Utilizing people sources, government resources, and XanEdu.
- Publisher resources; evaluating web resources.
- Audio/video resources, asynchronous communication, video-conferencing.
- Syllabus design, interactivity, cohort group activities.
- E-mail and discussion forums.
- Integrating resources and activities into course design.
- Assessment.

Journal articles, book chapters, and case studies are provided with copyright permission for use in specific courses through XanEdu. (www.xanedu.com) The mentors receive syllabus templates and electronic copies of Assignment Cover Sheets. The student website includes course web pages that may be accessed by students (password protected) currently enrolled in the course, mentors teaching the course, and students who completed the course within the last year. These web pages allow for adding readings, PowerPoint presentations, Word documents, Excel files or other course related documents. The page includes a class discussion forum. Burge points out that students expect participation and a sharing of different perspectives that demonstrate application of knowledge, the willingness to risk sharing tentative ideas, and showing interest in educational experiences of other students. Equally important elements include: response with constructive feedback, encouragement, identifying students by name, and the creation of a sense of community. Focused messaging, Burge goes on to define, as the use of concise statements that avoid messages that do not contribute to the discussion (Burge, 1994). In the NCU class discussions, mentors or students may create and contribute to folders on course related topics. Posting URLs that contribute pertinent information supports and encourages further discussion. "An essential component of CMC [computer mediated conferencing] is its ability to lessen students' feelings of isolation and to create a learning community" (Barsun, 2000, p. 20).

The mentor web site provides information on mentoring, course-related subject guides, reference tools, and access to First Search. Links to articles on distance learning and student-centered education encourage faculty mentors to improve instruction through an understanding of distance learning principles.

The Director of Information Resources works with department chairs and faculty mentors to integrate information literacy into the University curriculum and provides instructional design support to faculty mentors. An online assessment web page provides information that encourages mentors to incorporate assignments demanding higher level thinking skills and research. The ELRC web site for mentors includes a request form for tailoring information skills to a course or topic. The reference librarians provide one-on-one sessions with students to help them establish research strategies. Sometimes, a student decides that not enough resources are available and will attempt to use that as an excuse to a mentor. Mentors contact the ELRC staff who work directly with the student to acquaint them with resources, how to access the material, and consequently, provide the message that the student is not "off-the-hook" for an assignment. Interaction between the reference librarians and mentors assures integration between resources and specific course outcomes.

PROMOTION OF THE ELRC

The primary promotion of the ELRC and its services occurs through the web sites. The three web sites tailor resources and services to students, faculty mentors, and the general public. The ELRC provides a monthly online newsletter, a "Tip of the Week," and "Tips and Tricks" in the Dissertation Center. Mass emails to students, faculty mentors and/or staff provides information on new resources, or strategies for research. ELRC website content must be updated regularly. The staff must respond promptly to questions and comments, create an educational community that relies on library services and resources, and plan ahead for future needs (Sanchez, 2000).

The ELRC survey results mirrored many of Lee's (1999) findings on evaluation of library usage. At Northcentral University survey findings indicated:

- Students use a variety of libraries for their coursework: ELRC, public libraries, local academic libraries, and corporate libraries.

- Students identified the following services as important: reference, document delivery, database access, and full-text articles.
- Students were able to obtain research assistance as needed.
- Students desire additional full-text databases and other online resources.
- Students prefer using electronic services as compared with in-house lending collections.
- ELRC provided instruction in methods of effective research.
- ELRC provided instruction on evaluation of web resources.

In a total online learning environment the ELRC works to build a community of students, mentors and staff who view the virtual library, as a useful, responsive part of the University. The ELRC staff works to establish such a community through its policies, resources, and interactions of with all its patrons.

CONCLUSION

Students and faculty mentors believe that most resources may be acquired online in full-text format. John Barnard points out that "prior to these developments, students accepted the fact that they needed to travel to an academic or public library to fulfill most of their course-related information needs. These students are now coming to expect remote access to information for a variety of reasons" (1999). "It would seem that most assignments requiring more in-depth information sources can be met, in the experience of many students, more quickly and efficiently via full-text databases or document delivery services afforded through virtual universities' Web-based electronic libraries. Most librarians resolve themselves to a new reality where there appears to be a fundamental shift in the minds of many graduate students) particularly busy professional working adults) relative to the importance of a library in their education?" (Garten, 2001, p. 5). But not all documents are available online. For an in-depth coverage of research topics, the virtual libraries must provide databases to locate books, dissertations, and other support materials available through interlibrary loan. Ongoing evaluation of the online collection will lead to the purchase of additional full-text resources and curriculum specific e-books appropriate to the academic level. With the global reach of NCU, offering coursework to any qualified candidate regardless of location, NCU is committed to providing quality online resources and interlibrary loan. Continual evaluation maintains the balance between accessibility and affordability of resources while retaining academic excellence.

Northcentral University concentrates on putting students first in distance education by providing dynamic student support systems including library services.

"Often there are anxieties and stress related to time, returning to school, meeting the demands of the course, and adjusting to the various technologies they must be able to use. In other words, the . . . librarian will spend more time anticipating users' needs, and helping them be prepared to do their own research" (Black, 2000). The distance-learning environment dictates a multi-faceted role for the staff and serves patrons who seek an environment on their desktops rich with information, instruction, and assistance available anywhere, anytime. Although virtual delivery of library services may differ from traditional libraries, the same "best practices" that govern all libraries guide the development of a virtual library. "Both models serve important needs in a learning society and neither can take the place of the other. What we can do is learn best practices from each other and share what we discover as, together, we learn how to more effectively employ advances in information technology to our students' benefit" (Garten, 2001, p. 19).

Virtual libraries will continue to develop and grow. As globalization continues in the economic sector, the globalization of library services will continue to expand to address student needs. "The advantages of the new technological tools in delivering distance service are obvious. We are able to offer our distance learners far more options and avenues. This, in turn, provides convenience, eliminates barriers of distance and isolation, saves the learner time, streamlines procedures and document deliver, makes communication easier, and can be used to provide library instruction in a way that was not previously possible" (Black, 2000). Since Thomas Jefferson's contribution of books to the Library of Congress, libraries in the United States continue to adjust to the needs of their patrons. Jefferson preferred arranging his books by subject using Lord Bacon's table of science, from that point on the Library of Congress expanded and changed collection development, access, and organization. Libraries are dynamic entities. The existence and progress of virtual libraries presents another branch of a continuing, information flow.

REFERENCES

ACRL guidelines for distance learning library services. (February 4, 2002). from: http://www.ala. org/acrl/guides/distlrng.html

Barnard, J. (1999). Web accessible library resources for emerging virtual universities. *The Journal of Library Services for Distant Education, 2* (February 4, 2002), from: http://www.westga.edu/ ~library/jlsde/vol2/JBarnard.html

Barsun, R. (2000). Computer mediated conferencing, e-mail, telephone: A holistic approach to meeting students' needs. In: P. S. Thomas (Ed.), *Ninth Off-Campus Library Services Conference Proceedings, April 26–28, 2000* (pp. 19–27). Mount Pleasant, MI: Central Michigan University.

Beagle, D. (1998). Asynchronous delivery support for distance learning: A strategic opportunity for libraries. *Journal of Library Services for Distance Education*. Retrieved June 5, 2002, from: http://www.westga.edu/~library/jlsde/vol1/2/DBeagle.html

Besser, H. (2002). The next stage: Moving from isolated digital collections to interoperable digital libraries. *First Monday*, 7(6). Retrieved June 11, 2002, from: URL: http://firstmonday.org/issues/issue7_6/besser/index.html

Black, N. E. (2000). Emerging technologies: Tools for distance education and library services. In: P. S. Thomas (Ed.), *Ninth Off-Campus Library Services Conference Proceedings, April 26–28, 2000* (pp. 29–35). Mount Pleasant, MI: Central Michigan University.

Burge, E. J. (1994). Learning in computer conference contexts: The learners' perspective. *Journal of Distance Education*, 9(1), 19–43.

Campbell, K. (1999). Learner characteristics and instructional design. *Academic Technologies for Learning* (February 4, 2002), from: http://www.atl.ualberta.ca/articles/idesign/learnchar.cfm

Coffman, S., Kehoe, C. A., & Wiedensohler, P. (Eds) (1998). *The Internet-plus directory of express library services: Research and document delivery for hire*. Chicago: American Library Association.

Fichter, D. (2000). Making your library website sticky. *Online*, 24, 87–89.

Garten, E. D. (2001). Online and for-profit graduate education: A challenge of understanding and accommodation for academic librarianship. *Technical Services Quarterly*, 19(3), 1–20.

Lee, A. (1999, July). Delivering library services at a distance: A case study at the University of Washington. *The Journal of Library Services for Distance Education, 2* (February 4, 2002), from: http://www.westga.edu/~library/jlsde/vol2/1/Alee.html

RUSA Access to Information Committee (2000). Guidelines for information services. Prepared by the Standards and Guidelines Committee, Reference and User Services Association, 1990, under the title, Information Services for Information Consumers: Guidelines for Providers. Revised 2000 by the RUSA Access to Information Committee. Approved by the RUSA Board of Directors, July 2000. Chicago, IL: American Library Association. February 4, 2002. From: http://www.ala.org/rusa/stnd_consumer.html

Sanchez, M. (2000). Eight ways to sticky sites (February 4, 2002), from: http://www.efuse.com/Plan/sticky-sites.htm

LIBRARY SERVICES FOR OVERLAPPING DISTANCE LEARNING PROGRAMS OF TWO HIGHER EDUCATION SYSTEMS IN WASHINGTON STATE

Harvey R. Gover

INTRODUCTION

The global proliferation of distance learning programs has become a major phenomenon of our times. So rapid is the growth rate of distance learning options, that statistics on them are rendered out-of-date at the moment of publication. As soon as innovations in media and automation technologies have appeared, their new capabilities have been adapted to distance learning applications, fueling the growth of distance learning programs, and providing marketing tools for the promotion of newly upgraded or newly created distance learning programs and institutions. Rapid growth in a highly competitive market has led to the duplication and overlapping of new distance learning options both within institutions and across institutional and geographical boundaries.

A major emphasis of this study is the importance, for all personnel involved in decision making processes within higher education systems, particularly for those with responsibility for future planning and development, of taking a global view of the systems, particularly those based in the same geographical region

Advances in Library Administration and Organization
Advances in Library Administration and Organization, Volume 20, 83–122
Copyright © 2003 by Elsevier Science Ltd.
ISSN: 0732-0671/PII: S073206710220005X

and competing for the same student population. Further, the study undertakes to demonstrate the vital importance to developmental planning for one's own institution of familiarity with the work of individuals having similar roles in other educational enterprises within ones own community, region, and state. With the race to provide distance learning options, this is nowhere more true in planning for higher education than in the development of distance learning programs. To optimize the benefit of these programs over the long term to both the institutions and their clientele, regional planning, coordination, and system-wide communication within and across institutions and systems are necessary. The importance of taking into account differences in institutional profiles and internal cultures should also be evident from the material presented in the study. Another purpose of this study is to provide an initial prototype for the assemblage of the kinds of data relevant to planning distance learning programs and library services to support these programs. Pulling together such information from a wide range of disparate sources provides documentation for grounding the decision making and planning processes.

In this study, an overview is provided of the distance learning programs, and their supporting library services offered by the Community Colleges of Spokane (CCS) district and the Washington Sate University (WSU) system, two systems of higher education sharing some geographical territory in the state of Washington, USA. Although some overlapping of programs exists both within and between these two systems, their distance learning programs and corresponding library services will be seen to be largely coordinated through inter-institutional cooperation, as well as through unique intra-institutional adaptations designed to support the provision of library services.

THE STATE

Washington State, with a population of just over 5,894,000, is located in the far northwestern corner of the contiguous United States. It is bordered to the south by the U.S. state of Oregon; to the east by the U.S. state of Idaho; to the north by the Canadian province of British Columbia; and to the west by the Pacific Ocean. The state covers 66,582 square miles or 176,600 square kilometers, making it the twentieth largest state in the U.S. Close to rectangular in shape, the state is about half the size of Japan, three fourths the size of Great Britain, and 40% the size of California. At its widest point from north to south, the state extends 235 miles or 380 kilometers, and from east to west, 345 miles, or 555 kilometers (Access Washington, 1998–2002).

Washington State is divided from south southwest to north northeast by a wide swath of the Cascade mountain range, more than a quarter of the width of the state, with lush greenery and concentrated population to the west of the Cascades, and to the east, other smaller mountain ranges, arid lands, and sparse population. The overall sparseness of population across most of the state is due to fully more than half of its lands being mountainous. Even the comparatively populous section of the state west of the Cascades has its Olympic mountains on the peninsula just west of the greater Seattle area. The northeastern corner of the state is covered by southwestern hills and peaks of the Elkirk Mountains that progress north, northwest into Canada from northwestern Idaho. Near the geographical center of the state are the Rattlesnake and Saddle mountains, and the northern most peaks of the Blue mountains run east and west to cover the far southeastern corner. Such geographic conditions with sparse population and difficulty of transportation are typical of those of the American west and have engendered some of the earliest development of distance learning in the United States (Dively & McGill, 1991).

These geographical and demographic contrasts have influenced the distribution of institutions of higher learning in the state. Figure 1, Distribution of Community College Campuses in the State of Washington (Washington State Board, n.d.), provides a clear illustration of this phenomenon with 62% of the colleges concentrated on the west side around the complex of inland waterways known as Puget Sound in the greater Seattle metropolitan area.

In contrast, a quick overview of the WSU facilities shown later in Figs 3, 4, and 5 demonstrates a more even distribution across the state than is true for the community colleges. With its main campus on the sparsely populated east side, WSU breaks the pattern of population distribution for the state, bringing students east over the Cascades to enroll in its programs. Through the more even

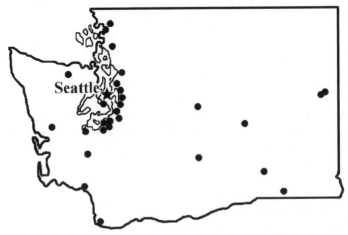

Fig. 1. Distribution of Community College Campuses in the State of Washington.

distribution of its campuses, learning centers, and telecommunications sites, WSU also undertakes to compensate for population imbalances in its distance learning offerings (WHETS, 2001).

DEFINITIONS

Opening with a full definition of distance learning as the term is used in this study is necessary, since that term is so often understood to refer only to courses taken remotely via correspondence, video, or the Internet. The relationship between the terms distance learning and distance education also requires some clarification. Distance learning is used here in lieu of, and as a general, somewhat broader synonym for distance education.

Distance learning in this context follows the scope and definition of distance learning as it is found in the *ACRL Guidelines for Distance Learning Library Services* (*ACRL Guidelines*, 2000). Accordingly, distance learning here refers to any program of instruction in which the students and the instructor are not simultaneously present in a single classroom on the main campus of a school, college, or university. For example, if the students and instructor are both simultaneously present in a classroom on a main campus, but are also electronically linked via video or online with other students individually, or with students in a group or groups in other classrooms at other sites, then the term distance learning applies. Similarly, if the students and instructor are simultaneously present in a classroom on the main campus, but the class is recorded to be played for students taking the course via videotape or other means, then the term distance learning applies to future uses of the recorded version of the course.

The term distance learning also applies even when students and the instructor are present together in a classroom, if that classroom is located at a learning center or on a branch campus or at any other facility which is geographically removed from the main campus, and which exists expressly to bring higher education to students away from the main campus. Thus, learning centers and branch campuses are distance learning units within their institutional systems. The distinctions between learning centers and branch campuses can be subtle. As learning centers grow in size and functionality they begin to take on more of the identity of branch campuses. Likewise, as branch campuses grow in size and complexity, taking on separate identities from the original main campus, their identity as distance learning units correspondingly diminishes, adding to the ambivalence of the terminology. The so called virtual institutions, which have no physical classroom facilities, and therefore no campuses, and which make all their course offerings available electronically, are entirely distance learning institutions.

With the rapid proliferation of distance learning options, students have found themselves selecting from a bewildering array of choices, while academic librarians have raced to stay on the leading edge of technological applications for providing library services to these programs (Kirk & Bartelstein, 1999). Tailoring unique library and information services for distance learning programs within an environment of duplication and overlapping of course offerings has further added to the challenges of these librarians. Prototypes of these processes are examined in the two systems of higher education covered in this study. Described here are unique adaptations used to bring library services of academic merit to the distance learning programs these two systems offer.

THE SYSTEMS

The Community Colleges of Spokane (CCS), encompassing the state community college District 17, one of thirty-two such districts in the state of Washington, includes five entire counties and portions of a sixth covering over 12,302 square miles. The district extends south from the northeastern corner of the state to more than three fourths of the distance down its eastern border, as shown in Fig. 2 (Community Colleges of Spokane, 2002).

As noted earlier, the WSU system is dispersed across the entire state, including the CCS, as shown later in Figs 3, 4, and 5. Large-scale overviews are made of the units within each system, the types of distance learning options offered by each unit, and the corresponding kinds of distance learning library services provided.

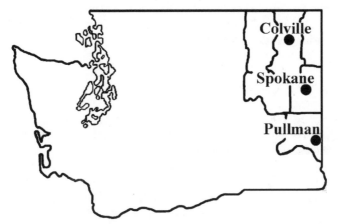

Fig. 2. Community Colleges of Spokane District.

One of the advantages of this study is that a relatively small number of institutions are covered in a relatively small and sparsely populated region, facilitating the processes of overview, description, and comparison. More heavily populated areas with many more and much larger institutions generate an even more numerous and complex assortment of distance learning options. Such areas present far more complex, overlapping models, making the processes of sorting out and reporting the patterns of options far more complex. Bryant (2001, p. 58), in describing such complex, overlapping programs provided the metaphor of ". . . a map of the Los Angeles freeway system with multiple routes, each with its own advantages, to the same location," with that location being the acquisition of learning and the attainment of a certificate, diploma, or degree.

The overviews in this study of the CCS and WSU systems will show that the distance learning options and their library services, while often well coordinated, overlap both within each system and across the two. Overlapping within each system is due to the development of separate distance learning programs at different times within different system units, with each unit offering distinct distance learning options, often to the same students and to the same student population pools. Under these circumstances, students occasionally opt for enrolling simultaneously in more than one distance learning option, and in more than one unit of the system.

Overlapping of distance learning options across the two systems is due to some sharing of geographical territory, as well as the provision of electronic access to some course options not subject to geographical limitations. Students, then, not only can enroll in more than one unit option or program within either system, but also in unit options from both systems. An additional phenomenon are those students who are enrolled on one of the CCS main campuses in Spokane or on the WSU main campus at Pullman, and are simultaneously enrolled in one or some distance learning options of their own or some other institution.

The Community Colleges of Spokane (CCS) District

As seen earlier, Fig. 2 shows the boundaries of the CCS within the state of Washington. The cities of Spokane and Pullman, both located within the CCS, are also shown on Fig. 2 to demonstrate the geographical relationships of the cities to the CCS and to each other. Also shown within the CCS on Fig. 2 is Colville, a town with a population of just under 5,000 people in the mountains eighty-five miles or 137 kilometers driving distance north-northwest of Spokane that has learning centers located in the same building for both the CCS and the WSU systems. The Spokane Falls Community College unit of the CCS operates a library in the CCS learning center there. Through the WSU learning center, Colville is a site as well for the WSU Washington Higher Education Telecommunication System, or WHETS, which will be described in more detail later. As noted earlier, Fig. 5, which is presented later, shows all the WHETS locations in the state.

Eastern Washington University

The presence of Eastern Washington University (EWU), still another institution of higher learning located within the boundaries of the CCS, should also be noted at this point. EWU is located in Cheney, a town of just under 9,000 population not quite twenty miles or 32 kilometers driving distance west southeast of Spokane. EWU is a regional, state-supported university with a fall 1999 enrollment of 8,261 students and a full time equivalent (FTE) of 8,050 (Eastern Washington University, 2001). Although a thorough examination of EWU is outside the scope of this study, it must be noted that EWU and WSU share physical facilities at their Spokane branches. EWU is also one of the four institutions which make up the Spokane based Intercollegiate College of Nursing (ICN), along with WSU, Whitworth College and Gonzaga University, two Spokane private institutions. In addition, as will be seen again later, EWU participates in WHETS.

Another major interaction between EWU and WSU, with significant impacts on their distance learning initiatives, is their sharing of Griffin, their online library catalog. Griffin features an online request button for most materials that can be borrowed, enabling students of both institutions to request books from each other's libraries. Griffin is in turn linked to Cascade, the online joint catalog for all the state supported universities of the state. Cascade provides a request item option for all students of the participating institutions. The request item options of Griffin and Cascade are particularly beneficial to distance learning students who are frequently in isolated settings.

The Community Colleges of Spokane (CCS) Institutions

Located within the city of Spokane are the three major CCS institutions plus two branch campuses of the WSU system. The three institutions of the CCS in Spokane are Spokane Community College, Spokane Falls Community College, and the Institute for Extended Learning. The two WSU branch campuses in Spokane are WSU Spokane and the Intercollegiate College of Nursing (ICN). Both WSU branch campuses in the city share programs and facilities with EWU.

The CCS offers two-year college degrees or one-year certificates in approximately 145 professional, technical, liberal arts, and social sciences disciplines. The CCS charges tuition and fees that range from about one-half to one-tenth of those of other pubic and private colleges and universities in the area (Community Colleges of Spokane, 2001). According to the CCS Web pages, the Spokane Community College unit has one of the largest two-year professional and technical enrollments in the state, as well as a broad liberal arts program. The ninety-eight acre campus of ten major buildings is located five miles east of the city center on the Spokane River (Spokane Community College, 2001). As described in the CCS Web pages, Spokane Falls Community College has two-year professional and technical programs, plus a broad liberal arts program, with many of its graduates transferring to four-year colleges and universities. The Spokane Falls campus of 118 acres is located along the western edge of the city on the Spokane River (Spokane Falls Community College, 2001).

Another CCS unit covered in its Web pages is the Institute for Extended Learning, which provides off-campus instruction and specialized programs at more than 100 locations throughout the CCS, including traditional degree and certificate programs, basic education, community-based non-credit courses, and customized programs to meet the special needs of its constituents. The Institute also develops and utilizes innovative delivery systems to overcome barriers to education while serving the CCS six-county area (Institute for Extended Learning, 2001).

During the 1999–2000 academic year, Spokane Community College had an FTE enrollment of 5,594 students; Spokane Falls, 4,037; and the Institute, 3,022. Student average age for Spokane Community College was 30.3 years, for Spokane Falls, 26.2 years, and for the Institute, 42.8 (Community Colleges of Spokane, 2001).

The Community Colleges of Spokane (CCS) Learning Centers

In addition to its campus locations, the CCS has two administrative office buildings at other locations and the following centers scattered across the city:

- Adult Education Center Head Start/AEC.
- Business Training and Applied Technology Center (BTATC).
- Apprenticeship and Journeyman Training Center.
- District Services.
- Felts Field.
- Geiger Corrections Center.
- Head Start/Bancroft Center.

- Head Start/Bethel AME Center.
- Head Start/Northeast Community Center.
- Head Start/West Central Community Center.
- Hillyard Center.
- Small Business Development Center.
- Head Start/East Central Community.
  (Community Colleges of Spokane, 2001).

The Business Training and Applied Technology Center (BTATC) listed above is the CCS building that houses the Training and Education Coordinating Center (TECC) and several other programs which link the training needs of businesses within the six-county service district with the considerable training resources of the CCS. TECC coordinates programming, scheduling, and marketing for all CCS programs offered to business and industry, while also serving as the site for many CCS training programs for business, government, and nonprofits. Many of these programs are provided on site at business facilities (Community Colleges of Spokane, 2001).

These listings of the individual CCS centers both within and outside Spokane are given above and below to indicate the intense level of involvement of the CCS district in the life of the city and surrounding rural areas. The following sites are maintained outside the city:

- Colville Center
  985 S Elm
  Colville
- Fairchild Center
  6 W Castle St, Suite 120
  Fairchild Center, FAFB
- Head Start/West Plains Community Center
  13120 W 13th St
  Airway Heights
- Newport Center
  501 N Newport Ave
  Newport
- Pine Lodge Pre-Release
  1 Pines Rd
  Medical Lake
- Republic Center
  970 S Clark Ave
  Republic
  (Community Colleges of Spokane, 2001).

- Whitman County Center
  Community Center
  Pullman
- Pend Oreille County Center
  Community Building
  Ione
  (Lloyd, 2002).

As noted earlier, the CCS Colville Center is in the same building as the WSU Colville (or Northeast Washington) Learning Center. As noted earlier and described later, the CCS maintains a library in its Colville Center. A further indication of the deep involvement of the CCS in the life of the surrounding community and region is its use of over 700 community volunteers to serve on seventy-four program advisory committees (Community Colleges of Spokane, 2001).

The total of 12,653 FTE state-supported college and distance learning students for the CCS in 1999–2000 does not begin to reflect the total unduplicated headcount of 50,016 students reached by the district in the very broad range of instructional programs offered throughout all its facilities. Students range in age from the over 1,400 children listed in the programs below to the over 8,000 senior citizens enrolled in 670 classes during the year. In between these two age groups, the CCS offers customized business and computer training classes for more than 6,300 workers throughout the region (Community Colleges of Spokane, 2001).

The CCS operates one of the state's largest child-care programs, offering full-time and part-time day care, as well as part-time evening child care, and enrolling:

- 654 children in Head Start programs;
- 550 children in Early Childhood Education Assistance Programs (ECEAP);
- 210 children in Early Head Start programs.
  (Community Colleges of Spokane, 2001).

CCS Distance Learning Programs and Initiatives

Spokane Community College
The Spokane Community College (SCC) Learning Resources Center (LRC) coordinates the college's distance learning courses, which include video taped and Internet formats, and two-way interactive video classes offered through the state's K-20 network, and correspondence courses. Blackboard is used for some Internet courses. The LRC is administered by the Division of Instructional Services and Telecommunications, which also coordinates the Library, Media

Services, Instructional Technology, and Distance Learning (Spokane Community College, 2001).

The SCC Library provides a "Library Services for Distance Learning: Frequently Asked Questions" Web page for distance learning students with links to the online book and media catalog, periodical indexes, and other resources (Spokane Community College, 2001). The catalog, a joint project shared with Spokane Falls Community College, features a Request Item button. Borrowing privileges are reciprocal, and catalog users may choose either to have the item mailed directly to them or held for pick up. An online interlibrary loan request form is also available, and students have the option of either having materials mailed to them or held at the library for pick up. For distance learning student questions, there is also a toll-free number and an "Ask a Librarian" Web page (Spokane Community College, 2001).

Spokane Falls Community College
Spokane Falls Community College (SFCC) offers both video taped and Internet distance learning courses. The video course tapes may be viewed via cable or may be rented. The Internet courses are of three types:

- SFCC Online Courses,
- WashingtonOnline or WAOL courses,
- Community Colleges of Spokane courses that utilize the WAOL system.

WAOL is a cooperative effort among units of the Washington State Community and Technical Colleges system that allows students who live in the state of Washington and elsewhere to take online courses from instructors from various colleges throughout the state. It is possible for SFCC students to sign up for a WAOL class that is taught by an instructor in a different part of the state and also to chat with students from elsewhere (Spokane Falls Community College, 2001).

In addition to the shared online book and media catalog with its request item capabilities, the SFCC library has an online reference request form with a projected twenty-four hour turnover. A toll-free number is offered for questions requiring a more immediate response. Likewise, there is an interlibrary loan information page and request form. A "Library Services for Distance Learners" page is linked from the "Information about the SFCC Library" page. It should be noted at this point that the SFCC library provides distance learning library services both for SFCC students and for students of the Institute for Extended Learning. Accordingly, the SFCC library is linked from the Institute Web pages (Lloyd, 2002; Spokane Falls Community College, 2001).

Institute for Extended Learning
As its name implies, the Institute for Extended Learning is a major distance learning entity for the CCS. The Institute describes itself as ". . . a network of innovative services, offering traditional and non-traditional education and customized training throughout the . . . district" (Institute for Extended Learning, 2001). Although we have already noted several of the following bulleted items within the context of the CCS as a whole, all of them are presented here to indicate that they originate with the Institute and to convey the full scope of the Institute's accomplishments. The following is from the Institute's Web pages: "As a result of our people and partnerships:

- Over 44,000 duplicated and 21,000 unduplicated people were served.
- We produced 3,100 state-supported annualized FTEs (full-time equivalent) in 1997–1998. Our FTE allocation is larger than 11 other community and technical colleges in the state system.
- We generate over $15 million in contracts and grants – which is more than twice our $6 million state allocation.
- We employ (sic) over 900 full-time and part-time people during the past year.
- Nearly 2,000 adults graduated from GED, high school completion, and English as a Second Language programs.
- We serve approximately 4,000 adults per year in the Adult Basic Education division.
- We teach more than 900 immigrants and refugees per year.
- More than 4,200 seniors (55 and older) participated in classes at over 21 centers throughout the area.
- We help more than 425 families enhance their parenting skills each year in our Parent Cooperative Preschools.
- Close to 200 widows and widowers are served each year in our Solo Strategies workshops.
- We provide guidance each year to 150 dislocated workers seeking new careers.
- We serve more than 1,300 preschool children per year in our Head Start/ECEAP (Early Childhood Education and Assistance) and Early Head Start programs.
- The SBDC provided individual counseling to 450 businesses and had 900 participants in noncredit workshops.
- Through our Help Line more than 2,950 callers received information and referrals.
- More than 1,700 noncredit classes are offered at more than 80 off-campus sites.
- Through Project Self-Sufficiency, more than 70 participants learned how to make the transition from public assistance to productive employment; and 44 students were enrolled in Change Point!

- People Accessing Careers and Education (PACE) enrolled 300 students last year in their work employment program and classes.
- Last year, over 4,000 individuals enrolled in classes offered by the Corrections Programs.
- The Colville Center is the only educational institution in the state offering instruction via an audio teleconference system. They are the first to offer full motion interactive video classes in four counties.
- We deliver educational programs at approximately 100 sites annually.
- Through a cooperative agreement with WSU we extend classes leading to a Baccalaureate Degree by television to Stevens, Ferry and Pend Oreille counties. Last year 14 completed their degrees.
- More than 12,000 adults enroll each year in Community Services noncredit classes held in local high schools throughout the district."
(Institute for Extended Learning, 2001).

Spokane Falls Community College Distance Learning Library Services

As delineated in the SFCC Web pages, the SFCC Library supplies focused distance learning library services for both SFCC and the Institute. "Distance Learning Library Services and the Community Colleges of Spokane," the 1999–2000 Annual Report of the SFCC Distance Education Librarian, Diane Lloyd, presents an overview of the library and media services provided to the students attending CCS classes throughout the "Northern Counties" of the District. These services constitute a major segment of the SFCC distance learning library services. Lloyd's Report notes the professional support services she supplies to the Library Technician responsible for running the CCS Colville Center Library, a full-service library staffed by one full time classified staff member and numerous workstudy students (Lloyd, 2000).

All the information services to the "Northern Counties" Lloyd performed herself, unless otherwise specified. Not only does Lloyd's Report constitute a valuable checklist of these services, but it also provides a vivid example of the extraordinarily heavy workload that distance learning librarians typically face. As will be seen in Lloyd's circumstances, the provision of distance learning library services is often an add-on to other challenging levels of position responsibilities. Inevitably, these differing categories of responsibilities grow at varying rates and tend to compete for the librarian's time and attention, crowding each other out and adding to the pressures and frustrations of the job.

Lloyd opens her Report with a quote from the 1989 *ACRL Guidelines for Distance Learning Library Services*:

Traditional on-campus library services themselves cannot be stretched to meet the library needs of distance learning students and faculty who face distinct and different challenges involving library access and information delivery. Special funding arrangements, proactive planning, and promotion are necessary to deliver equivalent library services and to maintain quality in distance learning programs. Because students and faculty in distance learning programs frequently do not have direct access to a full range of library services and materials, equitable distance learning library services are more personalized than might be expected on campus (Lloyd, 2000).

Services Coordinated by the Distance Education Librarian

SFCC has assigned responsibility for the coordinating of library services to one full-time librarian housed at Spokane Falls. Currently the Distance Education Librarian:

- Visits sites and centers on a regular basis.
- Selects materials.
- Manages collections.
- Provides training and information to extension library technician, extension staff, extension teachers, and
- Provides reference assistance/instruction sessions to students, faculty and staff.

These tasks comprise one third of the Distance Education Librarian's assigned duties, as the Librarian is also expected to teach and provide reference service to students on the SFCC campus, and to manage the library's media collection. In reality, the growing demands of this service require at least 50% of the Librarian's work hours.

Services Provided for 1999–2000

Site visits by Distance Education Librarian:

- Colville-15 trips, 21 library research classes taught during site visits.
- Newport-6 trips, 10 library research classes taught during site visits.
- Republic-3.
- Inchelium-4.
- Colfax-1.
- Total visits-29.

Sites visits require leaving Spokane at 5:30 a.m. returning after 6:00 p.m.

Requests for Library/Media Materials and Services

Subject requests for material-81

Subject requests generally require thirty minutes to fulfill; a librarian must determine what material is available to satisfy the student's request and then ensure that the material is forwarded to the student in a timely fashion. In addition to these individual requests, when preparing for orientation classes, if the Librarian has student topics ahead of time, she and the SFCC staff attempt to presearch the topics to locate something relevant to take to the student.

Interlibrary loan requests filled-89 (June 1999–March 2000).

Book requests filled:

With the new circulation system, students can request items themselves from the SFCC catalog online as they are searching the catalog. Circulation staff then retrieve and mail them.

Video requests filled-158 (These items are borrowed from the SFCC collection.)

Additional library services provided:

- Preparation time for classes taught at IEL sites.
- Selection of materials for the IEL Center library at Colville.
- Collection maintenance at Colville Center Library.
- Ordering and processing materials.
- Ordering library materials for IEL students using the Interlibrary Loan system.
- One-on-one consultation with students regarding their topics and the time spent researching and locating materials for them.
- Trouble shooting over the phone with students needing assistance using the SFCC Library homepage and indexes.
- UPS shipping for books and videos sent to IEL students and sites.
- Film rental when a faculty member needs a film that must be rented from a film rental library.

Access to resources:

- ProQuest Direct: This full text periodical index provides access to articles from over 1000 periodical titles to students not only when they are at the centers but also from their home computers. This eliminates the need to request articles from SFCC and allows instant access. This represents a tremendous increase in service over what was previously available. Previously, SFCC mailed or faxed articles to students after they had identified them in our print-based indexes.
- Gale Literary Databases: These databases provide full text biographical and critical information on authors and their work. Previously, students had to request material to be copied and mailed from SFCC. A major factor in our decision to subscribe electronically to this service was to provide better service to extension students.
- Art Index.

Technical support:

SFCC Media staff make regularly scheduled trips to each IEL site in order to examine and service audiovisual and satellite equipment. Media staff deal with problems at the Spokane County sites on an "as needed" basis. At least once a quarter, the staff also travels to Colville to provide services on-site. In addition, at least one trip per year is scheduled to visit Chewelah, Inchelium, Newport, and Republic.

Total visits per year: 10

SFCC Media staff repair equipment sent to SFCC from the IEL sites.

SFCC Media staff support the K-20 link to the Northern Counties, which is used to deliver classroom instruction as well as other conferencing services. Not funded is the SFCC Media staff maintenance of the SFCC library web pages, which provide students with access to the book catalog, periodical indexes, and Internet search guides (Lloyd, 2000, 2002).

The Washington State University System

The WSU system is a land grant university system having the main campus in Pullman, on the eastern border in the lower eastern quadrant of the state, and four branch campuses. The locations and distribution of the WSU campuses is shown in Fig. 3. The following are major attributes of the main campus in Pullman:

- Ranked among the top research universities in America according to the Carnegie Foundation for the Advancement of Teaching.
- One of just two Northwest universities ranked among the top 50 public universities in America by *U.S. News & World Report.*
- 150+ fields of study – the broadest selection in the state.
- Many academic programs ranked among the best in the nation – and in the world.
- Ranked the No. 1 Most Wired University in the West for high-tech services by Yahoo Internet Life.
- Three faculty elected to the National Academy of Sciences, the nation's highest honor for scientific researchers.
- Small classes, averaging 10 to 19 students.
- Most students' high school GPAs higher than 3.4.
- Only major public research university in the country to require an approved writing portfolio for graduation.
- A fully accredited institution, with many departments and colleges accredited by professional associations.
- One of the most respected Honors Colleges in the nation.
  (Washington State University, 2001).

In Fig. 3 only three locations are given for the four branch campuses, since two branch campuses, as noted earlier, WSU Spokane and the ICN, are both located in

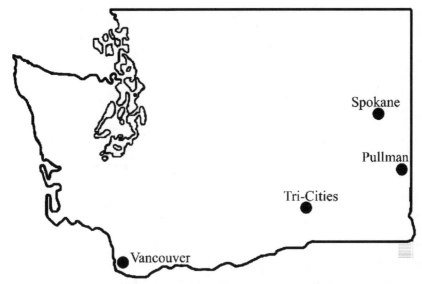

Fig. 3.   Washington State University Campus Locations.

Spokane, seventy-six miles, or 122 kilometers, driving distance north of the main campus. Another, WSU Tri-Cities, is in the southeastern section of the state, in the city of Richland, which is 143 miles or 230 kilometers driving distance south southwest from Pullman. The fourth, WSU Vancouver, in the southwestern corner of the state, is 354 miles or 570 kilometers driving distance from Pullman. Figure 3 shows the locations of the main campus and the four branch campuses (State Map, 2001). The distance learning programs of the WSU campuses and library services to them will be covered later.

The distance learning facilities of the WSU system also include ten Learning Centers scattered across the state. Figure 4 shows the distribution of the Learning Centers (Learning Centers, 2001). Also serving or interacting very closely with the WSU distance learning programs are many of its nine statewide service operations, including WHETS; thirty-three statewide research units and programs; and five agricultural research and extension centers across the state (Washington State University, 2001).

Washington Higher Education Telecommunication System (WHETS)
Much of the WSU system, including its campuses and learning centers, is connected for distance learning and other purposes by an interactive compressed digital television network mentioned earlier and known as the Washington

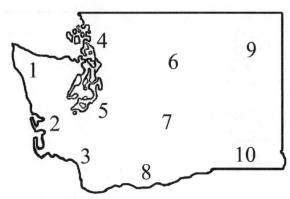

Fig. 4. Washington State University Learning Centers.

Higher Education Telecommunication System or WHETS. As observed in the preceding paragraph, WHETS is one of the nine WSU statewide service programs summarized into one entry there. Figure 5 shows WHETS locations throughout the state (WHETS, 2001).

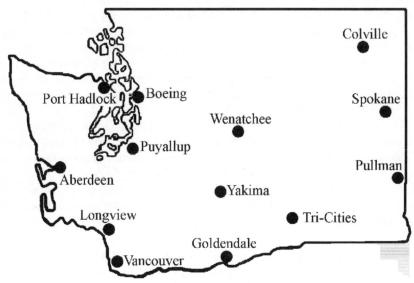

Fig. 5. Washington State University Washington Higher Education Telecommunication System (WHETS) Locations.

Through WHETS, WSU classrooms are linked electronically across the state by two-way video and audio interaction. In addition to delivering academic courses, WHETS is used for video conferencing among sites. Faculty and administrative meetings, student advising conferences, and staff development programs are other examples of how people use the system when they work or study at different locations (WHETS, 2001). WSU Libraries faculty meetings are telecast via WHETS so that library faculty at the branch campus libraries may attend, participate, and vote on issues affecting themselves. Faculty of the branch campus libraries also conduct meetings among themselves via WHETS.

Besides the five WSU campuses, other institutions and centers from around the state are connected to WHETS. The following sites also receive and deliver academic programs via WHETS: Wenatchee Valley College, Seattle Central Community College, Yakima Valley Community College, Central Washington University, and the University of Idaho in Moscow (WHETS, 2001).

In addition, business-related sites are also connected to WHETS through partnerships outside higher education. The Boeing Company in Seattle has partnered with the WSU College of Engineering and Architecture to receive a graduate program in engineering management at eight sites in the Puget Sound area via the Boeing Education Network (WHETS, 2001).

Another WHETS partnership outside academe entails the interaction of still another Spokane distance learning unit with the WSU system, the Spokane Intercollegiate Research and Technology Institute (SIRTI). SIRTI receives five WSU engineering degree programs via WHETS, bringing to Spokane professionals the resources of a research university, while enabling WSU faculty to interact with industrial scientists and faculty from other universities (WHETS, 2001).

As the WHETS Web site so eloquently states:

Access to higher education is a major issue in the state of Washington. The state ranks in the upper third of the nation for students completing two years of higher education, but in the lower third for students completing a bachelor's degree. The need for more upper-division education delivered to place bound students provides much of the impetus for the state's investment in the Washington Higher Education Telecommunication System. WHETS serves as a national model for providing distance education – by design (WHETS, 2001).

Enrollment Distributions for Washington State University

Tables 1 through 5 show the relative sizes of the various WSU units and programs by supplying the 1999–2000 enrollment figures for all. These enrollment figures are given in both headcount and FTE, or full-time equivalent values. During that academic year, the enrollment for the ICN was counted as part of the off campus enrollment for Pullman, so ICN figures are included, though not separately identified, in the Pullman off campus enrollment totals in Tables 1 and 3, while

Table 1. Washington State University Enrollment by Campus for Fall 1999.

Campus	Headcount		FTE	
	On Campus	Off Campus	On Campus	Off Campus
Pullman	15,914	1,722	16,532	1,087
Spokane	486	118	435	47
Tri-Cities	1,083		612	
Vancouver	1,503	18	1,013	10
Totals	18,986	1,858	18,592	1,144

Source: Fulkerson, 2001.

Table 2. Washington State University Pullman Off Campus FTE
Detail for Fall 1999.

Campus	DDP	ICN	SCHRA	Misc. Other
Pullman	678	358	15	36
Spokane	2			45
Tri-Cities				
Vancouver				10

Source: Fulkerson, 2001.

the separate FTE figures are given for the ICN in the breakdown of Pullman off campus FTEs in Tables 2 and 4.

However, because ICN includes class offerings scattered across the state, a separate breakdown for all ICN location headcounts and FTEs is given in Table 5, in order to show the relative size of the ICN Spokane campus to its other locations and to other WSU and CCS units. The separate count for ICN is also provided, because ICN is treated in this study as a branch campus of the WSU system, although it is not regarded as such by the main Pullman campus.

Table 3. Washington State University Enrollment by Campus for Spring 2000.

Campus	Headcount		FTE	
	On Campus	Off Campus	On Campus	Off Campus
Pullman	14,713	1,690	15,353	997
Spokane	446	99	349	33
Tri-Cities	1,025		580	
Vancouver	1,441	13	906	11
Totals	17, 625	1,802	17,188	1,041

Source: Fulkerson, 2001.

Table 4. Washington State University Pullman Off Campus FTE Detail for Spring 2000.

Campus	DDP	ICN	SCHRA	Misc. Other
Pullman	311	361		325
Spokane	2			31
Tri-Cities				
Vancouver				11

Source: Fulkerson, 2001.

Closely related to the issue of the ICN as a branch campus are the On Campus and Off Campus designations used in Tables 1 and 3 for the Spokane and Vancouver branch campuses. For the purposes of this study and in accordance with the definition of distance learning in use, the branch campuses are considered to be entirely off campus, being away from the main campus, and therefore distance learning units, even though specified as having both on campus and off campus counts in the tables. That units off the main campus, such as branch campuses, can also have their own "off campus" designations, off off campus, in effect, is indicative of the levels of complexity and ambiguity with which one must deal in attempting to establish uniform definitions and usages of terminology for research on distance learning programs.

WSU Branch Campus Programs and Libraries

Intercollegiate College of Nursing
The Branch Campus. The names of the ICN participating institutions have been given earlier in the study. The ICN offers the upper division undergraduate

Table 5. Washington State University Intercollegiate College of Nursing Enrollment for 1999–2000.

	Fall 1999		Spring 2000	
	Headcount	FTE	Headcount	FTE
Spokane	384	359.19	302	279.74
Tri-Cities	17	13.07	21	10.60
Wenatchee	0	0	0	0
Yakima	7	5.07	85	60.80
Vancouver	96	50.50	79	49.00
Totals	504	412.30	487	400.14

Source: Pringle, 2001.

and graduate course work in nursing for EWU, WSU, and Whitworth College. Gonzaga University students participate in the Bachelor of Science in Nursing program only. The ICN is the first and the largest combined public and private nursing education consortium in the United States. The ICN is accredited by the National League for Nursing through 2004 (ICN, 2002).

Founded in 1968, the ICN is a leader in distance learning, with students studying on their campus in Spokane; at the Tri-Cities and Vancouver branch campuses; and at a separate nursing building adjacent to the WSU Yakima Learning Center. In the WSU system, the ICN is the largest volume user of time on WHETS, benefiting students at all sites (ICN, 2002).

The ICN is proud of its reputation for quality education. ICN Bachelor of Science in Nursing graduates consistently achieve one of the highest rates of passage of first-time candidates on the National Council Licensure Examination (NCLEX) for baccalaureate-prepared registered nurses in Washington State. ICN graduates from both the undergraduate and graduate programs are highly sought after for their excellence in nursing practice (ICN, 2002).

The Branch Campus Library

The Betty M. Anderson Library is a Resource Library for the Pacific Northwest Region of the National Network of Libraries of Medicine (NN/LM). Its membership in the NN/LM provides access to library collections across the United States (Betty M. Anderson Library, 2002). Library faculty provide telephone and e-mail consultation to distance students to smooth their use of electronic resources. Staff, including one at the College's Yakima satellite, provide reference assistance and document delivery throughout the system. The Library's collections in Spokane include 10,000 volumes and 200 paper journal subscriptions, and support students at all locations and provide depth to the nursing materials held in the other branch campus libraries. The Library separately funds access throughout the WSU system to the database for CINAHL, *The Cumulative Index to Nursing and Allied Health Literature* (Pringle, 2002).

Hours per week of assigned Reference Desk duty and other direct patron contacts were asked of the two full-time librarians working in the Anderson library as an informal measure of workload for these distance learning librarians. Each is assigned ten hours per week. Each averages another five hours per week for distance and drop-in service on demand. During the 1999–2000 period covered by the study, each contact with a distant student involving access to electronic resources consumed about an hour, with time required for the student to test procedures, report status, and make changes to the remote system, add software, etc. A subsequent change in proxy servers has greatly reduced the time required for each student to make changes, allowing access to the WSU online services and thereby reducing the amount of time required for individual professional assistance (Pringle, 2002).

Washington State University Spokane

The Branch Campus. Established in 1989 as an urban branch campus, WSU Spokane offers a learning and research community that provides around 500 local area students hands-on opportunities for professional growth and academic excellence. Students range from full-time, traditional undergraduates to working adults juggling their studies with family responsibilities and community involvement. The average student age is thirty-two, and the campus is approximately 58% female, 42% male. (Washington State University Spokane, 2001) As shown earlier, the 1999–2000 enrollment figures for the branch campus are given in Tables 1 through 4.

WSU Spokane is currently divided between two campus locations, one in downtown Spokane and one at Riverpoint, a new development on the Spokane River projected to be the permanent home of the branch campus. Classes are offered in three different buildings: at the downtown location, at the Riverpoint location, and in the SIRTI building, which is adjacent to the Riverpoint campus. Campus growth is planned for the Riverpoint location, where a new science building is nearing completion (Washington State University Spokane, 2001).

Academic programs include the following:

Undergraduate Degrees and Fields of Study:

- Architecture;
- Computer Engineering;
- Construction Management;
- Interior Design;
- Landscape Architecture;
- Real Estate.

Graduate Studies:

- Architecture;
- Computer Science;
- Criminal Justice;
- Design-Build Management (M.S. Arch.);
- Dietetics;
- Educational Leadership & Counseling Psychology;
- Electrical Engineering;
- Engineering Management;
- Health Policy & Administration;

- Human Nutrition;
- Interior Design;
- Landscape Architecture;
- Speech & Hearing Sciences;
- Technology Management;
- Teaching.

Professional Programs:

- Architecture;
- Construction Management;
- Educational Administration;
- Interior Design;
- Landscape Architecture;
- Pharmacy;
- Dietitian Studies;
- Doctoral Programs;
- Doctor of Pharmacy (Pharm. D.).

Certificates and Professional Credentials:

- Educational Leadership: Principal's Credentials;
- Educational Leadership: Superintendent's Credentials;
- Graduate Certificate on Aging;
- School Psychology Certification;
- Dietitian Studies.
  (Washington State University Spokane, 2001).

Although enrollment figures for 1999–2000 are available for the WSU students at the Spokane branch campus, there are no similar figures for the EWU students. For EWU in 1999–2000, enrollment for course offerings at the Spokane site were not counted separately from courses offered on the main campus. Up to this point, the EWU course offerings in Spokane were not regarded as distance learning, nor were the Spokane facilities treated as separate distance learning facilities (Buxton, Enrollment, 2001).

Stemming in part, no doubt, from its own institutional culture, the EWU view and definition of distance learning follow that of the state of Washington itself which restricts the term to courses offered with no direct interaction between instructor and student, the narrowest definition of the term. This perception is reinforced by the fact that there is no separate state funding for the EWU Spokane operation, as there is for the WSU Spokane, Tri-Cities, and Vancouver operations.

The Branch Campus Library

The library facility for WSU/EWU in Spokane is known as CALS or the Cooperative Academic Library Service. CALS provides on-site library services to the Spokane based faculty, students, and staff of the two universities.

Typical of branch campus libraries, CALS maintains small collections, emphasizing access to information by electronic means through the main campus libraries. Requests for materials from individual students may be sent to CALS via fax, courier services between the two universities, Ariel scanning, and by mail. However, direct access to full-text articles through Griffin with on-site printing and downloading, is by far the most popular option. As with other remote, authenticated Griffin users, CALS users may also call up and print full-text articles in Griffin away from the branch campus.

In addition to electronic access options, CALS acquires books and journal titles at faculty request to support the curriculum in Spokane. In 1999–2000, the collection of paper resources included approximately 12,000 book titles and 400 journal titles. Since CALS is a joint effort of EWU and WSU, it is relevant to note the breakdown of shared funding for CALS materials and staffing. However, an exact breakdown of library holdings and the proportions contributed by each of the two cooperating universities is not available.

EWU materials housed in CALS are purchased by EWU bibliographers in the main campus library. No exact records are kept on how much EWU spends annually for library materials for CALS, and since EWU does not consider CALS a branch campus library, no separate budget line exists out of which the EWU CALS materials are purchased. Librarians on the EWU main campus indicated that a great deal of difficulty would be involved in figuring out how much had been spent in 1999–2000 on library materials that ended up being shelved in CALS (Buxton, Funding, 2001).

CALS staffing, however, does lend itself to institutional definitions. The WSU employees include one faculty librarian and three staff who are on full-time, twelve-month contracts. EWU supplies one faculty librarian who is on a ten-month contract, and one half-time staff member. CALS also has 0.7 FTE student assistants who are paid by WSU (Buxton, Funding, 2001).

In response to the question of reference desk duty hours for CALS librarians, David Buxton (2002), WSU's CALS librarian responded that the concept did not at that time exist at their branch campus library, because their limited physical facilities do not allow for having a separate reference desk, per se. There is a service counter with the librarian's office right behind it, so, in his words, "I'm on the desk whenever I'm in my office." The EWU librarian does not have a separate office, but rather a chair and a personal computer workstation at the service counter, so that person is "on the desk whenever she is at work."

Washington State University Tri-Cities
The Branch Campus. Located on the banks of the Columbia River in north Richland, and close to the other two Tri-Cities of Pasco and Kennewick, WSU Tri-Cities is a unit of the Tri-Cities Science and Technology Park on the southern boundary of the Hanford Nuclear Site. The Tri-Cities campus traces its origins back to the General Electric School of Nuclear Engineering, founded in 1945. Since the 1960s, the campus had been jointly operated by several institutions until it became the exclusive responsibility of WSU in 1989. The 1999–2000 enrollment figures for the campus are given in Tables 1, 3, and 5.

The 1,300 students who take classes at the Richland campus and at the Yakima and Wenatchee learning centers are served by over thirty full-time resident faculty and a pool of more than 350 adjunct faculty drawn from the Hanford "brain trust" of highly qualified scientists and professionals (Washington State University Tri-Cities, 2001).

WSU Tri-Cities gives students an opportunity to earn bachelor's and master's degrees from a premier research university; prepares an increasingly diverse work force for changing technologies, benefiting economic diversification and employee recruitment, retention, and advancement efforts; attracts grants and research projects to the region that only a research university can, infusing the local economy; and assists the agricultural community through research and extension activities, course offerings, and a close relationship with the nearby WSU Prosser Agricultural Research Station (Washington State University Tri-Cities, 2001). WSU Tri-Cities offers degrees in the following areas:

- Biology, MS;
- Business Administration, BA, MBA;
- Chemistry, MS;
- Communication, MA;
- Computer Science, BA, BS, MS;
- Counseling Psychology, Ed.M.;
- Education, BA;
- Education, Master in Literacy Education, Ed.M;
- Education, Master in Teaching, MIT;
- Educational Leadership, Ed.M., Ed.D.;
- Electrical Engineering, BS, MS;
- Engineering Management, M EngMgt;
- Environmental Engineering, MS;
- Environmental Science, BS, MS;
- General Science, BS;
- Liberal Arts, BA;

- Management Technology, MTM;
- Master in Teaching, MIT;
- Materials Science & Engineering, MS;
- Mechanical Engineering, BS, MS;
- Nursing, BSN.

Beyond these degree programs, additional courses are also offered in agriculture, biology, business, chemistry, education, computer science, chemical, electrical, environmental, and mechanical engineering, environmental science, the liberal arts, management, mathematics, statistics, and a variety of other disciplines (Washington State University Tri-Cities, 2001).

The Branch Campus Library

The Max E. Benitz Memorial Library is the branch campus library serving WSU Tri-Cities and is housed there as a unit of the Consolidated Libraries of the Consolidated Information Center. The libraries which constitute the Consolidated Libraries are: the Benitz Library, the Hanford Technical Library, the U.S. Department of Energy (DOE) Public Reading Room, and the Business Information Center (a combined project of WSU Tri-Cities and the U.S. Small Business Administration, designed to assist in the start-up of new small businesses in the southeastern corner of the state). (Max E. Benitz Memorial Library, 2001.)

The Benitz Library includes an on-site collection of 718,000 books, periodical issues, and microfiche, housed in combination with the collections of the Hanford Technical Library. As a branch campus facility of the Washington State University Libraries, the Benitz Library functions primarily as a gateway to the much more extensive library collections on the main campus through Griffin and with all the other institutions whose library holdings are included in Cascade (Max E. Benitz Memorial Library, 2001).

The Benitz Library has one full-time librarian. The Director of Information Services for the campus is also a librarian and contributes a portion of his time to library duties. For 1999–2000 ARL statistics purposes, the Director of Information Services counts himself as three tenths of an FTE, making the professional level staffing 1.3 FTE. Support staff consists of 3.8 FTE, and there are also two student assistants (Benitz Library ARL Statistics, 2001).

With such sparse staffing, the one full-time librarian is scheduled for three consecutive evenings per week and Saturdays, maintaining a high level of contact hours with students and other patrons. These reference desk shifts typically average eighteen to twenty-two hours per week. However, it is the distribution of the hours during the week more than the total number of hours that is the greater challenge. In addition to these scheduled hours of desk duty, there is an average of ten additional hours per week when the librarian is on call for e-mail and phone reference and is on call when the Reference desk is otherwise not covered by WSU personnel. The impact on other aspects of the librarian's duties is incalculable (Gover, 2002). Most other reference desk hours are covered by one support staff member with a similarly challenging number of hours and distribution of hours during a typical work week.

Washington State University Vancouver

The Branch Campus. WSU began offering courses in southwest Washington in 1983 as part of the Southwest Washington Joint Center for Education. In 1989, the University formally established WSU Vancouver as a branch campus. Currently the campus offers junior, senior, and graduate level courses. Students may pursue one of WSU Vancouver's thirteen bachelor's and seven master's degrees. WSU Vancouver offers degrees in the following areas:

Undergraduate Degrees and Fields of Study:

- Biology, B.S.
- Business Administration, B.A.
  - Accounting
  - Business Administration
  - Finance
  - General Business
  - Human Resources
  - Management
  - Management Information Systems
  - Marketing
- English, B.A.
- Electronic Media and Culture
- Human Development, B.A.
- Manufacturing Engineering, B.S.
- Nursing, B. S.
- Psychology, B.S.
- Public Affairs, B.A.
- General Studies
- Humanities, B.A.
- Social Sciences, B.A.

Fields of Study:

- Aging
- Anthropology

- Biology Business
- Community Studies
- Criminal Justice
- Early Childhood Education
- Electronic Communications and Culture
- Electronic Media and Culture
- English
- Environmental Science and Regional Planning
- History
- Human Development
- Human Resource Management
- Natural Resource Sciences
- Political Science
- Pre-Law
- Pre-Medicine
- Professional Writing
- Psychology Sociology
- Womens Studies.

Graduate Degrees and Fields of Study:

- Business Administration, M.B.A.
- Engineering Management, M.E.M.
- Mechanical Engineering, M.S.M.E.
- Nursing, M.N.
  - Community Health Nursing
  - Psychiatric/Mental Health Nurse Practitioner
  - Family Nurse Practitioner
  - Acute Care Nurse Practitioner
- Public Affairs, M.P.A.
  - Public Administration
  - Applied Policy Studies
  - Health Policy and Administration
- Technology Management, M.T.M.
- Education and Teaching
- Education, Ed.M.
  - Elementary Teacher option
  - Secondary Teacher option
  - Diverse Learners option
  - English as a Second Language endorsement
  - Special Education endorsement

Education Administration:

*   Secondary Education Certification, as part of Ed.M. or as fifth year program
    *   Biology
    *   English
    *   History
    *   Social Studies
*   Teaching, M.I.T.
    *   K-8 Elementary Certification

Certificate Programs:

*   Accounting Aging
*   Engineering Management
*   Finance
*   Health Care Policy
*   Human Resource Management
*   Management Information Systems
*   Manufacturing Engineering
*   Professional Writing.
    (Washington State University Vancouver, 2001).

The Branch Campus Library

WSU Vancouver's library has more than seven hundred journals in hardcopy and over 1,100 full text online journals and newspapers, a core collection of more than 14,000 books, and access to more than sixty major bibliographic databases. The library participates in several local and regional library consortia, including PORTALS, the Portland (Oregon) Area Library System and the Cooperative Library Project in Washington. The library also houses the Environmental Information Cooperative Library (Washington State University Vancouver Library, 2001).

The WSU Vancouver Library has an advantaged staffing situation compared with the other WSU branch campus libraries. Its staff includes an FTE of four librarians, three support staff, and four student assistants (Vancouver Library ARL Statistics, 2001). With their professional staffing level, their librarians report reference desk duty hours ranging from five to fifteen hours per week. There are some additional contact hours online or on the phone with distant students, but exact records are not kept of these hours.

WSU Learning Centers

The distribution of the WSU Learning Centers is shown in Fig. 4, using the numbers assigned to them in the listing below. As indicated in the following goals, the WSU

Learning Centers follow a mission very similar to the branch campuses in bringing higher education to even more geographically isolated areas:

- Make higher education degrees locally accessible for time- and place-bound adults.
- Increase opportunities for lifelong learning through non-credit, certificate, and professional development programs.
- Enhance the possibility of participation in higher education for those with limited income.
- Contributing to WSU becoming a national leader in distance education.

Learning Center recruitment activities, August through December, 2000, indicate their level of involvement in local communities:

- Recruiting Inquiries – 1,618.
- Formal Presentations – Presentations to 3,769 people.
- Presentations to Freshman and Transfer Students – 37 presentations to 900 people.
- Community Service Activities held in Learning Centers – 178 events.
- Recruiting Booths at 24 Fairs with 511,247 in attendance.
- Participation in Community College Events and Presentations.
  (Learning Centers, 2001).

As can be seen from the following activities listings, nine of the ten centers have strong interactions with local area community colleges. The Learning Centers are numbered in accordance with their numerical designations on Fig. 4:

(1) North Olympic Peninsula:
   - Location – large, centralized location for hosting events.
   - Coordinator – local community educator for twenty years.
   - Philosophy – "Do what it takes; education is everyone's future."
(2) Grays Harbor and Pacific
   - Close partners with Grays Harbor Community College, especially with the Collaborative Teacher Education Program.
   - Close partners with Quinault Indian Nation.
   - Close partners with the child care community.
   - ... Bringing credit and non-credit educational offerings to its rural area.
(3) Cowlitz and Wahkiakum
   - Close partners with Lower Columbia Community College.
   - 2 + 2 programs in teaching and business.
   - Partner with community agencies to present computer classes and satellite training programs to thousands of residents.
(4) Skagit, Island and San Juan

- Strong partnership with Skagit Valley College campuses/centers in Skagit Island, and San Juan counties with regular visits to each location.
- Developing relationship with Skagit Valley Latino/a community.
- Connection with FarWest Cougar alumni association.

(5) Pierce County at Salishan
- Located in a multi-cultural community and urban housing development.
- Bi-monthly visits to community colleges and military bases.
- Strong partnership with Tacoma Housing Authority.
- Support early college awareness programs and SAT/ACT practice test.

(6) North Central Washington
- Contact with: Wenatchee Community College faculty & staff, including WSU alumni Chamber of Commerce, ESD, and other community agencies and businesses.

(7) South Central Washington
- Numerous contacts with community organizations.
- Strong partnership with Yakima Valley Community College.
- Working with Latino and Native American students.

(8) Klickitat County
- Sole point of contact for Yakima Valley Community College and WSU in Goldendale.
- Community college classes and non-credit offerings available at LC.

(9) Northeast Washington
- Strong ties to high schools and Spokane Falls Community College centers in Ferry, Stevens, and Pend Oreille counties.
- Affiliated with American Association of University Women.
- Recruiting for and supporting 4-H Cougar track scholarship.
- Working on Career Day/College Knowledge event for Spring 2002.

(10) Southeast Washington Strong partnerships with:
- Walla Walla Community College;
- local businesses;
- community organizations.
  Interactive Television Courses:
- BSN;
- MN – Psychiatric Nurse Practitioner;
- Special Education Certification.
  (Learning Centers, 2001).

WSU Distance Degree Program

In addition to the programs of the branch campuses, Learning Centers, and WHETS, the distance learning offerings of the WSU system include the Distance

Degree Program (DDP), with courses offered via video tape and the Internet. The DDP program is based on the main campus in Pullman, but the students are scattered across the state and frequently interact with nearby WSU learning centers and branch campuses. The situation with DDP students is further complicated because these students are also often being enrolled in other WSU course offerings via WHETS, a learning center, or a branch campus. Whether or not DDP students are enrolled in additional courses based at a Learning Center or on one of the branch campuses, they frequently interact with personnel at nearby WSU learning centers or branch campuses, especially the branch campus libraries which house reserve collections of the DDP video tapes and proctor exams for DDP students.

DDP degrees are offered in the following disciplines:
Degrees Requiring No Site-based Participation:

• Bachelor of Arts in Social Sciences;
• Bachelor of Arts in Business Administration;
• Bachelor of Arts in Criminal Justice;
• Bachelor of Arts in Human Development;
• Bachelor of Science in Agriculture: TADDA.

Degrees Requiring Site-based Participation:

• Bachelor of Arts in Education (teaching certificate).

Graduate & Professional Degrees at a Distance:

• Bachelor of Science in Nursing (BSN) for Registered Nurses;
• Master of Science in Agriculture;
• Master of Engineering Management;
• External Doctor of Pharmacy;

Certificate Program:

• Professional Writing Program.

Collaborative Teacher Education Program (CTEP).

CTEP enables students to earn a bachelor's degree and elementary (K-8) certification through a combination of interactive telecommunications, locally taught courses, and extensive field experience in local schools. CTEP is a full-time, two-year, cohort-based program delivered entirely on site at WSU Pullman, WSU Vancouver, Clark College, Centralia College, Lower Columbia College, and Grays Harbor College. To be eligible, students must have an Associate of Arts degree or higher, as well as specified prerequisite courses. All prerequisites are offered through local community colleges (Distance Degree Program, 2001).

Distance Degree Library Services (DDLS)
History of DDLS. DDLS was established in 1993 to support a specific group of WSU distance students who were enrolling in semester-based courses through the Distance Degree Program. At that time these library services were paid for and maintained by DDP and included a half time classified staff position, supervised by the User Education unit in Holland Library. GenEd300, then "Univ300," a basic library and research skills course, was also established at this time to help distance students with research.

In 1998, the Libraries received additional funding from the University to support a part-time librarian and a part-time classified staff position. In 2000, the Libraries added a part-time librarian position to DDLS, making the librarian position full-time.

Philosophy and Services
In accordance with *ACRL Guidelines*:

- All students who are enrolled in the WSU Extended Degree Program can receive personalized library service.
- DDLS promotes library instruction with GenEd300, and other online self-help modules.
- Services available include Internet access to databases, reference assistance, borrowing WSU-owned books and other circulating materials, computer searches of Library holdings, database searches, and photocopies of non-circulating materials.

DDLS Support and Services to DDP Students

- Prompt retrieval and checkout of requested sources.
- Students contacted if an item cannot be sent.
- Free first-class mailing for fast delivery of source materials, such as books and other circulating materials with students paying return postage for books.
- Database access and searches on assignment-related topics.
- Free photocopying of any materials that do not circulate, including reference materials, microfilm, journal articles, and newspapers.
- Twenty-four hour toll-free telephone access for requesting materials.
- Requesting materials via e-mail.
- The DDLS Web site includes a variety of resources online.

Delivery of Materials

- Library Materials will be mailed within six working days.
- Journal, magazine, and newspaper articles will be photocopied free for DDP students.

- Photocopied materials need not be returned to DDLS.
- Materials which circulate (books, CDs, etc.) will be checked out to students. All items are mailed first class to ensure fast delivery. Students are responsible for the cost of returning circulated materials.
- The Self-Renewal option is now available to all students.

(Distance Degree Library Services, 2001).

Staffing and Function of DDLS

Jane Scales, WSU DDLS Librarian provided the following details about her program:

DDLS has invested heavily in its Web presence <http://www.wsulibs.wsu.edu/electric/library>. The Website addresses student needs on a number of fronts: technical assistance, general research instruction, delivery services, and assignment-specific resources.

Above all, students need to access library databases. The DDLS Web site has been designed to facilitate this access by helping students "conFig." their Web browsers and to establish a library PIN, or personal identification number, which functions as a password that enables students to both access the databases and take advantage of other online services such as book requests and recall. Most recently, attempts to improve this service have resulted in the online "EZ-GUIDE" which incorporates a Java script that automatically identifies the student browser and browser version and then guides users to instructions specific to their browser.

Another illustration of how DDLS is helping students access databases is the construction of an online form by which students can request that a NetLibrary account be set up for them. NetLibrary, as an online database of electronic books is just the type of resource especially useful for distance students. Unfortunately, NetLibrary only allows WSU affiliates to establish an online account from a prescribed set of WSU IP addresses. Distance students who are using home computers are unable to establish their account even though they are legally licensed users of NetLibrary. DDLS has enabled the establishment of NetLibrary accounts for this group of library users by setting them up in-house. After a distance student requests an account via our online form, a time-slip student working for DDLS can set it up, and then e-mail the student his or her account password.

DDLS works one-on-one with students. A typical student interaction with the unit lasts for several days with two to four contacts. Interactions vary significantly as we make extensive efforts to maintain a relevancy in the academic life of distance education students. Our focus is public service. DDP students, who are often physically isolated from an academic environment, seem to consider their contact with the WSU Libraries as one of the few social encounters with the University available to them. These remote students enjoy and thrive on this personalized attention (Scales, 2001).

Summary of WSU Distance Learning Library Services

Table 6 provides a quick display of the types of distance learning course options offered in the WSU system and the corresponding library services provided to support them. With the DDP video tape and Web courses, the DDLS is the primary provider of library services as described above. However, DDP students are also served on a walk-in basis in the learning centers and branch campus libraries in their vicinity. In the branch campus libraries, course tapes are made available and tests are proctored.

ECLS, the Extended Campus Library Services, is a distance learning library services unit, similar to DDLS, operated by the WSU Pullman Libraries Interlibrary Loan operation (Pullman ILL) on behalf of three of the branch campus libraries. ECLS is funded proportionately by these three of branch campus libraries, WSU Spokane, WSU Tri-Cities, and WSU Vancouver, to provide their students document delivery of paper copy of journal articles and other materials which cannot be requested through Griffin Request Item. Pullman ILL also provides floor space and library faculty supervision for the one ECLS paraprofessional and student assistants at no additional cost to the branch campuses.

Pullman ILL, as it appears in Table 6, refers to the provision of document delivery of journal article photocopies and other materials that cannot be requested in Griffin Request Item to students at the learning centers, including students taking WHETS classes away from the branch campuses. Since these students are not enrolled in DDP, they are not eligible for DDLS. Likewise, since these students are not enrolled on the branch campuses, they are not eligible to use the ECLS unit for document

Table 6. WSU Distance Learning Options and Corresponding Library
Service Providers.

Distance Learning Option	Library Services Providers
DDP video tape	DDLS and Branch Campus Libraries
DDP Web based	DDLS and Branch Campus Libraries
WHETS	ECLS, Pullman ILL, Branch Campus Libraries
Live Learning Center Courses	Pullman ILL and Branch Campus Libraries
Live Branch Campus Courses	ECLS and Branch Campus Libraries

Table 7. Washington State University Libraries Services Provided Distance Learning Students.

Services To Distance Learning Students	Library Services Providers
GenEd 300	Pullman and Vancouver Branch Campus Librarians
Electronic Reserves	Branch Campus and ICN Personnel
Library Use Instruction Live in Classroom/Library	Branch Campus Librarians
Library Use Instruction via WHETS	Branch Campus Librarians and DDLS Librarian to Classes in Multiple Locations, including Pullman
Reference Services	Branch Campus Librarians and DDLS Librarian Via E-Mail
Test Proctoring for DDP Students	Branch Campus Library Personnel
Circulation Services	Branch Campus Library Personnel and DDLS
Document Delivery	Branch Campus Library, DDLS, ECLS Personnel
Interlibrary Loan	Branch Campus Library and Pullman ILL Personnel

delivery. Pullman ILL voluntarily provides document delivery services for these students.

Table 7 displays six services provided to distance learning students by the WSU Libraries and the Libraries units providing each service. GenEd 300, as mentioned in the description of DDLS, is a separate, one credit library skills and information literacy course offered at the locations shown.

Tables 8 and 9 supplement Tables 6 and 7 by summarizing the cataloging and indexing services of Griffin and the cataloging services of Cascade. "Direct Remote Internet," as used in Tables 8 and 9, refers to accessing Griffin directly on the Internet, using its URL, as opposed to accessing Griffin as it is provided on computers inside the EWU or WSU libraries, or in other campus or learning center facilities.

Table 8. Washington State University Libraries Griffin Cataloging and Indexing Services Used by Distance Learning Students.

Griffin Services	Access
Searching EWU/WSU, Book Collections by Author, Title, Author/Title, Subject, Keyword	Remote via Internet and Direct, All WSU Locations
Direct Searching, Electronic Journal Titles	Remote via Internet and Direct, All WSU Locations
Direct Searching, Paper Journal Titles	Remote via Internet and Direct, All WSU Locations
Indexing and Full Text Newspapers, Magazines, Journals	Remote via Internet and Direct, All WSU Locations
Request Item for Books	Remote via Internet and Direct, All WSU Locations

Table 9.   Washington State University Libraries Cascade Cataloging Services
Used by Distance Learning Students.

Cascade Services	Access
Searching State University Book Collections by Author, Title, Author/Title, Subject, Keyword	Direct or Linked From Griffin
Title Searching, Paper Journal Holdings	Direct or Linked From Griffin
Request Item for Books	Direct or Linked From Griffin

ADMINISTRATIVE OVERVIEW AND CONCLUSIONS

One observation that comes readily to mind in looking back over the material in this study is that these educational programs offered by the CCS district, the WSU system, and all the other institutions with which they interact to provide instruction and other related services, are not so much overlapping efforts as they are coordinated activities designed to meet the educational needs of targeted groups of individuals who use them. This is the first study to assemble this information in one place, and the extent to which this is the result of inter-institutional planning as opposed to fortuitous circumstances that have developed as pragmatic attempts to meet perceived needs is a question to be explored through further research. Much of what has been viewed in this study was coordinated by the Washington Higher Education Coordinating Board (HEC Board). Further study is needed to identify and define the work of the HEC Board. Further study should also address more closely the programs of Whitworth College and Gonzaga University in Spokane.

That both Diane Lloyd and Jane Scales cited the *ACRL Guidelines* in their respective reports is noteworthy. Lloyd's intent in including the quotation from the *Guidelines* does not make it clear as to whether she intended to demonstrate the extent to which her program meets or fails to meet the expectations expressed in the passage. It is ironic that Diane Lloyd used in her Annual Report the same quote, warning against the stretching of traditional library resources and services to meet the needs of distance learners, since she herself is stretched as a professional to provide the number and quality of services that she does. Although the *ACRL Guidelines* mention resources in the most general and generic sense, they do not address this problem of stretching human resources to meet user needs. An ongoing theme throughout this study has been to note the reference and other user contact hours of the distance learning librarians involved. These hours were not reported for Scales (2002), as she and her one staff member have not been keeping statistics on client contacts. Suffice it to say that both Scales and her staff member are on call throughout their hours on duty. National surveys are clearly needed on work loads of academic librarians in general and distance learning librarians in particular.

An additional factor not addressed in this study is the competition in any geographical setting from electronic course offerings of institutions at a great distance from those that are regionally clustered. There is an urgent need for further study on how individual institutions factor in the availability of remote competitors for their students in their own individual and regional inter-institutional planning.

REFERENCES

Access Washington (1998–2002). STATE FACTS; Geography. Retrieved June 25, 2002, from http://access.wa.gov/government/awgeneral.asp#geo/

ACRL Guidelines for Distance Learning Library Services (2000). Association of College and Research Libraries of the American Library Association. Retrieved June 27, 2002, from: http://www.ala.org/acrl/guides/distlrng.html/

Benitz Library ARL Statistics (2001). ARL statistics questionnaire, 1999–2000. Max E. Benitz Memorial Library. Washington State University Tri-Cities. Unpublished Report.

Betty M. Anderson Library (2002). Intercollegiate College of Nursing. Washington State University College of Nursing. Retrieved January 11, 2002, from: http://nursing.wsu.edu/library/index.asp/

Bryant, E. (2001). Bridging the gap. *Library Journal, 126*(16), 58–60.

Buxton, D. (2001). Re: EWU fall 1999 enrollment figures. E-Mail reply message to Harvey Gover received November 2, 2001.

Buxton, D. (2001). Re: Funding sources for CALS. E-Mail reply message to Harvey Gover received November 21, 2001.

Buxton, D. (2002). Re: Number of reference desk duty hours per week. E-Mail reply to Harvey Gover received March 18, 2002.

Community Colleges of Spokane (2001). Campuses, 1999–2000. Retrieved June 30, 2001, from http://ccs.spokane.cc.wa.us/

Community Colleges of Spokane (2002). CCS Overview. (With District Map). Retrieved June 27, 2002, from http://ccs.spokane.cc.wa.us/Overview/default.htm

Distance Degree Library Services (2001). Distance Degree Programs. Publications. Services. Library Services. Retrieved November 17, 2001, from http://www.distance.wsu.edu/pubs/handbook/services.asp#library

Distance Degree Program (2001). Distance Degree Programs. Washington State University. Retrieved November 18, 2001, from http://www.distance.wsu.edu/

Dively, D., & McGill, M. (1991). State planning and implementation of educational telecommunications systems in the West. Boulder, CO: Western Interstate Commission for Higher Education. (ERIC Document Reproduction Service No. ED342375).

Eastern Washington University (2001). Eastern Washington University. Retrieved June 25, 2001 from http://www.ewu.edu/

Fulkerson, C. (2001). Re: Enrollment stats needed for another article. E-Mail message to Harvey Gover received October 31, 2001.

Gover, H. (2002). WSU Libraries faculty professional activity report. January 1, 2001–December 31, 2001. Unpublished report.

ICN; Intercollegiate College of Nursing (2002). Washington State University College of Nursing. Retrieved January, 2002, from http://nursing.wsu.edu/index.asp/

Institute for Extended Learning (2001). IEL Institute for Extended Learning. Retrieved June 17, 2001, from http://ielhp.spokane.cc.wa.us/

Kirk, E. E., & Bartelstein, A. A. (1999). Libraries close in on distance education. *Library Journal, 124*(6), 40–42.

Learning Centers (2001). Learning centers. Washington State University. Retrieved June 20, 2001, from http://learningcenters.wsu.edu/

Lloyd, D. (2000). Distance learning library services and the Community Colleges of Spokane. An Annual Report of the Spokane Falls Community College Distance Education Librarian, submitted May 12, 2000. Edited by Mary Ann Lund Goodwin, Assistant Dean for Learning Resources May 23, 2000. Edited by Diane Lloyd August 2, 2001, for a Pacific Northwest Library Association Conference presentation to be given by Harvey Gover, August 10, 2001.

Lloyd, D. (2002). Here are some corrections. E-Mail message to Harvey Gover received June 28, 2002.

Max E. Benitz Memorial Library (2001). Max E. Benitz Memorial Library. Washington State University Tri-Cities. Retrieved January 12, 2002, from: http://www.tricity.wsu.edu/dis/maxben.htm/

Pringle, R. (2001). Re: ICNE enrollments for 99–00. E-Mail message to Harvey Gover received November 1, 2001.

Pringle, R. (2002). Re: Revised . . . draft. E-Mail message to Harvey Gover received July 1, 2002.

Scales, J. (2001). Report to Harvey Gover on DDLS. Unpublished report.

Scales, J. (2002). Re: Number of reference desk duty hours per week. E-Mail message to Harvey Gover received March 22, 2002.

Spokane Community College (2001). Spokane Community College. Retrieved June 17, 2001, from: http://www.scc.spokane.cc.wa.us/

Spokane Falls Community College (2001). Retrieved June 17, 2001, from: http://www.sfcc. spokane.cc.wa.us/; soon to be http://www.spokanefalls.edu/

State Map (2001). Washington State University. State Map. Retrieved September 2, 2001, from: http://www.wsu.edu/campusmap/1statemap/statemap.html/

Vancouver Library ARL Statistics (2001). Washington State University Vancouver Library. ARL statistics questionnaire, 1999–2000. Unpublished Report.

Washington State Board for Community and Technical Colleges. (n.d.). College System Maps. Retrieved June 27, 2002, from: http://www.sbctc.ctc.edu/Maps/maps.htm/

Washington State University (2001). Washington State University; Taking you anywhere you want to go. Retrieved June 27, 2001 from: http://www.wsu.edu/

Washington State University Tri-Cities (2001). Washington State University Tri-Cities. Retrieved November 2, 2001, from: http://www2.tricity.wsu.edu/

Washington State University Vancouver (2001). Washington State University Vancouver. Retrieved November 17, 2001, from: http://www.vancouver.wsu.edu/

Washington State University Vancouver Library (2001). Washington State University Vancouver Library. Retrieved November 17, 2001, from: http://www.vancouver.wsu.edu/vis/infoserv.htm/

WHETS, Washington Higher Education Telecommunications Network (2001). WHETS; Bridging the gap. Retrieved June 25, 2001, from: htttp://www.ett.wsu.edu/WHETS/ information.asp#ITEM6/

THE ATTRIBUTES OF INFORMATION
AS AN ASSET

Charles Oppenheim, Joan Stenson and
Richard M. S. Wilson

INTRODUCTION

The resource-based view of information was central to the development of an "information economy." It was economists such as Machlup (1962) and Porat (1977) who pioneered the idea of an "information economy." Cooper (1983, p. 12) identified Machlup as the first proponent of an "information economy," a new sector of the economy made up of:

> ... a group of establishments – firms, institutions, organisations, and departments, or teams within them, but also in some instances, individuals and households that produce knowledge, information services or information goods, either for their own use or for use by others (Machlup, 1962, p. 228).

Porat (1977) took an alternate approach to that of Machlup (1962) in focusing, not on the producers of knowledge, information services or goods, but on the information activities themselves. Porat's (1977) fundamental unit of analysis were information activities and these comprised the building blocks of an "information economy." These information activities included:

> ... all the resources consumed in producing, processing, and distributing information goods or services (Porat, 1977, p. 2).

The "information economy" itself has been characterised by a flexibility and dynamism which has raised awareness of the importance of information. However,

Advances in Library Administration and Organization
Advances in Library Administration and Organization, Volume 20, 123–147
ISSN: 0732-0671/PII: S0732067102200061

these two approaches to the "information economy" have resulted in development of a wide and often contradictory range of attributes of information. In particular, the value of information has been extremely difficult to identify or to quantify. As a result, the role of information in improving business performance has been largely unrecognised. Too often senior managers have focused on the costs of information rather than the benefits.

The aim of this paper is to explore some of the issues surrounding the identification of attributes of information and the recognition of these attributes by senior executives. The identification of information as an asset is proposed as a method to enable the recognition of significant attributes of information by senior executives. Attributes of information from the information science and management literature are discussed. Further attributes are identified in an interview with a senior executive from a large consumer goods company in the U.K. The purpose of the interview was to identify those attributes of information that were considered significant by this senior executive. Repertory grid analysis was used. This technique was pioneered by the psychologist George Kelly (1955). Although originally developed for quite different purposes, this technique has frequently been used as a tool in management development and change (Easterby-Smith et al., 1996, p. 12). Some examples of applications of repertory grid are job analysis, employee selection, task analysis, performance appraisal and management and development training and needs (Easterby-Smith et al., 1996, p. 13).

A RESOURCE-BASED VIEW OF INFORMATION

The resource-based view of information has its origins in economic necessity. Black and Marchand (1982, p. 205) traced the rise of a resource-based view of information from the mid-1970s, when the U.S. Federal Government realised that the rising cost of processing information was becoming unsustainable. The U.S. Government addressed this by setting up a Commission on Federal Paperwork, which stated that:

> ... as a resource, data and information can and must be managed just as we manage human, physical and financial resources. Data and information must be subject to the same budgetary, managerial and audit disciplines as any other resource (Black & Marchand, 1982, p. 207).

Information was recognised as a resource to be subject to active management just like any other resource. Most importantly for libraries and information services, the resource-based view of information led to the popularisation of the idea of a life cycle process for information. This was epitomised by the development of Information Resource Management, or IRM, a management concept which argued that information should be treated as an organisational resource that has a life cycle of creation, distribution, use and disposal. This meant that maintenance and investment in information resources were brought to the foreground. The focus on managing information actively to retain its currency and relevance was a substantial step.

The resource-based view of information was defined in the late 1980s by Cornelius Burk and Forest Horton (1988) in their seminal book on corporate information. They sought to map information as a corporate resource. Burk and Horton (1988, p. 18) argued that nine basic similarities between information and other traditional managed resources existed and that many organisations were under utilising their most valuable resource.

There was, however, some criticism of the resource-based view of information. Burk and Horton's (1988) approach focused on the information activities of organizations and the productivity of information resources in relation to their costs. The potential of information as a strategic or competitive tool in itself was not highlighted. The focus on information activities and the costs involved in producing and using information meant that managers' attention was not directed towards the outcomes of information activities but towards regulating inputs. However, it is interesting to discuss the similarities that Burk and Horton (1988) identified between information and traditional resources, as many of the attributes of information traditionally identified are based on this resource-based view of information.

Burk and Horton's Nine Similarities Between Information and Traditional Resources

(1) *"Information is acquired at a definite measurable cost"* (Burk & Horton, 1988, p. 18). This statement is true for externally acquired information. However, information that is produced internally often makes up the more significant part of the information resource that an organisation holds. The existence of valuable information stores, that are produced internally and fed by individual ideas and expertise means that often the more important information present in an organisation cannot be quantified. Quantifying externally acquired information does not then help to identify the more significant or perhaps valuable information in an organisation. An understanding of the importance of internally generated information has been highlighted by the concepts of knowledge management and intellectual capital.

Knowledge Management can be defined as:

> The systematic organisation of organisational knowledge to make it easier to share and apply throughout the business (Skyrme, 1997, p. 503).

Intellectual capital can be defined as:

> The possession of knowledge, applied experience, organisational technology, customer relationships and professional skills that provide us with a competitive edge in the marketplace (Edvinsson & Malone, 1997, p. 368).

These two concepts have encouraged senior managers to look beyond the information gathered from external sources and to focus on the integration of various types of knowledge, information and expertise into business processes and into the production of services and goods. There are, of course, multiple definitions of information and knowledge, but it is beyond the scope of this paper to cover these in detail. For the purposes of this research study, information is seen as a prime component of knowledge. A different definition of information and knowledge as proposed by Elizabeth Orna (1999) is a useful working definition, as it reflects the importance of communication and of people:

> Information is what human beings transform knowledge into when they want to communicate it to other people (Orna, 1999, p. 8).

Or:

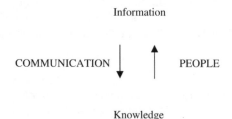

(2) *"Information possesses a definite value, which may be quantified and treated as an accountable asset"* (Burk & Horton, 1988, p. 18). This argument is again problematic. Definite value assumes that all those who use the information would or could place a similar value on it. However, the value of information is subjective. For example, information that cost nothing may prove very valuable to a particular user and information that cost a great deal may not be used at all. As Eaton and Bawden (1991, p. 163) point out, "the value of information is not quantifiable," its value depends on "context and use." More importantly, Eaton and Bawden (1991) also argue that such concentration on quantifying information value actually detracts from the dynamic role which information plays in organisations.

The identification of information as an accountable asset is also difficult. The Accounting Standards Board (ASB) gives the accounting definition of an asset in the U.K. as:

> ... rights or other access to future economic benefits controlled by an entity as a result of past transactions or events (Wild, Creighton & Creighton, 2000, p. 12).

The words "rights or other access" emphasizes that an asset is not a particular item of property itself, but rather reflects the benefits deriving from ownership, occupation or use of the asset (Davies & Paterson et al., 1997, p. 97). Therefore, information may be defined as an asset if it can be shown to give future benefits. However, to be recognised as an asset for accounting purposes, control becomes the critical factor. Control in the context of the recognition of an asset means the ability to obtain economic benefits and restrict that of third parties. If an asset cannot be "separately identified from the business as a whole, it cannot be individually controlled by the entity, and it is not an asset" (Davies & Paterson et al., 1997, p. 97).

Since information is typically diffused through all aspects of the business (Davenport, 1993, p. 79), it cannot be sold separately and so cannot be controlled. This means information is not capable of being recognised by an accountant as an asset. For example, a business may, in principle, sell a database as a separate asset. Yet, the information included in that database may have been collected and organised by many different people and from many sources. Unless these can also be separated and sold, then arguably the database is not an asset. To sell the database would indeed, in many cases, mean selling the entire business.

The criteria for recognizing an asset in accounting terms are limiting. Many assets, which are recognised, would not meet the strict definitions of an accounting treatment. There are, however, some convincing arguments for the identification of information as an asset as a method to encourage senior managers to recognise the importance of information to their businesses. The identification of information as an asset in this context points to the "future economic benefits" which information can bring rather than to a conventional accounting treatment. This was highlighted in the U.K. by the publication of the Hawley Report (KPMG/IMPACT, 1994) which was produced by management consultants KPMG with the backing of the Confederation of British Industry (CBI). It argued that information is a vital resource and proposed that someone at board level should be responsible for its management.

The key finding of this report stated:

> ... all significant information in an organisation, regardless of its purpose, should be properly identified, even if not in an accounting sense, for consideration as an asset of the business. The board of directors should address its responsibilities for information assets in the same way as for other assets, e.g. property, plant (KPMG/IMPACT, 1994, p. 23).

The Hawley Report (KPMG/IMPACT, 1994) recommended that information assets should be identified and classified by value and importance, and that skilled resources were needed to manage and harness them. This was to ensure information assets were providing the maximum business benefit. Information assets were defined as:

> ...data that is or should be documented and which has value or potential value (KPMG/IMPACT, 1994, p. 23).

Dr Robert Hawley, the chairman of the committee that produced the Hawley Report, pointed out that many intangibles (like brands, people and intellectual property) had received attention in the business literature (Hawley, 1995, p. 237). This meant that boards of directors were at least aware of most of them – and aware that attention should be paid to them. In contrast, very few organisations recognised the value of information. The Hawley Report (KPMG/IMPACT, 1994) positioned this recognition of the importance of information as being pivotal. If boards of directors were not paying attention to information, then there was, at best:

> ...a lack of consistency in strategic understanding, planning, budgeting, management and control, and at worst, the very existence of the organisation can be under threat (Hawley, 1995, p. 237).

The benefits of identifying information as a vital asset for business was further developed by the publication of *Information as an asset: the invisible goldmine* (Reuters, 1995) which reported the results of 500 telephone interviews with senior managers in U.K. companies. The main conclusions of this report were that one in four U.K. companies said that information was its most important asset; half thought it was more important than trade names and registered trademarks; and one in ten valued its information more than its staff. However, more than 40% of respondents said their companies had not awakened to the value of their information.

The results showed that companies wanted to capitalise their expenditure on information, yet some 25% of the respondents said they could not capitalise information assets because they found it too hard to identify what the value of the assets was (Reuters, 1995, p. 5). These reports seem to indicate that organisations would benefit from defining information as an asset, even if not in a conventional accounting sense.

In the U.S., attempts to identify and define information as an asset have also emerged. For example, McGinn (1993, p. 40) promoted the view that the management of a library would benefit from a treatment of information as an asset. McGinn argued:

When public tax monies are used to purchase information delivery products (CD-ROM's, electronic databases) then the products become the "information assets" of the community in the same manner that police cars, computers, school buildings, and other items purchased with public dollars become – and are considered for legal, accounting, and community development purposes – assets (McGinn, 1993, p. 40).

From a business perspective, John E. Framel, President of IR Concepts, an information management, planning and consulting firm in the U.S. argued that managing information costs and technologies as assets had benefits in achieving a total management approach. This approach integrated all information and technologies into the total organisation (Framel, 1990, p. 13). The purpose of managing information as an asset was:

... to achieve maximum value and return from expenditures made (Framel, 1990, p. 13).

This approach should not be confused with accounting developments in the U.S. such as Government Accounting Standards Board (GASB) 34 (1999). GASB 34 is currently applicable to businesses in the U.S., but the standard has now been extended to public sector bodies. This is being heralded by accountants as a major change in the U.S. Government's requirements for financial reporting (Hennen, 2001, p. 48). Under established rules, public bodies in the U.S. included the capital cost of infrastructure only once in an agency's annual financial report (in the year in which the cost is incurred). GASB 34 will require public sector bodies, such as public libraries, to report infrastructure costs like buildings, library systems and even books in their financial reports (Hennen, 2001, p. 48). This is intended to reflect the long-term value of such investment and, of course, allow for their depreciation.

Long-term planning for infrastructure needs is being brought to the forefront by GASB 34, which is being introduced in three phases between June 2001 and June 2003 (Hennen, 2001, p. 48). However, the new accounting treatment cannot really reflect the value, for example, of a prized national collection housed in a historic building that has been built up over many years by innumerable dedicated staff. What it does do is point to the future, and the need for investment to be allocated to libraries' infrastructure in line with traditional infrastructure investments such as roads and railways.

(3) *"Information consumption can be quantified"* (Burk & Horton, 1988, p. 18). The consumption of information can be quantified but this tells us little about how any information consumed creates value for the organisation. Information can also be consumed more than once, it is not consumed by its use, rather, it is expanded. Hall (1981, p. 150) is one of many authors who identified the consumption of information as an attribute that is not shared by other economic goods:

the consumption of information means we cannot manage information like any other resource. It is not lost when given to others and does not deplete on use. Sharing and transmission may actually cause it to increase to both parties (Hall, 1981, p. 150).

(4) *"Cost accounting techniques can be applied to help control the cost of information"* (Burk & Horton, 1988, p. 18). Again this is applicable to externally acquired information, which has a historical cost, but it does not help in quantifying the cost of internally produced information. Such an approach may also reduce the innovative and creative possibilities of information because it looks to the past but tells nothing about future benefits. It is also interesting to note that historically, information has in itself rarely been the primary focus of transactions or an object of exchange in its own right (Boisot, 1998, p. 72). This makes it difficult to apply techniques such as cost accounting to information because such techniques were never developed with information in mind.

(5) *"Information has identifiable and measurable characteristics"* (Burk & Horton, 1988, p. 18). These measurable characteristics can help to define its value and include:
    (a) Quality of the information itself.
        Degree of accuracy, comprehensiveness, credibility, relevance, simplicity and validity.
    (b) Utility of information holdings.
        Degree of intellectual and physical accessibility, ease of use, flexibility and presentation.
    (c) Impact on productivity of organisation.
        Contribution to improvement in decision-making, product quality, efficiency of operation, or working conditions, time-saving and promotion of timely action.
    (d) Impact on effectiveness of organisation.
        Contribution to new markets, improved customer satisfaction, meeting targets and objectives and promoting more harmonious relationships.
    (e) Impact on financial position.
        Contribution to cost reduction or cost saving, substitution for more expensive resource inputs, increased profits and return on investment" (Burk & Horton, 1988, p. 93).

The first two characteristics, quality and utility, can be seen to be inherent to information as an entity in itself. They can be identified and measured according to a set criterion within a particular context or organisational setting. However, the remaining three characteristics are not so readily identifiable or measurable. The main difficulty is that information, although useful, may in all likelihood be only a tiny factor in any productivity or effectiveness improvements. Or it may not. The difficulty is that, while information underpins improved productivity and effectiveness, it cannot be easily separated from all the other elements that impact on these areas. It is also extremely difficult to demonstrate any financial benefit from information directly, for these very reasons.

Financial or economic characteristics of information are particularly problematic. Indeed, some "economic" characteristics of information are notable because of their non-economic properties. Poirier (1990, p. 266) points out that the:

> ... concept of information as a resource like energy or water is not a sustainable analogy, because it doesn't always obey the laws of physics: it is diffuse, compressible and extendable; it can be shared or consumed more than once; it is long-lasting and does not necessarily decrease with use (Poirier, 1990, p. 266).

Arrow (1984, p. 142) argues that information is not an economic good because it cannot properly enter into the process of economic exchange. This is because it cannot be made appropriable; information once transferred becomes the possession of both buyer and seller.

> ... information is inappropriable because an individual who has some can never lose it by transmitting it (Arrow, 1984, p. 142).

This means that the same information can benefit both the giver and receiver. Unlike a traditional economic good like, for example, a car, information can never really become the sole possession of the receiver. If I have an idea and I share it with another person, then, not only does that person benefit, but I can still retain and benefit from that idea. As a result, the financial benefits of information may be seen more in the sharing and communication of information than in increased return on investment.

(6) *"Information has a clear life-cycle: definition of requirements, collection, transmission, processing, storage, dissemination and disposal"* (Burk & Horton, 1988, p. 18). While information does have a life cycle, that is far from clear. Information may, at different stages of its life, become useful to varying projects and may be used at the same time for a variety of purposes. Information, which may be identified as ready for disposal in one situation, may become critical in another. The life cycle approach is useful but should not detract from the reusability of information, which may be one of its more important attributes.

(7) *"Information can be processed and refined so that raw materials (e.g. Databases) are converted into finished products (e.g. Published directories)"* (Burk & Horton, 1988, p. 18). This is certainly true, but the process of moving from a database to an organized and accessible directory is human. Raw materials have to be transformed by human cognition, and the cost of this

transformation cannot normally be quantified even if the raw material and finished product can.

(8) *"Substitutes for any specific item or collection of information are available, and may be quantified as more or less expensive"* (Burk & Horton, 1988, p. 18). Substitutes for information that are lost or destroyed *may* be available, but it is unlikely that every item in a collection would have a readily available substitute. More significantly, the intellectual effort involved in designing and creating a collection of information means that it is almost impossible to replicate especially if the original was built over a number of years.

(9) Finally, *"choices are available to management in making trade-offs between different grades, types and prices of information"* (Burk & Horton, 1988, p. 18). Choices may be available, but there is no certainty that the choices made will be the correct ones. A large expenditure on externally acquired information may result in little benefit while a small expenditure on organising internally generated information may bring exceptional but unexpected benefits for a business.

RESOURCE-BASED OR KNOWLEDGE-BASED ORGANISATION

The characteristics identified by Burk and Horton (1988) reflect an economic view of the organisation. The organisation is seen as an economic entity the behaviour of which in external markets is the key element (Grant, 1996, p. 109). Organisational theory, on the other hand, sees the organisation as a complex system that encompasses multiple individuals and analyses both internal structures and the relationship between units and departments (Grant, 1996, p. 109). The primary goal of organisational theory is to explain an organisation's performance and the determinants of strategic choice (Grant, 1996, p. 110). A third view of the organisation is that of a knowledge-creating entity where the primary purpose is to integrate existing specialist information and the knowledge of its members into goods or services (Grant, 1996, p. 120). This view is especially prevalent at the moment because of the popularity of the ideas associated with knowledge management.

The resource-based view of information is a strong one, but as it arises from an economic view it is potentially at odds with views associated with a knowledge-based organisation. What it does do is focus attention on information as a valuable resource and places it within a management framework that is familiar to senior managers. We argue that a resource-based view of information and its definition as an asset is useful because it changes the perception of managers towards information, even if it does not result in any valuation being made. Despite all the difficulties outlined above, such recognition is fundamental to the creation of a knowledge-based business.

OUR RESEARCH – AIMS AND OBJECTIVES

The main aim of our research is to explore the ways in which information has value for organisations and to explore how the management and measurement of attributes of information assets can enhance organisational effectiveness. We are currently identifying the issues involved in managing, identifying and measuring attributes of information assets.

Methods

The major methods being used are guided personal interviews with senior executives in information-intensive U.K. organisations. Senior executives are those who make up the senior management team in an organisation such as Managing Directors, Finance Directors and Personnel Directors. Many have a direct influence on the management of information within their organisations and on budgeting decisions relating to information management. Guided interviews with experts in the accounting and information profession and with representatives of their professional and regulatory bodies are also being undertaken. A number of case studies with information-intensive U.K. organisations are also being compiled. An information asset and attribute scoring grid has been developed for use in these case studies along with a guided interview schedule.

Analysis

The main analysis for this research will comprise concept mapping of guided interviews using a qualitative data analysis tool, ATLAS Ti. Analysis so far has included the use of the repertory grid (Kelly, 1955) to identify the attributes of information as an asset considered significant by five senior executives in information-intensive U.K. organisations.

Findings

Our findings will identify those attributes of information as an asset which are considered significant by senior managers. The measurement of the effects of attributes of information as an asset on organisational effectiveness will indicate the extent to which information is critical to business success. From interviews analysed to date, it is clear that linking the business benefits of managing information to commercial objectives is key to senior managers recognition of the value of information in their organisations. This may be an area of future research that we will have to address.

OUR RESEARCH – INFORMATION AS AN ASSET

The Hawley Committee recommended the identification of information as an asset (KPMG/IMPACT, 1994). Its Chairman, Dr Robert Hawley, former Chief Executive of Nuclear Power plc, argued that the failure of organisations to address their information resource and its value could result in substantial risks (Hawley, 1995, p. 237).

The Committee recommended treating information as an asset because:

> ... every board of directors can relate to managing and reporting assets (Hawley, 1995, p. 237).

The Committee argued that the first step in benefiting from the information held and used by organisations was a formal process of identification. It claimed that a number of information types or assets were consistently identified across organisations. These information assets were:

Market and customer information, e.g. regional utilities have large amounts of data on every household in their region; trade names and marks.

Product information, e.g. the depth of knowledge in particular technologies which support particular products such as fluid and thermal dynamics in the aerospace industry; this includes both registered and non-registered Intellectual Property Rights (IPR).

Specialist knowledge and information for operating in a particular area, which is often in people's heads, e.g. retailing know-how amongst managers of grocery supermarkets who find that even closely associated areas of retailing difficult to move into. Since the publication of the Hawley Report, retailers in the U.K. have become very successful in expanding their markets into associated consumer durables and goods. Specialist knowledge is now being addressed in part by knowledge management techniques, but, at the time of the Hawley Report, knowledge management was not a well-established concept.

Business process information that underpins the workings of the business, e.g. economic, political, share price and other information in which the equity market trades.

Management information, particularly that on which major policy, competitive decisions or strategic plans will be based, e.g. economic statistics, or cost base information.

Human Resource information, e.g. skills databases, particularly in project-based organisations such as consultants who need to be brought together to support a client project. These days knowledge management attempts to address this area.

Supplier information, e.g. agreements or networks of contacts for services or product development.

"Accountable" information, i.e. legally required information, including shareholder information or information to deal with public issues, e.g. information to defend health and safety cases or environmental pollution evidence (KPMG/IMPACT, 1994, pp. 9–10).

These eight information assets formed the basis of a discussion forum held by us in London with a group of senior British information managers in January 2001. The discussions were intended to review and update the information assets identified by the Hawley Committee and to clarify them for the purposes of our further research. A small number of attributes of information as an asset were also presented and debated. The information managers were members or guests of the Aslib Information Resources Management group, a special interest network focused specifically on the management of information resources (see http://www.aslib.co.uk/members/contact.html).

REVISING THE LIST

We made two changes to the original listing by Hawley of the information assets before presenting them to the information managers' discussion forum. These were:

(1) *"Market and customer information"* was renamed *"Customer information"* to reflect the widening application of customer information to inform all aspects of business.
(2) *"Competitor information"* was added to differentiate this asset from management information as a whole. Highlighting competitive advantage gained from information assets requires its identification as a separate information asset.

The recommendations from the information managers' discussion group were as follows:

Specialist knowledge: This term was considered confusing and out of place – especially as it brought all of the requirements to identify and define "knowledge" within the process. While recognising the importance of "knowledge," it was felt that concentration on types of information or information assets would provide a firmer foundation for later work.

"Accountable" information: This term was not understood by the information managers as referring to legal information, for example health and safety information in legal cases. This was identified as one of the most important information assets, one often only identified under pressure of legal action. Renaming the asset as *"Legal and Regulatory"* was recommended.

Human resource information: This was regarded as an outdated term. The argument was that "people are not resources for an organisation; they are of course people." The term *"People management"* was recommended instead.

Organisational information: This asset was suggested as an important information type. It was not included in the Hawley Report (KPMG/IMPACT, 1994), but now is increasingly recognised by organisations as essential to organisational learning and change management.

> Organisations must be aware of the features of their organisational culture that they most value . . . and look at those features that make a negative contribution to corporate well-being (Orna, 1999, p. 131).

Of the remaining information assets, *Business process information* provided the most debate. Some participants argued that business process information should not be regarded as an information asset at all. Others pointed out that organisations like Cisco, the American technology giant, were packaging and selling their business processes, making such information a financial asset. The arguments for including business processes among the information assets outweighed the arguments against.

The revised list of information assets based on the Hawley information assets and the discussion forum with information managers now form the columns of our proposed matrix of information assets (Fig. 1).

The next stage of the research study was to identify the attributes of information that relate most strongly to each of these types of information asset.

ATTRIBUTES OF INFORMATION AS AN ASSET

Despite the wealth of work in identifying attributes of information, it has always been unclear what it is about information that managers really value.

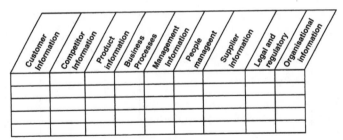

Fig. 1. Matrix Information Assets.

The information science literature has described characteristics of information in three ways. The first of these sees information as an entity in itself which has attributes of quality (for example, accuracy, comprehensiveness and credibility) and attributes of utility (for example, ease of use, accessibility and flexibility) (Burk & Horton, 1988, p. 93). The second approach identifies attributes that are inherent to the nature of information (for example, information improves productivity by improving decision-making, and information improves effectiveness by enabling better relationships with customers and partners) (Burk & Horton, 1988, p. 93). Finally, information has economic attributes that make it unique (Arrow, 1984, p. 142).

We argue that the attributes of information traditionally identified can be applied to the information assets identified by the Hawley Committee. This is because information is the prime ingredient of all the assets we identified. These attributes, when recognised, may act as pointers to significant information assets for managers. One of the aims of the project team was to investigate whether the traditionally identified attributes of information were indeed recognised and understood by managers.

First of all, we attempted to find out which of the attributes might be seen as most significant to each information asset by asking the discussion group of senior information managers to score attributes of information assets against the Hawley categories of information assets. The senior information managers were presented with a number of attributes of information based on broad categories of quality, utility, productivity, effectiveness and economy (Burk & Horton, 1988, p. 93). These attributes included, for example, accuracy, currency and accessibility. They were then asked to score the attributes on a one to five scale against each of the information assets, with one being the least important attribute for that particular information asset, and five being the most important (Fig. 2).

There was a good deal of difficulty encountered. The ability of an attribute to change in importance as the situation changed was identified as a major issue, and this difficulty remains in our research study. There was very little

Attributes	Customer Information	Competitor Information	Product Information	Business Processes	Management Information	People management	Supplier Information	Legal and regulatory	Organisational information
Accessible									
Expandable									
Current									
Accurate									
Sufficient									

Fig. 2.   Matrix Attribute Scoring Grid for Information Managers.

consistency found in the results overall, with a wide range of scores resulting in little consensus. What was clear was that presenting attributes in this way was not working, even with a group of information managers who might have been expected to be familiar with them. The attributes presented were seen as confusing and in need of contextualisation.

The scoring mechanism itself was also found wanting as an asset that consistently scored a one on all the attributes would outweigh an asset that scored a five on just one attribute and zero on all the others. This would inevitably lead to misrepresentation of the views of the senior information managers. Numeric weighting of scores was also seen as confusing. The information managers argued that a more visual scoring mechanism based on a gold, silver and bronze Olympic medal system was needed. The argument was that the temptation to add up numbers was high and that the abstract nature of information required a more visual approach. The idea that any manager, with or without experience of managing information assets, could immediately see which information assets were considered significant and which were not was convincing. This Olympic scoring approach is currently being developed by the project team for use in further case studies for the project.

INTERVIEWS WITH SENIOR EXECUTIVES

The aim of the next stage of the research was to investigate whether those attributes of information identified in the information science literature were those considered significant by senior executives. If they were not, this might explain why the importance of information was not recognised at senior executive level (Abell, 1994). To investigate this, and bearing in mind the information managers' experience, we needed the senior executives to describe attributes of information assets without prompting from the interviewer. This, it was hoped, would result in a range of attributes being identified independently that could then be compared with the traditional attributes. The problems of contextualisation would be eliminated as the attributes would be described by the executives themselves. A method was therefore needed which would allow the attributes to be elicited with the minimum input from the interviewer. The method chosen was the repertory grid technique.

Repertory Grid Technique

The repertory grid technique was developed by George Kelly (1955) as a method of identifying how individuals construe elements of their social world. Kelly was an American psychologist and psychotherapist and one of the founders in the 1950s of the Association for Humanistic Psychology (Stevens, 1996, p. 162). Kelly proposed a theory called "Personal Construct Theory" which assumed that humans are basically "scientists" who mentally represent the world around them and who formulate and test hypotheses about the nature of reality. Humans are continually exploring and developing an understanding of their world and, in doing so, they develop cognitive maps that then define and limit their behaviour. By discovering the personal maps of individuals, it is possible to understand their views of the world and possibly alter their maps and change behaviour (Easterby-Smith et al., 1991, p. 85).

Kelly's (1955) work had a particular appeal to clinical psychologists in the U.K., where training had tended to be experimental and research led. These psychologists often encountered difficulties when faced with the complex problems of their clients' own experience. The repertory grid method, in particular, made it possible to chart the nature of each person's world view as she or he experienced it; and did this from each person individually (Stevens, 1996, p. 162). It is as a result, much more widely used in the U.K. than in the U.S. where Kelly a worked.

Applications of repertory grid technique are now wide and varied. As well as management development and change (Easterby-Smith et al., 1991, p. 12), they have also been used in clinical and educational settings (Beail, 1985) and in classification studies (Dillon & McKnight, 1990).

One of the benefits of repertory grid is that it has been identified as a useful method to reduce observer bias (Stewart et al., 1981, p. 4). Observer bias has long been recognised as a major problem in conducting research. The interviewer's background, history and experience give him/her expectations about the world so that he/she recognises familiar things. The problem with this is that there is a tendency to turn less familiar things into those that resemble what the interviewer knows. Observer bias can have serious consequences, as shown in a widely used example quoted by Stewart et al. (1981) of a schoolteacher whose class was randomly split into two groups. The teacher was told that all the children had been tested and that Group A children were brighter than Group B children (although no difference in fact existed). At the end of term the children were re-tested and it was found that Group A children scored more highly than Group B (Stewart et al., 1981, p. 4).

The repertory grid technique itself has three main components:

- elements, which define the area to be investigated;
- constructs, which are the ways in which the person groups and differentiates among the elements;
- linking mechanisms, which show how each element is judged on each construct. These are usually a set of observations and the constructs or criteria by which those observations are rated (Beail, 1985, p. 2).

Repertory grids can enable an interview to be carried out in some detail, and reduce observer bias, but this depends very much on how the grids are administered. For example, when choosing elements, there are three strategies which can be adopted to generate elements and each has its own advantages and disadvantages. These strategies are:

(1) The interviewer provides the elements.
(2) Free response, this is where the interviewee names a list of elements spontaneously with the interviewer providing only a broad class from which to draw.
(3) Using eliciting questions, with the answers to the questions forming the elements (Stewart et al., 1981, p. 35).

Either of the last two strategies puts the interviewer within reach of eliminating observer bias. However, this does mean that if there is a particular element which the interviewer needs to introduce, (for example, a particular brand of product which is being compared to others), then it cannot be assumed that the interviewee will introduce this element. With the first strategy, where the interviewer supplies the elements, the problem is that some or all of the elements may not be familiar to the interviewee, thus reducing the usefulness of the distinctions subsequently made.

When selecting elements, there are some general rules that can be followed. Elements selected are most often people, objects, events and activities, in other words nouns and verbs. Elements should also be homogenous, that is classes of elements should not be mixed and should not be sub-sets of other elements. For example, "Making presentations" and "Making presentations to the Managing Director" would be inappropriate. Elements should not be evaluative; terms such as "Leadership" and "Communicating" fall into this area.

An important point to remember when selecting elements is the repertory grid's basis in Personal Construct Theory. Personal Construct Theory asserts that humans can only understand what is meant by "good" by also understanding what is meant by "bad." This means that the elements must allow contrasts to be made between them. This is important for the elicitation of constructs. Constructs reflect how the individual views the world. The process for eliciting constructs is based on presenting triads and appears simple but can quickly become more complex. For example, if we take three words representing elements, such as, SHEEP COWS PIGS and write them on three separate cards, we can ask in what way any two of them are similar and the third different. The answer might be that Sheep and Cows eat grass and Pigs eat swill. These answers would then form a bipolar distinction so that we have:

Eats grass – Eats swill

These bipolar distinctions represent the dimensions the interviewee uses when he/she is thinking about the elements, and these dimensions are the constructs. The elicitation becomes more complex when we replace elements like sheep and cows with elements like my mother, myself, and my boss (Stewart et al., 1981, pp. 11–13). The constructs elicited for sheep, cows and pigs may be similar for many interviewees but those elicited for my mother, myself, and my boss are likely to be widely differing. By using these triadic comparisons and asking for both a similarity and a difference the method allows equal focus on both poles of the construct. This means that a construct is not just composed of a phrase and its semantic opposite; it is also contrast (Stewart et al., 1981, p. 17). Each end of the bipolar construct can be made equally clear. This is much more difficult to achieve when elements do not have a "good" and "bad" contrast, as in the information assets, resulting in possibly more opposites being produced than bipolar constructs.

There were three main steps followed in conducting the repertory grid interviews. The findings of one of these interviews are reported here. These were: Step 1, the identification of elements or information assets; Step 2, administering the grid and Step 3, analysing the grid. These are dealt with below and are supplemented by further discussion on the repertory grid method.

Step 1. The Identification of Elements or Information Assets
The nine information assets presented were based on the Hawley assets and reflected the revisions recommended by the discussion forum of senior U.K. information managers described earlier. These formed the elements in the repertory grid exercise.

Step 2. Administering the Grid

The participants were given prepared sets of combinations of three information assets, or triads, printed on 6 × 4 index cards. The cards had no additional contextual information as this had been provided before the exercise and we wanted to encourage a focus on the elements themselves. Participants were then asked to identify two of the information assets in the triad that they considered similar and one information asset they considered different. They were then asked to describe why the two they selected were similar and why the remaining one was different. Then a second set of five cards with the numbers one to five was presented. The two assets identified as the same were placed at number one and the one asset identified as different was placed at five. Participants were then given the six remaining information assets and asked to position them in relation to the constructs, or attributes they had identified for the triad. This gave a result for all the nine information assets in relation to the attributes proposed. The numbers one to five carry no inherent meaning but simply provided a way in which the executives can position the elements in relative terms.

In all, four triads were used:

123 Customer information, Competitor information, Product information.
456 Business processes, Management information, People management.
789 Supplier information, Legal and regulatory, Organisational information.
159 Customer information, Management information, Organisational information.

With these nine information assets it would have been possible to present at least nine different triads of information assets. However, time constraints meant that only a limited number of four triads were completed by each executive. The length of time taken to complete a repertory grid has been identified as a major drawback of this method with a twenty by ten matrix taking up to one and a half hours to complete (Easterby-Smith et al., 1991, pp. 84–87). It was clear also that the executives found it difficult to think of information assets in such a formal way and they subsequently reported that they felt challenged by the process but that it was "fun" overall.

Step 3. Analysing the Grid

There are five principal methods of analysis for repertory grid. These are: frequency counts, content analysis, visual focusing, cluster analysis and principal-component analysis. The first two methods are concerned with analysing the content of the grid. Thus, frequency counts simply count the number of times a construct or element is mentioned. Content analysis involves selecting a number of categories which the constructs or elements fit into and then assigning individual constructs and elements to them (Stewart et al., 1981, pp. 47–48). Visual focusing, cluster analysis and principal-component analysis show not only the content but also the interrelationships between the constructs and the elements (Stewart et al., 1981, p. 46).

The tool used to analyse the senior executives' grids was WebGrid II http://tiger.cpsc.ucalgary.ca/, which is a Web-based version of repertory grid technique for building conceptual models (Gaines & Shaw, 2001, p. 2). It is based on the concept of revealing the meanings in a grid by re-sorting it so that like elements are placed together and like constructs are placed together as in visual focusing (where the analysis is conducted by eye).

WebGrid II is based on the FOCUS program developed at Brunel University by Gaines and Shaw (Stewart et al., 1981, p. 57). FOCUS works in the same way as visual focusing but allows correlations to be made. It uses variations of cluster analysis. This makes the analysis much more sensitive and able to deal with five to nine point scales. FOCUS looks first at the elements and searches for correlations between them. When it finds a correlation, it joins the elements together and creates a new element, which it then prints on a vertical scale between 50 and 100 points. It continues to search until all the elements are covered. The programme then re-sorts the grid and prints the complete dendogram or tree diagram (Easterby-Smith et al., 1991, pp. 84–87) with the inter-correlations on the bottom. The same process is carried out on the constructs. The grid is then re-sorted so that similar constructs are placed together. The constructs, in this case, were sorted using a rating scale of one to five. In WebGrid II, the "FOCUS" button is used to sort the grid, and thus bring similar elements and constructs together. Element dendograms are printed to the bottom right of the grid and construct dendograms are printed to the upper right of the grid, along a vertical scale ranging, in this case, from 60 to 100.

Interview with Head of Knowledge Management – Company C

Company C was represented by its Head of Knowledge Management. The company is a large consumer goods organisation that has a long-established and well regarded research and development ethos. Aligned to this is an active knowledge management function. The organisation's main information assets were brand related and there is a long history of managing such assets. The interview was conducted by telephone in early 2001 and comprised a general interview (reported elsewhere) on the identification and management of information assets and the repertory grid exercise. The grid for Head of Knowledge Management – Company C is shown in Fig. 3.

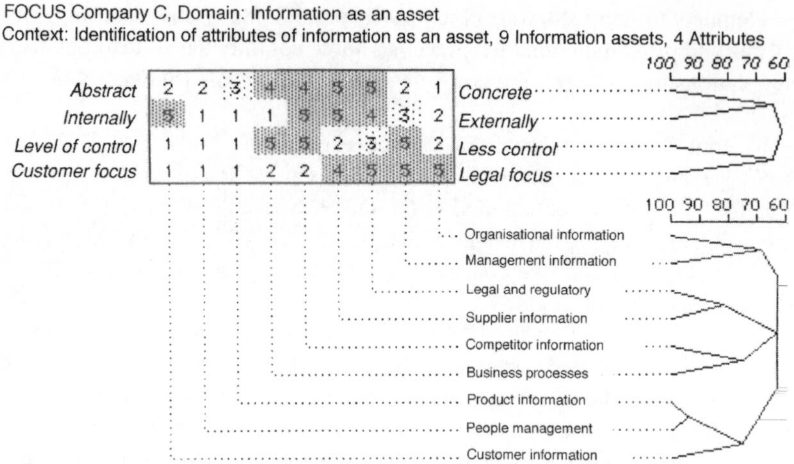

FOCUS Company C, Domain: Information as an asset
Context: Identification of attributes of information as an asset, 9 Information assets, 4 Attributes

Fig. 3.   Head of Knowledge Management – Company C.

For Head of Knowledge Management, Company C the information assets clustered into four main groups:

Group one contains *Legal and Regulatory* and *Supplier Information* matching at 81% and showing that little distinction was made between these two information assets by Head of Knowledge Management, Company C.

Group two contains *Business Processes* and *Competitor Information*, which matched at 75%. These assets differed on only one attribute (Internally-Externally), on which they were poles apart (see Fig. 3, attribute dendogram to the upper right of the grid).

Group three contains *Product Information*, *People Management* and *Customer Information*. *Product Information* and *People Management* were strongly linked and matched at 94%. They only differed slightly in one construct (Abstract-Concrete). This indicates the strong role of employees in developing and delivering this organisation's products as construed by this executive. *Customer Information* is linked with *People Management* at 75%. Head of Knowledge Management, Company C, seems confident in his organisation's management of customer information but is unsure of his organisation's employees' management. *Customer Information* and *People Management* differed only on one attribute (Abstract- Concrete) which occupied different poles. (See Fig. 3, attribute dendogram to the upper right of the grid.)

Group four, *Organisational Information* and *Management Information*, matched at 69% and then matched with *Groups one, two and three* at 62%.

The Head of Knowledge Management, Company C, (see Fig. 3) focused mainly on the information assets as entities in themselves. Information assets were described as *Abstract-Concrete* and *Customer Focus-Legal Focus*. He did not describe attributes in terms of value or in terms of productivity or effectiveness. What is clear is that the attributes identified were not those traditionally identified in the information science literature. They were much more specific to the individual executive's own perceptions of the various relevance of the information assets. As such, they may be a better indicator of what attributes may be recognised by senior executives.

CONCLUSION

The identification of attributes of information that are relevant and understood by senior managers is a critical step in enabling the recognition of information as a valuable business resource. The resource-based view of information though presenting a number of difficulties is useful in providing a framework for the management of information. However, the knowledge-based view of the organisation is becoming more common (Grant, 1996) and requires a less mechanistic approach to the creation and utilisation of information and knowledge. This means that many of the assumptions found in a resource-based view need to be re-examined. In particular, the focus on information activities needs to be re-assessed in terms of usefulness.

However, because of the abstract nature of information and knowledge it is useful to retain some elements of the resource-based view. The identification of information as an asset, we argue, enables an abstract concept to be recognised by senior executives who are familiar with managing traditional assets such as inventory and property. The key to the value of information may lie in measuring or tracking attributes of information. However, the first step is identifying those attributes that are relevant today. We have attempted to do this by using the repertory grid method to facilitate the open identification of attributes of a range of information assets. Further work for the project will involve carrying out case studies in a small number of information-intensive U.K. companies to investigate current business approaches to the identification and management of information assets and their attributes. The challenge for library and information professionals is to identify those attributes that can help managers recognise significant information that can improve business performance.

REFERENCES

Abell, A. (1994). *An information policy for Business Link Hertfordshire*. Hertfordshire: University of Hertfordshire Press.

Arrow, K. J. (1984). The economics of information. In: *Collected Papers of Kenneth J. Arrow: The Economics of Information* (Vol. 4). Oxford: Blackwell.

Beail, N. (1985). An introduction to repertory grid technique. In: N. Beail (Ed.), *Repertory Grid Technique and Personal Constructs: Applications in Clinical and Educational Settings* (pp. 1–24). London: Croom Helm.

Black, S. H., & Marchand, D. (1982). Assessing the value of information in organisations: A challenge for the 1980s. *The Information Society Journal, 1*(3), 191–225.

Boisot, M. H. (1998). *Knowledge assets: Securing competitive advantage in the information economy*. Oxford: OUP.

Burk, C., & Horton, F. (1988). *Infomap: A complete guide to discovering corporate information resources*. Englewood Cliffs, NJ: Prentice-Hall.

Cooper, M. D. (1983). The structure and future of the information economy. *Information Processing and Management, 19*(1), 9–26.

Davenport, T. H. (1993). *Process innovation: Reengineering work through information technology*. Boston: Harvard Business School Press.

Davies, M., Paterson, R., & Wilson, A. (1997). U.K. *GAAP: Generally accepted accounting practice in the United Kingdom*. London: Macmillan.

Dillon, A., & McKnight, C. (1990). Towards a classification of text types: A repertory grid approach. *International Journal of Man-Machine Studies, 33*, 623–636.

Eaton, J. J., & Bawden, D. (1991). What kind of resource is information? *International Journal of Information Management, 11*(2), 156–165.

Framel, J. E. (1990). Managing information costs and technologies as assets. *Journal of Systems Management, 41*(2), 12–18.

Easterby-Smith, M., Thorpe, R., & Lowe, A. (1991). *Management research: An introduction*. London: Sage.

Easterby-Smith, M., Thorpe, R., & Holman, D. (1996). Using repertory grids in management. *Journal of European Industrial Training, 20*(3), 3–30.

Edvinsson, L., & Malone, M. S. (1997). *Intellectual capital: The proven way to establish your company's real value by measuring its hidden brainpower*. London: Piatkus Publishers.

Gaines, B. R., & Shaw, M. L. G. (2001). *WebGrid: Knowledge modeling and inference through the world wide web*. Available at: http://tiger/cpsc.ucalgary.ca/ Accessed 31/01/02.

Grant, R. M. (1996). Towards a knowledge-based theory of the firm. *Strategic Management Journal, 17* (Winter) (Special Issue), 109–122.

Hall, K. (1981). The economic nature of information. *The Information Society, 1*(2), 143–166.

Hawley, R. (1995). Information as an asset: The board agenda. *Information Management and Technology, 28*(6), 237–239.

Hennen, T. J. (2001). Do you know the real value of your library? *Library Journal, 126*(11), 48–50.

Kelly, G. A. (1955). *The psychology of personal constructs* (2 vols.). New York: Norton.

KPMG/IMPACT (1994). *Information as an asset: The board agenda*. London: KPMG/IMPACT Group.

McGinn, H. F. (1993). Good business: Information assets. *The Bottom Line, 7*(Fall), 40–41.

Machlup. (1962). *The production and distribution of knowledge in the United States*. Princeton NJ: Princeton University Press.

Orna, E. (1999). *Practical information policies* (2nd ed.). Aldershot: Gower.

Poirier, R. (1990). The information economy approach: Characteristics, limitations and future prospects. *The Information Society, 7*(4), 245–285.

Porat, M. U. (1977). *The information economy: Definition and measurement.* U.S. Department of Commerce, Office of Telecommunications Special Publication 77–12 (1). Washington DC: U.S. Government Printing Office.

Reuters (1995). *Information as an asset: The invisible goldmine.* London: Reuters.

Skyrme, D. J. (1997). *Creating the knowledge-based business.* London: Business Intelligence Ltd.

Stevens, R. (1996). The reflexive self: An experiential perspective. In: R. Stevens (Ed.), *Understanding the Self* (pp. 147–218). London: Sage.

Stewart, V., Stewart, A., & Fonda, N. (1981). *Business applications of repertory grid.* London: McGraw-Hill.

Wild, K., Creighton, B., & Simmonds, A. (2000). *GAAP 2000: U.K. Financial reporting and accounting.* London: Deloitte & Touche.

MANAGEMENT EDUCATION FOR LIBRARY AND INFORMATION SCIENCE

John M. Budd

INTRODUCTION

Direct, administer, manage. All of these are words applied to those who lead libraries, and they are usually applied interchangeably. But not only do they have unique definitions, they each carry a distinct implication for library managers and the organizations they lead. "Direct" means to provide a forward-thinking grounding for action in an organization (and this word's meaning is most closely synonymous with "lead"). "Administer" suggests dispensing or carrying out, for instance, policy. The word is in some ways distant from the creation of policy or direction. "Manage" frequently is limited to the performance or overseeing of tasks on a daily basis. None of these words is false or pejorative when applied to the library, but each is limited in some important ways. The genuine work of guiding actions in libraries is actually an iterative balance of all three of the functions denoted by these words. If the terms are conflated in the everyday usage of our profession, from where does the confused usage come? Is understanding of the aforementioned balance common in practice? How clearly is the range and complexity of action communicated in educational programs? (Terminology presents some problems; for ease of expression and reading, the whole complex of action will be referred to as management, understanding that the usage here encompasses all requisite connotations.)

Advances in Library Administration and Organization
Advances in Library Administration and Organization, Volume 20, 149–163
Copyright © 2003 by Elsevier Science Ltd.
All rights of reproduction in any form reserved
ISSN: 0732-0671/PII: S0732067102200073

The last question, with all its attendant implications, is what concerns us here. If we grant that the guidance of action in libraries entails many skills, decisions, and understandings, what is the role of library and information science (LIS) education in preparing people to assume leadership positions in professional organizations? This question necessarily involves exploring what is being done in LIS programs, what can be done, and what should be done. Also, necessarily, the exploration must be accompanied by some relation to what is being written and said about management in libraries. Current thought and opinion is varied, with some studies and other writings emphasizing some elements of management and others emphasizing different elements. Some research has been conducted in our field and in others, but very often writings on management could best, and perhaps most generously, be classified as informed opinion.

A bit of background on LIS education may be helpful here. At present there are 56 master's programs in North America that are accredited by the American Library Association (ALA). Some of the 56 programs also include undergraduate offerings, but those offerings are, in the main, focused on information technology and its use; undergraduate courses may not introduce students to the full complexity of libraries as organizations. Students entering master's programs do not tend to have undergraduate backgrounds that include the study of management, and while many students do have work experience, those experiences may not involve management in the broad sense employed in this paper. The nature and structure of LIS education is such that, at the master's level, it provides students with an introduction to the profession and its work, and an introduction to the skills required to prepare for entry-level jobs. Educational programs also provide some more specialized introductions to organizational function, information content, and the communities they will work in and those they will be expected to serve.

What follows is an examination of educational content of master's programs, insofar as that is possible from information provided by the programs themselves (including available course syllabi). The place of management and the content of courses is scrutinized along with our professional discourse. Educational content and writings on management are looked at in order to see the extent to which there is agreement/consonance or disagreement/dissonance. The totality of management content is examined in light of possible and desirable educational approaches to the topic and their expected outcomes. In other words, the formal investigation will not be divorced from personal observation and suggestion; I will offer thoughts, along with rationale, regarding educational content.

COURSES IN LIS PROGRAMS

The simplest measurement possible is the calculation of programs that require a management course of all students. The Web sites of ALA-accredited programs in the U.S. and Canada were consulted to ascertain requirements and other information. These sites were selected because they are the public statements of curricular information, and they tend to be the most up-to-date sources of requirements and syllabi. Of the fifty programs for which information is available, 28, or 57%, explicitly require a management course. Another 12 programs (24%) offer such a course but it is not required. Five programs do not offer a generic management course, but do have a set of courses organized by type of library (academic, public, etc.). Five programs do not appear to have a management-related course. That said, there may be courses in the curricula of those five programs that address management topics. What is difficult to identify from this single measure is the number or proportion of graduates who have taken some kind of course as part of their programs intended to prepare them for management in libraries or other information agencies.

More telling is an examination of the course syllabi for management courses in LIS master's programs. Twenty-four syllabi were available for perusal. These documents provide varying amounts of information about particular aspects of the courses, including overall approach, readings, assignments, and descriptions of particular functions and tasks, along with ways of thinking about management. One simple indicator (which may, however, be deceptive) is the required readings for the course. I begin with this indicator because it illustrates the variability of course content quite clearly. A considerable number of texts are mentioned in syllabi, but only three are mentioned in more than one syllabus. The more frequently mentioned required text is *Library and Information Center Management*, by Robert Stueart and Barbara Moran. This text is required in eight courses. Next in frequency, with six occurrences, is *Management Basics for Information Professionals*, by G. Edward Evans and others. The only other book that has two mentions is *Management: Skills and Application*, by Leslie W. Rue and others. Seven course syllabi indicate that a readings packet (an assortment of readings available from library reserve or for sale) is required. In those syllabi that include complete reading lists, a variety of types of readings are mentioned. Readings from LIS are about as numerous as those drawn from other fields (primarily management). An inference that can be drawn from the readings is that students are exposed to different ways of thinking about management and of behaving in management positions.

The assignments that are required in these courses can also be examined, although they are not always included in the syllabi. Further, many assignments

Table 1.   Assignments in Management Courses.

Assignment	Frequency
Case Study/Analysis	9
Literature Review/Bibliography	6
Plan (Mission, etc.)	6
Budget	5
Evaluation	3
Grant Proposal	2
Leader Profile	2
Library Profile	2
Memo	2
Personal Philosophy Statement	2
Resumé	2
Organizational Observation	1
Personnel Assignment	1
Policy Statement	1
Staffing	1
Strategic Plan (distinct from Plan)	1

are (necessarily) rather vague. Syllabi indicate that students will write short or long papers, respond to scenarios, and address issues of the students' choosing. Some syllabi provide lists of potential topics of these assignments, but the lists tend to mirror the course topics. Table 1 provides a list of the more explicit assignments; given the variability of some assignments, this list should not be over-interpreted.

The case study (where a specific case is presented for analysis) is the most frequently occurring assignment, with nine mentions. A literature review of bibliography, and a planning assignment (that can include writing a mission statement, goals, and objectives) are tied for second with six occurrences each. Next is a budget assignment, which is included in five syllabi. Several of the assignments are what might be called "detached;" that is, they are not tied to particular organizations (or even types of organizations) and they do not address specific problems or decision opportunities that can occur in libraries. Literature reviews, book review, philosophy statements, leader profiles, etc. fit into this category. Other assignments, such as evaluations, budgets, plans, and case studies are more grounded in specific situations. From a pedagogical point of view, a mix of the two types of assignments is likely to be most effective. Assuming that many students in such a course will have limited or no prior experience in/knowledge of libraries as organizations, beginning with the more generic and moving to the more specific will enable students to most fully understand the complexities of organizations and their management.

Perhaps more telling than anything else in the syllabi is the content of the courses offered by LIS programs. The available syllabi include course topics, which may indicate the actual experience of the students in these courses. As can be expected, there is a considerable variety of content, perhaps reflecting that variance is a function of the experiences, backgrounds, knowledge, and inclinations of the instructors. Table 2 presents a list of the topics and the frequency of occurrence in the syllabi.

A few topics appear to be fairly common to the LIS courses: planning (including mission, goals, and objectives) appears in 23 syllabi; human resources (including personnel appraisal and assessment) and budgeting/fiscal management appear 17 times each; leadership is included in 15 syllabi; management theory and thought, and evaluation/measurement appear 14 times each; and communication occurs 13 times. One two-part caveat needs to be explicit here: the appearance of a topic in a syllabus is not necessary an indication of depth of coverage of the topic, and the absence of a topic does not necessarily mean the topic is not covered.

One thing that is evident from the course syllabi is that, for the most part, management courses are oriented towards upper-level positions in libraries and information agencies. Topics such as budgeting, directing, control, personnel appraisal, and the like presume that the students will become, at the very least, department heads in organizations. It may very well be true that many who take these courses as students will, from the outset, be in decision-making positions in small libraries. Given that many special and public libraries are small operations, with few staff members, some graduates will almost immediately have to develop budget requests, purchase technology (on a small scale), and present the needs of the library to library boards or administrators. One question that arises is whether the management courses are oriented to such smaller, less complex organizations. What may be needed by people going into smaller environments that serve smaller (and perhaps more homogeneous) communities is content designed to teach practitioners how to make personal contacts with individuals in order to understand what they want and need from the library. It may be that other courses in the programs' curricula relating to services and operations address the needs of these kinds of environments more effectively than those focusing on management.

Many people who graduate from LIS programs do not immediately have sophisticated decision-making or supervisory duties. They may enter organizations as reference, or cataloging, or serials librarians and may be primarily responsible for functional duties. What might they need most to do their jobs well? Beyond functional competencies, perhaps they need to understand how to work with student assistants or volunteers; how to communicate within and across functional lines; how to plan on a micro-, rather than on a macro-level; and

Table 2. Syllabus Topics.

Topic	Frequency
Planning	23
Human Resources/Personnel Appraisal	17
Budgeting/Fiscal Management	17
Leadership	15
Management Theory/Thought	14
Measurement/Evaluation	14
Communication	13
Staffing/Development	12
Control	11
Change/Innovation	10
Decision Making	10
Supervision/Directing	10
Organizing	9
Information Technology	7
Marketing/PR	6
Physical Facilities	5
Environment	4
Motivation	4
Authority	3
Organizational Behavior	3
Organizational Culture	3
Organizational Design/Structure	3
Politics/Political Context	3
Power	3
Responsibility	3
Style (Management/Leadership)	3
Trends and Issues	3
Cooperation (Interinstitutional)	2
Ethics	2
TQM/CQI	2
Customers	1
Fund Raising	1
Information Policy	1
Knowledge Management	1
Strategic Management	1

how to comprehend the political structure and workings of the entire environment (including both the library and the parent organization). Given that libraries are complex organizations, decision making is likely to involve several dimensions, including fiscal implications of decisions made, service outcomes, and the morale of personnel. Both management and the assessment of managers entail critical evaluative elements; master's programs present an early opportunity to help students with the critical thinking necessary for success as managers and as professionals.

The concerns just mentioned illustrate a specific challenge faced by both LIS programs and libraries as organizations. What is the essential distinction between education and training? This is a concern that is not frequently addresses explicitly either in programs' curricula or in the professional literature. One notable exception is Glen Holt's detailed exposition of the kinds of training that libraries can and should be responsible for, plus the costs associated with that training. He cautions colleagues that training is expensive, but ignoring training is even more expensive in services not offered, community needs not met, and resources not attracted (Holt, 1999). Training tends to be (and probably needs to be) locally determined; only a given library can accurately and effectively identify the kinds of services and access that the library's community wants and needs, plus the skills and competencies needed by staff (professional and other) to meet community needs. However, understanding why particular training may be necessary, what the training will accomplish, and what to do with those skills that result from training is the province of education. To an extent, LIS master's programs can begin the training of managers by creating experiences that are as authentic as possible. Such experiences can help students understand both the processes of management and its outcomes. Along with the training, though, should come education grounded in thought and theory, especially theory that is explicitly aimed at action in organizations. The concerns related to training and education point to some specific purposes of LIS programs and their curricula. Before addressing those purposes directly, it would be helpful to take a look at the LIS literature on management issues.

WHAT DOES THE LITERATURE SAY?

The first thing that should be mentioned here is that very little in the professional literature specifically addresses education for management. There are some individual works that do touch on topics that are included in course content. As is apparent from Table 2, the topics "authority" and "responsibility" are not frequently featured (at least not prominently featured) in syllabi. Further, the two topics are not always co-mentioned (that is, a syllabus may mention authority, but not responsibility). To at least one author, authority and responsibility are of great importance. Phillip Jones (2000) (who uses "accountability" rather than "responsibility," but obviously is speaking of responsible behavior) bemoans the absence of these topics in management literature generally, and library literature specifically. In particular, he points to the apparent absence of accountability and authority in team-based organizations, and wonders how decisions are made and what consequences follow from those decisions. Since authority, accountability, and responsibility are not prevalent in management course syllabi, one might wonder if the courses deserve to be criticized, along with the LIS literature.

The idea of responsibility or accountability is also connected with ethics – another topic that occurs infrequently in course syllabi. The library profession does not ignore ethics, but generally compartmentalizes ethics in the category of intellectual freedom, service quality and effort, and access to information. A connection between ethics and management is not common in the literature, and occurs only rarely in management courses. A search of the database, *Library Literature and Information Science Full Text*, limited to the years 1999–2002 (other topics are searched in this database, with the same date limits, and will be referred to throughout this section), yields only one article on authority and management (Jones's), none on responsibility and management, and none on ethics and management.

As is mentioned above, planning is the topic that occurs most frequently in course syllabi. Planning does not, however, occur with great frequency in the professional literature. A search in the Library Literature database indicates that 55 articles include planning and management. It may be that the concept of planning has been addressed for many years and is now what we might call "textbook knowledge" (that is, the topic is so imbued throughout educational and organizational content that it need not be the focus of a great amount of published work). One article that addresses strategic planning (McClamroch et al., 2001) points to an aspect of thought that has limited planning efforts, and really all management activities – the assumption of rationality. The authors, in writing about planning in one organization, recognize that previous planning processes assumed that all individuals in the organizations, and indeed the process itself, is rational in the narrow sense that everyone reasons before acting, and that the reasoning is grounded in the collective, rather than the individual, interest. What is missing from the article is an apprehension of the historical infusion of this narrow definition of rationality, from scientific management forward. Some schools of management thought have, for at least a century, predicated decisions and action on simple calculations of costs and benefits, without recognizing the individual and personal motivations people may have for what they do. Some syllabi situate management theory and thought in the historical context broadly, but it is not readily evident from syllabi if the course content addresses the foundations of this kind of rationality (based in holdovers of particular Enlightenment thought traditions). That is, it is not clear if the management thought referred to in the syllabi is connected with its psychological, cognitive, social, and ethical implications. Such a historical foundation would enable students to understand more fully the nature and practice of management today.

Leadership is a topic that recurs in the literature; the search already described yields 134 items on leadership. The vast majority of those pieces are aimed at identifying leaders or specific characteristics that acknowledged leaders demonstrate (that is, the pieces tend to be a bit superficial). There is apparent interest in the topic. Leadership is frequently included as a course topic; it is a broad subject that could be treated in a number of ways. One recent publication briefly addresses education for leaders (Honea, 1997). While human relations is generally taken to be the bulk of managerial work, simple interaction with members of the organization is not sufficient to assert leadership. Honea contends that several other things are required. First, the leader must have a deep understanding of the array of operations and functions of, and within, the library. The second thing that is required is the kind of self-awareness (which should include honest appraisal of oneself and of others) that results in a moral imperative that informs all work of the library. From an educational standpoint, such an approach to leadership takes on a particular character that in some important ways transcends the usual leadership rhetoric that emphasizes vision and communication. One example of that usual approach is "Library Leadership in Times of Change" (Dusky, 2001). The article speaks of transformation leadership that energizes, provides vision, engages in communication, and also adds elements of the learning organization (Senge, 1990), although learning organization rhetoric does not explicitly rely on leadership. The management course, if it is to develop people who exhibit these characteristics, must include discussion of "good" and "right" in an organizational context.

Some items in the literature focus on frequently occurring topics, but in a somewhat different context. Todaro (2001) includes such areas as organizational culture, flexibility, teamwork, planning, etc., but in the context of social changes that have taken place in recent years. The article's basis is organizational effectiveness, which is integral to management education; the twist is that it does not define effectiveness as a static measure. Public service, information structures, user expectations, and the social milieu are some of the factors that have altered over time. Effectiveness, then, is a socially- and culturally-sensitive concept and is not subject to reified norms or standards.

The literature includes a considerable number of items on some topics related to management that are not prevalent in course syllabi. For example, the database search reveals that there are 235 pieces from 1999 to 2002 on "knowledge management," but the topic is mentioned in only one syllabus. Again, it is important to caution not to read too much into these data; some programs may include knowledge management in other courses. Total Quality Management (TQM) or Continuous Quality Improvement (CQI) are mentioned in only two syllabi; while CQI is not represented as such in the literature, 39 articles on TQM

Table 3.   Topics in the Professional Literature.

Topic (Search Term)	Frequency
Knowledge Management	235
Budgets and Budgeting	145
Leadership	134
Customer(s)	108
Plans and Planning	55
Personnel Management	54
TQM	39
Strategic Plan/Planning	23
Organizational Culture	5
Learning Organization/Fifth Discipline	4
Bureaucracy	2
Peter Drucker (name)	2
Authority and Management	1
Organizational Theory	1
Ethics and Management	0
Management Theory	0
Organizational Communication	0
Responsibility and Management	0

were published. The explicit mention of customer or customers occurs in only one syllabus, but 108 articles include the term. Some of the more frequently occurring topics in syllabi are also recurrent in the literature; 145 articles were published on budgets and fiscal management and 54 were published on personnel management.

Some topics are featured in syllabi, but not in the literature; management theory and thought as search terms yield only one item, and organizational communication yields none. Table 3 lists some search terms and numbers of hits (1999–2002).

To reiterate, some of the differences between syllabi mentions and items in the literature may be due, in part, to the assumption that some topics are necessary for course coverage, but need not be addressed repeatedly in the contemporary literature.

PROPOSED COURSE CONTENT

The foregoing discussion has been based essentially on empirical information-the content of programs, course syllabi, and the professional literature. Ideal, or prototypical, course content is a more subjective matter. What follows is presented in the interest of beginning a dialogue, of starting conversation on the purposes of a management course. The first assumption guiding the content presented here is that a management course should be required of all LIS students. The second assumption is that someday most graduates of LIS programs will be in decision-making positions, but the likelihood of their first position being strictly managerial is rather low (expect in the cases of very small organizations). The third assumption is the genuine goal of such a course is to provide students with the intellectual, critical, and professional wherewithal to develop a deep understanding of the underlying and necessary thinking and action related to making decisions in complex organizations. A tie that binds the three assumptions is that a management course is foundational; it both educates students regarding the nature and operations of libraries as complex organization and begins the training process of professionals who may develop into managers and leaders. There is an overarching concern that envelopes the effort at designing course content: management is a communicative human action and success depends, not merely on analytical skill and logic, but on a pervasive recognition that libraries exist to meet human needs and are peopled with human workers.

Accepting the above assumptions and starting point, the first concern is the development of a set of objectives that a management course should help students achieve. The following is just such a set of objectives:

(1) Provide a background knowledge of management thought (N.B., the presentation of management thought), through the literature should draw from the most efficacious writings, regardless of the source; that is, works from LIS, management, public administration, and other fields could and should be included).

(2) Examine the organizational structure of libraries (this should be a critical examination, not simply accepting traditional or common structures in place today; the critical examination of structure should be based in the ultimate purpose of the library).

(3) Investigate the process, mechanism, and product of planning, including fiscal planning (the process needs to be grounded in the human aspect, first, of those who visit, use, and access information from, the library, and, second, of the library staff whose reason for being is meeting the fundamental goals of the organization).

(4) Look at the characteristics and functions of the manager (this includes a discussion of the personal qualities of people who are effective in managerial positions, such as the ability to analyze situations, reach decisions for the good of the organization and its users, communicate, and create an ethical foundation for life in the organization. It should also include information about the kinds of things that managers do in fulfillment of their roles).

(5) Evaluate the effectiveness of the library (this is closely related to planning, but also embraces flexibility in making and implementing decisions, gauging the impact of the library and what it does on its community, and recognizing that the community essentially determines what the library should be doing).

It should be clear from these objectives that the proposed management course is not a bag of tricks, a compendium of acronyms, or a set of rules that must be applied. Rather, this concept of management could better be called organizational ecology – it is not limited to a building and the people in it, but is a part of a community.

Building on these objectives, the next step is to develop content that can form the basis for thought, discussion, and action in the course. Here is a set of topics that fit into the course's purpose:

• Libraries' Parents
Information agencies are seldom completely autonomous. They are affiliated with a school, a college or university, a corporation, a law firm, a hospital, or a town or city. It would be very difficult to accomplish the agency's goals without an understanding of that parent.
• The Nonprofit Organization
Much of what we know about organizations comes, directly or indirectly, from the working of commercial, for-profit entities. The nonprofit environment is quite different, and the differences must be discussed.
• Bureaucracy
As we know, most libraries are, to a greater or lesser extent, bureaucracies; therefore, a key is to understand how they work and what bureaucracy does both to those within it and those on the outside, including investigation of potential benefits and limitations.
• Libraries as Complex Organizations
It is certainly no great revelation that libraries are complex. The first topics (above) point to sources of the complexity. Given the nature of information production, the diversity of our communities, and the variety of operations, we may ask if we can learn from work on systems theory. Contemporary thought on systems theory seeks to understand how elements of the organization – social, technical, functional, political, economic, etc. – interact and affect each other in complicated ways.
• Planning and Decision Making
People talk about planning a lot – so much so that it may have become more of a slogan than genuine action. Effective planning really informs us about the criteria and means by which we make decisions by codifying our vision,

setting a direction, and developing a strategy for addressing our goals. Beyond the planning, though, there are dynamics of decision making that rest in social structures as well as in data, and these must be considered.

- Fiscal Management
  Here's another topic that we can tire of quickly. But operational finances impinge upon daily action to such an extent that we have to understand where the money comes from, how budgets are formed, and where the money goes.
- Organizational Communication
  Communication may be something that we take for granted, but we become painfully aware of its importance when dysfunctions occur. A major challenge is to understand both the formal and informal modes and practices of communication, what open communication channels can accomplish, and how to develop those channels.
- Personnel Management
  A key to an effective organization is the recruitment, selection, development, and evaluation of personnel. Unfortunately, it is all too easy to adopt a mechanistic stance and treat people as though they are material resources, like books or furniture.
- The Management of Change
  I am putting discussion about change alongside personnel management because, while change has many sources and many implications, it affects people deeply, and has become a constant in our environments.
- Technology and Knowledge Management
  Technology is ubiquitous, but, as is the case with people, we may tend to reduce technology to some non-human mechanism that has narrowly-specified origins and uses. Technology is a human design, and is used by humans; the question that begs to be asked is how it fits into human organizations. Technology is sometimes at the heart of some definitions of knowledge management; the relation between technology and knowledge management should be explored here.
- Leadership
  Leadership is a lot like obscenity; we know it when we see it. What are the origins of leadership? Can it be developed? Perhaps most importantly, is it a component of every organization?
- Flexibility and the Learning Organization
  It is said that the most effective organizations are those that can most quickly adapt to the environment. One way organizations may be effective is to become "learning organizations;" that is, that the entire enterprise learn in ways similar to those that individuals use and find effective.
- Evaluation
  Ultimately, it is a responsibility of those in charge to assess the effectiveness of

the organization. There are a number of evaluation methods and tools that have been proposed in our field; we need to look critically at some of them.

Throughout a semester-long course on management there should be the pervasive and often revisited theme emphasizing the relation between authority and responsibility. Some one or some group needs to be in charge of making a decision related to a particular function or action in an organization. Responsibility must follow authority. That means that the person or group that has the authority to do or to decide something must have the associated responsibility for that action or decision. In this sense, the ethical life of the organization has to be consequentialist; responsibility is connected to the consequences of some action (allowing that unforeseen consequences are possible, but still should be considered).

CONCLUSION

As is stated above, this examination of the current state of management education and this presentation of one conception of a course is intended to be a starting point. Earlier on, it is stated that a management course can be foundational; it can provide students with a fundamental understanding of the nature of libraries as organizations, of the processes, functions, and operations of libraries, of the complexities of decision-making, of the social dynamics within libraries, and of the qualities of leadership. A management course can also initiate the training that is also necessary for developing professionals to assume managerial tasks and roles. It is evident from the examination presented here that not all LIS master's programs share the view that such a course should be foundational to every student's program. Granted, some of the content issues may be included in other courses, but it is an open question whether a more disjointed approach achieves the same educational and developmental goals that a discreet management embraces.

This analysis also indicates that there is at least some degree of agreement as to course content, as judged by the available course syllabi. Such elements as planning, fiscal management, personnel management, leadership, and evaluation are commonly represented in the syllabi. These topics are essential to management in practice and, so, should be included in a management course. Other topics, though, such as organizational culture, the political context of libraries, authority and responsibility, and ethics, are far less frequently mentioned explicitly in the syllabi. One possible interpretation of these minimal bits of information is that courses tend to focus considerably more on specific processes that arise in libraries, and less on the conceptual bases for addressing the processes. This interpretation should not be carried too far; the syllabi may not be absolutely reliable indicators of course content. Nonetheless, the topics highlighted in the syllabi do, themselves, communicate priorities of coverage. This analysis also indicates that the recent library literature likewise indicates priorities leaning towards process.

There is likely to be disagreement about specific elements of a course (witness the variability in existing course syllabi). There may also be some disagreement as to the order of course content based on the style and interests of the instructor. If there is any disagreement, however, regarding the purpose of such a course, including the assumptions according to which the course content was developed, then there needs to be a dialogue that includes all elements of librarianship. Given the ubiquity of management in all organizations, the conversation should begin as soon as possible.

REFERENCES

Dusky, K. L. (2001). Library leadership in times of change. *PNLA Quarterly, 65,* 16–20.

Holt, G. E. (1999). Training, a library imperative. *Journal of Library Administration, 29,* 79–93.

Honea, S. M. (1997). Transforming administration in academic libraries. *Journal of Academic Librarianship, 23,* 183–190.

Jones, P. J. (2000). Individual accountability and individual authority: The missing links. *Library Administration & Management, 14,* 135–145.

McClamroch, J., Byrd, J. J., & Sowell, S. L. (2001). Strategic planning: Politics, leadership, and learning. *Journal of Academic Librarianship, 27,* 372–378.

Todaro, J. B. (2001). The effective organization in the twenty-first century. *Library Administration & Management, 15,* 176–178.

AN EXAMINATION OF PSYCHOLOGICAL CHARACTERISTICS AND ENVIRONMENTAL INFLUENCES OF FEMALE COLLEGE STUDENTS WHO CHOOSE TRADITIONAL VERSUS NONTRADITIONAL ACADEMIC MAJORS

Bambi N. Burgard

INTRODUCTION

In the last twenty years, the women's movement has resulted in a greater representation of women in once male-dominated venues, such as the job force and higher education. Women currently represent nearly 43% of those in the United States labor market, and it is expected that four in every five women ages 25–54 will be employed by the year 2000 (Hoyt, 1988; U.S. Department of Labor, 1995). Despite women's increasing participation in the world of work, they continue to choose occupations that represent the stereotypically feminine range of occupations, meaning less pay and less status (Betz & Fitzgerald, 1987). For example, women are still underrepresented in engineering, architecture, and the physical sciences (Eccles, 1994; U.S. Department of Labor Women's Bureau, 1995). These gender-based occupational patterns are also evidenced

Advances in Library Administration and Organization
Advances in Library Administration and Organization, Volume 20, 165–202
© 2003 Published by Elsevier Science Ltd.
ISSN: 0732-0671/PII: S0732067102200085

in college enrollment; women continue to comprise the majority in academic majors that are considered traditionally feminine, such as early childhood, elementary, and secondary education, library science, nursing, and home economics, whereas men are the predominant majors in physics, chemistry, architecture, and engineering (Bartholomew & Schnorr, 1994; National Science Foundation, 1990).

This study used a social cognitive perspective on achievement and career decision-making in an attempt to explain college women's academic major choices. Social cognitive theory provides one explanation for individual differences in achievement-related behaviors, and researchers have applied social cognitive theory to understanding career choice behavior (Farmer, Wardrop, Anderson & Risinger, 1995; Gelso & Fassinger, 1992; Hackett & Betz, 1981). From a social cognitive perspective, an individual's behavior is shaped by their experiences in the environment. Accordingly, gender-based differences in career decision-making can be seen as attributable to the different environmental experiences afforded to girls and boys in our society. These experiences may directly affect behavior, such as occurs with imitation and modeling, and indirectly affect behavior by influencing an individual's psychological experiences (e.g. cognitions) of him or herself and the world.

This study focused on three environmental and three cognitive (psychological) variables that may have an impact on girls' career decision making. Environmental influences included in this study were family socialization experiences, the observation of role models, and parental support. Psychological characteristics included students' sex-role orientation, and levels of achievement and career motivation. Specifically, this research tested a social cognitive model of factors related to career decision-making such that environmental or socialization variables were seen as not only directly affecting an individual's career choice, but also as affecting the development of psychological characteristics which in turn influence career choice variables, and career choice as examined in the study.

Various theories have been used to explain differences between men's and women's career decisions (Holland, 1973; Super, 1957). According to Offermann and Beil (1992), however, women are too often viewed as "deficit" males within these theories, with researchers questioning why women do not act more like men. Eccles (1984) has pointed out that a better question may be "Why do women make the choices they make?" This study responded to this question by examining both the direct and indirect relationships between women's environmental influences, psychological characteristics, and career choice using a social cognitive framework.

It is well known that traditional majors such as elementary education, nursing, and library science generally limit students to female-dominated occupational roles, while students who pursue degrees in nontraditional fields such as engineering, architecture, and physics are propelled toward male-dominated, often higher paying and status occupations. However, much of the research to this point has simply examined the role of social characteristics and prior educational experiences in the career choices made by high school and college men and women. Furthermore, little attention has been given to the importance of career motivation as a psychological component in the career decision-making process.

REVIEW OF THE LITERATURE

Traditional Versus Nontraditional Career Choice

Rossi (1965) was one of the first researchers to suggest the usefulness of studying "career-oriented" women by comparing women pursuing traditionally female-dominated careers to those pursuing male-dominated careers. According to Almquist (1974), women who have chosen careers that have been historically male-dominated have been called pioneers, nontraditionals, and role innovators, and these terms are used interchangeably in the literature.

Achievement Motivation and Career Choice

Achievement motivation has not only been used in the study of gender differences, but also in the comparison of women in traditional and nontraditional careers. A number of researchers have found that women in nontraditional occupations possess higher levels of achievement motivation, compared to their traditional counterparts. Moreover, an achievement motivated individual is more likely than an individual with low motivation to demonstrate a high level of academic achievement, and strong academic achievement is usually required for traditionally male-dominated, often science-based career paths.

Traditional definitions of achievement motivation include masculine sex-typed qualities, namely competitiveness, individuality, and aggressiveness. Although these traditional definitions have been satisfactory in explaining the achievement behaviors of men, they fall short for women as women's achievement motivation appears to be influenced by their conceptualization of the feminine sex-role (Mednick, Tangri & Hoffman, 1975; Offermann & Beil, 1992). The feminine sex-role includes socially desirable, interpersonally oriented and nurturant traits such as care taking and being kind (Spence & Helmreich, 1978). Therefore, the exclusive emphasis of motivational constructs on task-oriented behavior may be incongruent with the social learning experiences of girls and women (Spence & Helmreich, 1983). Whereas men may evaluate their success in a domain against some internal or external criterion, some theorists suggest that women learn to develop strong affiliative and care-taking roles that contribute to their motivation and behavior. Motivation is often defined in task-oriented and competitive terms, yet research suggests that women also take relationship goals into account when evaluating an opportunity for action (Gilligan, 1982).

Given that achievement motivation, by traditional definition, is evidenced by psychologically masculine traits, it is often studied in conjunction with sex-role orientation. Both achievement motivation and sex-role orientation appear to be influenced by early family socialization experiences which have been found to affect the achievement motivation and career-related attitudes of boys and girls differently (Moss & Kagan, 1961).

Like early family socialization experiences, other background factors, such as family support, may influence the development of achievement motivation. For example, Farmer (1980) examined the environmental, background, and psychological variables related to optimizing achievement and career motivation for high school girls. In a study of 158 tenth-grade girls, she found that high achievement motivation and career choice were significantly associated with perceived support for achievement and career goals. Specifically, community support was included as an environmental variable, and Farmer found that those girls who perceived their teachers, peers, and families to be supportive of women combining home and work roles had higher levels of achievement and career motivation.

Based on the literature reviewed, it appears that women pursuing nontraditional careers, particularly those careers requiring a high level of academic achievement, demonstrate higher levels of achievement motivation than women pursuing traditionally female-dominated careers. In addition, it is important to note that an individual's sex-role orientation, socialization experiences, and perceived support appear closely related to their level of achievement motivation. Thus, this study included an examination of the achievement motivation, sex-role orientation, and parental support of women in traditional and nontraditional academic majors.

Career Motivation and Career Choice

Super (1957, 1976) presented a picture of the career-motivated individual that is similar to the person who is highly achievement-motivated. For example, the career-motivated person possesses similar characteristics, including persistence, preference for tasks of intermediate difficulty, and independence. However, Horner (1968) has suggested that such a model, whether of achievement or career motivation, is less useful when considering the achievement-related behaviors of females. Like theories of achievement motivation, Super (1976) emphasized that a theory of career motivation must account for both psychological and situational determinants. Therefore, studies of career motivation have often included an examination of factors such as self-confidence, sex-role orientation, home-career conflict, fear of success, risk taking, and family socialization (Fyans, 1980). However, the relationship between career motivation and a woman's choice of a traditional or nontraditional career has not been adequately studied.

Farmer (1985) has proposed a multidimensional model of women's career motivation, which takes into consideration the importance of background (e.g. gender), psychological (e.g. beliefs, self-concept), and environmental (e.g. parental support) influences. She suggested that career motivation develops through the interaction of the aforementioned influences and that career motivation contains three components: career aspiration which includes the average education level and salary of a given career; commitment, or the degree of commitment to a long-term career; and mastery motivation, or the motivation to achieve a challenging task.

Career motivation has received limited attention in the literature concerning traditional and nontraditional career choice among women. One component of career motivation, career aspiration, has been shown to relate to the pursuit of a traditionally male-dominated occupation such that women planning nontraditional careers demonstrated higher levels of career aspiration than women planning traditional careers (Murrell et al., 1991). The current study examines Farmer's (1985) career aspiration and career commitment in an effort to explore and clarify the role career motivation may play in career decision-making for women.

Sex-Role Orientation and Career Choice

From the vantage point of social cognitive theory, parents are a key influence in the development of gender roles (Crider, Goethals, Kavanaugh & Solomon, 1989). Parents model and reinforce what they regard as appropriate masculine and feminine behavior, and often socialize their children to adopt traditional gender roles. The socialization of gender roles is important in understanding the career choices of females in our society because the learning of feminine traits may be at odds with behaviors that are part of particular occupations (Betz & Fitzgerald, 1987; Rossi, 1965; Williams, Radin & Allegro, 1992). For example, males may be encouraged and rewarded for individuality, autonomy, and assertive and competitive behaviors. Females, however, may be discouraged from displaying such masculine sex-typed characteristics. Instead, they are praised for demonstrating feminine sex-typed traits such as dependence, affiliation, and vulnerability (Stein

& Bailey, 1973). Furthermore, women are valued according to their relationships with others, whereas men are valued for their individual successes (Gilligan, 1982).

As Bem (1975) has suggested, perhaps persons who view themselves as traditionally masculine or feminine tend to avoid sex-role incongruent behaviors, whereas androgynous individuals are more flexible in their behavior. Thus, in making career choices, women who are more androgynous may be better able to choose a major from a full range of options rather than being restricted by traditional definitions of "men's work" and "women's work." Furthermore, Long (1989) has indicated that sex-typed or gender-typed individuals avoid and are uncomfortable performing behaviors that are typically associated with the other gender because it is incongruent with their orientation. Farmer and Fyans (1983) examined the relationship between sex-role orientation, family socialization patterns, and female achievement, and they concluded that feminine and androgynous women may be highly achieving depending on perceived support. Therefore, when women perceive support from their significant others for their achievement behaviors, they may overcome their feelings of discomfort and believe that there is less chance that their interpersonal relationships will be negatively affected by their achievement. This finding relates to Spence and Helmreich's (1978) concept of personal unconcern. Spence and Helmreich (1978) suggested that women's achievement behaviors may be limited by their concern that their achievements may interfere with their relationships and have a negative impact on their friends and family.

The development of sex-role orientation by way of social learning appears to influence one's career choice. A woman who has learned to pursue and to feel comfortable engaging in activities that are not traditionally feminine may have a stronger motive to achieve in careers like architecture, engineering, and chemistry which are generally dominated by men, whereas women who have observed their role models in traditionally female roles may strive to achieve only in traditionally female areas. Women of a feminine sex-role orientation may be quite uncomfortable in a position that requires more stereotypically masculine or androgynous traits. The literature clearly suggests that sex-role orientation, and particularly psychological masculinity, shares a relationship not only with achievement and career motivation, but also with career decision-making. Therefore, this study investigated sex-role orientation as an important psychological factor in traditional versus nontraditional career choices.

Early Family Socialization and Career Choice

Social cognitive theorists believe people develop their sex-role orientation, achievement and career motivation through observing the behavior of the significant others with whom they identify. In addition to beliefs about self, individuals come to know appropriate sex role norms as a set of learned behaviors through the socialization process. Parents are the primary socialization agents, and women raised in a family where women held very traditional roles as housewives and mothers may be very comfortable competing and achieving in traditional women's roles, but less comfortable when forced to compete with men or to perform traditionally "male" tasks. Bailyn (1973) observed that achieving professional status may be more difficult for women than for men as a result of early family socialization experiences that enforce traditional gender role prescriptions. Conversely, the women who as young girls received messages from significant others that it is acceptable to share equal power with men and to achieve in stereotypically masculine domains may be more apt to pursue a traditionally male-dominated career. Thus, gender role socialization influences the personality development and subsequent career-related behaviors of young women (Paludi, 1990). According to Rossi (1965), "a childhood model of the quiet, good, sweet girl will not produce many women scientists or scholars, doctors or engineers" (p. 1201).

As evidenced in the literature, early family socialization experiences often lead individuals into traditional gender roles and influence their beliefs, attitudes, and behaviors. Thus, these socialization experiences not only contribute to individuals' achievement and career motivation and sex-role orientations, but also influence their career choices. In this study, the early family socialization experiences of women enrolled in traditionally male-dominated and traditionally female-dominated academic majors were measured to determine how they may have influenced the nontraditional career choices of women.

Influence of Role Models on Career Choice

The significant players in the socialization process are role models. Unfortunately, a lack of female role models in nontraditional careers continues to exist. Social cognitive theorists have emphasized the importance of role modeling in the development of learned behavior, and it has been suggested that same-sex models are the strongest and most attractive (Basow & Howe, 1979). Therefore, if role models are important to learning, particularly female role models for young girls, then the career development of women certainly may be impeded by a lack of women in certain career paths (Douvan, 1976). In accordance with social cognitive theory and because mothers provide a female role model, numerous researchers have examined the work roles and education levels of mothers in an effort to understand their influence on the career development of their daughters (Almquist & Angrist, 1970; O'Leary, 1974). The education level of father has also shown to be positively related to a woman's pursuit of a nontraditional occupation (Harmon, 1972). The impact of both same-sex and opposite-sex role models is an important factor to be considered in the career development of women, particularly when comparing women in traditionally male-dominated fields to those women in traditionally female-dominated careers.

Lemkau (1983) examined the background characteristics of traditional and nontraditional women with comparable education levels and found fewer distinguishing characteristics between the two groups than in past research. However, she found that, of those women in traditionally male-dominated careers, the presence of male role models was important. In other words, the support and positive influence of male figures, including fathers, boyfriends, and male teachers and professors, was more important for women in nontraditional careers than for women in traditional careers. Lemkau (1983) defined the traditional group so that it included those careers in which 75% of the workers were women: librarians, nurses, elementary teachers, and home economists.

In summarizing how role models influence women's career choices, it appears that both the mother and father play important parts in their daughters' career development. Lyson (1980) suggested that women following atypical career paths have been exposed to a wider and more enriching set of role models than women who are pursuing traditional careers. Studies have shown that women aspiring to nontraditional careers are more likely to have well-educated, employed mothers than women in traditional career paths. The working mother appears to serve as a significant model of sex-role attitudes and behaviors, and her participation in the work force is thought to influence her daughter's career achievement ambitions (Spenner & Featherman, 1978). Specifically, aspiring to a high-prestige career in a nontraditional field has been associated with having a working mother (Almquist & Angrist, 1970; Lemkau, 1979; Tangri, 1972). In terms of education, several researchers have indicated that having a college-educated mother is associated with nontraditional career orientation (Elder & MacInnis, 1983; Tangri, 1972). Father's education level also appears to be related to women's nontraditional career goals (Harmon, 1972; Tangri, 1972; Trigg & Perlman, 1976). Given the impact of both mother's employment and educational status and father's education level cited in the literature, this study attempted to determine the relative importance of these three factors in the career decisions of women in traditional and nontraditional majors.

Parental Support and Career Choice

Research has shown that women's educational and occupational choices are also influenced by the support they receive from the important people in their lives, including parents (Penn & Gabriel, 1976; Rehberg & Sinclair, 1970). Parents, as the primary socialization agents, may influence their child's career choice as they react to their personality traits, beliefs, and behaviors. Therefore, the role of parental support in career decision-making deserves attention as it has been found to be an important factor in a woman's nontraditional career choice. Haber (1980) found that women in male-dominated occupations experienced high levels of parental support, and Trigg and Perlman (1976) indicated that the traditional women in their study perceived their parents to be less supportive of career pursuits than did the nontraditionals. Standley and Soule (1974), in their study of women in nontraditional fields, found that 72% of the nontraditionals reported that they were the children of which their parents had been the most proud. Farmer et al. (1995) suggested that, because society does not give women clear messages about occupational roles, women may be more responsive to support given by significant others than are men who do receive clear messages about work roles.

In summary, women pursuing nontraditional career paths tend to perceive greater support for their career goals from their parents than women pursuing traditional careers, and parental support appears to be an important factor in the career choices of women. This study attempted to clarify the role that parental support plays in a woman's decision to pursue a career in a traditionally male-dominated field.

Research Questions

Three general research questions were investigated. First, do women enrolled in majors leading to a traditionally male-dominated career differ from women pursuing academic majors leading to a traditionally female-dominated career on a set of psychological variables, including components of achievement and career motivation, and sex-role orientation? Second, do the two groups differ in terms of environmental influences, including early family socialization, role model influences, and parental support for their chosen career path? Third, do women's psychological characteristics directly predict their career choice, and do their environmental characteristics both directly and indirectly predict their career choice?

Hypotheses

Several hypotheses were tested. First, it was hypothesized that psychological and environmental variables will distinguish women in the traditional major group from the women in the nontraditional major group. Second, for the psychological variables, it was hypothesized that women in the traditionally male-dominated major group will demonstrate higher levels of competitiveness, mastery, and personal unconcern than women in the traditionally female-dominated major group. Third, it was hypothesized that women in the male-dominated major group will have higher career aspirations and career commitment compared to women in traditionally female-dominated academic majors. Fourth, it was hypothesized that women in academic majors leading to traditionally male-dominated career paths possessed higher levels of masculinity and androgyny and lower levels of femininity compared to women in traditionally female-dominated academic majors. For the environmental variables, it was hypothesized that women in the traditionally male-dominated major group will demonstrate higher levels of parental support and will report fewer gender-congruent and sex-role stereotypical early family socialization experiences than will the traditional major group. Finally, for the environmental variables, it was hypothesized that, compared to women working in traditional majors, more women in traditionally male-dominated majors will have mothers in nontraditional careers, and both their mothers and fathers will have higher educational levels compared to the parents of the women in the traditional majors. Finally, it was hypothesized that psychological characteristics will directly predict an individual's career choice, and the environmental characteristics will both directly and indirectly predict career choice.

METHODOLOGY

Participants

Participants were 98 women enrolled in academic majors (e.g. elementary education, nursing, library science) leading to traditionally female-dominated careers and 109 women enrolled in academic majors (e.g. engineering, architecture, chemistry, computer science, physics) leading to careers in male-dominated fields. Traditionally, female-dominated fields are those which have at least 75% female workers, and traditionally male-dominated fields are those which have less than 30% female workers, based on U.S. Department of Labor statistics (U.S. Department of Labor Women's Bureau, 1995).

Procedure

At the time students agreed to participate, they were given a packet containing the Background Information Questionnaire, the Work and Family Orientation Questionnaire-2, the Career Commitment measure, the Personal Attributes

Questionnaire, the Early Family Socialization Measure, and the Parental Support
Questionnaire (see Appendix A through F).

Measures

Measurement of Achievement Motivation
The Work and Family Orientation Questionnaire-2 (WOFO-2; Spence &
Helmreich, 1978) provides a measure of four dimensions of achievement motivation: mastery, work, competitiveness, and personal unconcern (see Appendix B).
Only the mastery, competitiveness, and personal unconcern scales were used
in this study. The work scale was excluded because it has not been shown
to differentiate between groups expected to differ in achievement motivation
and its internal consistency is low with a Cronbach alpha of 0.39 (Spence
& Helmreich, 1978). Two of these scales (e.g. competitiveness and mastery)
relate to traditional male definitions of achievement motivation. The three item
mastery scale measures preference for difficult and challenging tasks. Four items
comprising the competitiveness scale evaluate one's desire to win in interpersonal
situations. The third scale, personal unconcern, is composed of three items that
assess one's lack of concern with the negative reactions of others to personal
achievement. Higher scores on this scale indicate less concern about the effects of
achievement behavior on significant others. Less concern suggests less fear about
the splitting of interpersonal relationships that may be caused by achievement
behaviors. The inclusion of this dimension recognizes the traditional feminine
value of interpersonal relationships as a determinant of achievement-related
behavior.

Measurement of Career Motivation
Two dimensions of career motivation were assessed: career commitment and
career aspiration. Career commitment was measured using the 16-item assessment constructed by Farmer (1985) (Appendix C). Those who score high on this
measure indicate that planning for a career is their major concern and view a
career as giving meaning to their life.

Measurement of Sex-Role Orientation
Assessments of masculinity (M), femininity (F), and masculinity-femininity
(M-F) were ascertained by the Personality Attributes Questionnaire (PAQ;
Spence & Helmreich, 1986). This self-report instrument is based on respondents'
self-perceptions of personality traits stereotypically believed to differentiate the
sexes yet considered socially desirable by both sexes. The Personality Attributes

Questionnaire measures not global masculinity or femininity, but self-assertive, instrumental traits (M) and interpersonal, expressive traits (F).

Early Family Socialization

Early family socialization experiences were measured using the four-item Sex-Role Enforcement subscale from the Parental Attitudes Questionnaire (Spence & Helmreich, 1978). A copy of the early family socialization scale is in Appendix E. Specifically, the respondents were asked to rank how characteristic certain parental attitudes toward sex-role stereotyped behavior were of their parents.

Role Model Influences

The participants were asked to complete a background information questionnaire which asked the participants, "While you were growing up, what was your mother's primary occupation?" (see Appendix A). In addition, the participants were asked to indicate their father's primary occupation for descriptive purposes. The questionnaire also requested that the participants indicate the education level (e.g. highest grade or highest degree completed) of both parents. Education level was coded for each parent from "one" (some high school) to "eight" (doctorate). Occupations of the mother were scored on a scale from "one" (very traditional) to "four" (very nontraditional) based on the percentage of women in the given career.

Parental Support

The participants' amount of parental support was assessed using an 11-item measure that includes items from the Parental Attitudes Questionnaire (Spence & Helmreich, 1978) and items written by the principal investigator (see Appendix F). The first seven items are from the Parental Attitudes Questionnaire and relate to the amount of support and encouragement the participants have received from their parents regarding their activities and achievements and the interest their parents have taken in their success. The last four items relate to the participants' perceived support for their college major choice and future career goal given by their mother and father.

RESULTS

Descriptive Analyses

Two hundred seven participants responded to this research, 98 (47%) in traditional academic majors and 109 (53%) in nontraditional career paths. The average age of

Table 1. Demographics of the Sample.

Variable	Frequency	%
Ethnicity		
Caucasian	179	86.5
African American	10	4.8
Asian American	6	2.9
Hispanic	8	3.9
Native American	1	0.5
Other	3	1.4
Year in College		
Freshman	12	5.8
Sophomore	21	10.1
Junior	52	25.1
Senior	109	52.7
Postgrad	13	6.3
Academic Group		
Traditional	98	47.3
Nontraditional	109	52.7
ACT Score		
14–18	5	2.7
19–23	48	26.1
24–28	73	39.7
29 or Above	58	31.5

participants was 24.5 years (SD = 7.17). As can be seen in Table 1 , the majority of the participants were Caucasian (87%) and in their senior year (53%). Seventy-one percent of the participants scored a 24 or above on the ACT college entrance examination.

Table 2 is a summary of the descriptive statistics of all psychological and environmental variables for the entire sample as well as for the two subgroups (traditional and nontraditional). Eyeballing the means, it appears that the women in the nontraditional group reported their mothers as having higher education levels than the women in the traditional group. Based on the descriptive results, it also appears that the traditionality of mother's career was comparable for the two groups. Compared to the traditional group, the women in the nontraditional group showed higher levels of competitiveness and mastery, which indicates a preference for challenging tasks. Furthermore, they demonstrated higher levels of career commitment and aspiration than their traditional group peers. For the environmental variables, the nontraditional group reported higher levels of

Table 2.   Descriptive Statistics of Psychological and Environmental Variables.

Psychological and Environmental Variables	Range	All Students (N = 207) (SD)	Traditional Students (N = 98) (SD)	Nontraditional Students (N = 109) (SD)
Competitiveness	4 to 28	14.12 (3.38)	13.43 (3.58)	14.73 (3.08)
Mastery	4 to 14	8.82 (1.94)	8.64 (1.84)	8.98 (2.03)
Personal Unconcern	7 to 15	11.36 (1.82)	11.52 (1.96)	11.22 (1.67)
Career Commitment	40 to 76	60.96 (7.30)	60.38 (7.23)	61.48 (7.37)
Career Aspiration	17.98 to 89.57	72.46 (10.15)	65.12 (9.31)	79.05 (5.11)
Masculinity	10 to 56	21.63 (4.06)	20.62 (3.51)	22.54 (4.31)
Femininity	10 to 75	25.38 (5.31)	26.39 (3.92)	24.47 (6.19)
Masculinity-Femininity	9 to 23	16.52 (2.70)	16.10 (2.64)	16.89 (2.72)
Parental Support	15 to 55	46.91 (8.13)	45.23 (9.77)	48.41 (5.94)
Early Family Socialization	4 to 20	14.77 (3.01)	14.43 (3.38)	15.08 (2.62)
Father's Education Level	1 to 8	4.39 (2.01)	4.19 (2.18)	4.58 (1.83)
Mother's Education Level	1 to 8	3.89 (1.86)	3.48 (1.81)	4.27 (1.84)
Traditionality of Mother's Career	1 to 4	1.35 (0.83)	1.23 (0.66)	1.46 (0.95)

parental support for the choice of academic major and career path as well as more flexible sex-role socialization experiences than the traditional group.

The simple correlations among the psychological and environmental variables are presented in Table 3. Significant positive relationships existed between competitiveness and masculinity, masculinity-femininity, and career commitment. Parental support correlated with the other environmental variables. Both masculinity and masculinity-femininity correlated with career commitment and career aspiration, and masculinity correlated with parental support. Mother's education level was significantly positively correlated with father's education level, and both mother and father's education level correlated with early family socialization.

Table 3. Correlation Matrix of Variables.

	1	2	3	4	5	6	7	8	9	10	11	12	13
1 Competitiveness		0.06	0.01	0.29**	−0.04	0.22**	0.28**	0.12	0.10	0.13	0.13	0.01	0.02
2 Mastery			0.09	0.08	−0.09	0.00	0.11	0.10	0.07	0.05	0.01	−0.13	0.01
3 Personal Unconcern				0.06	0.02	0.07	−0.06	−0.05	0.06	0.05	0.03	−0.01	−0.05
4 Masculinity					0.05	0.22**	0.23**	0.15*	0.20**	0.11	0.08	−0.02	0.07
5 Femininity						−0.02	0.05	−0.04	0.12	−0.06	0.02	−0.09	0.03
6 Masculinity-Femininity							0.19**	0.23**	0.01	0.04	0.05	0.09	0.02
7 Career Commitment								0.06	0.25**	0.20**	0.11	0.04	0.16*
8 Career Aspiration									0.16*	0.15*	0.11	0.08	0.07
9 Parental Support										0.25**	0.24**	−0.14*	0.37**
10 Mother's Education											0.55**	0.01	0.18*
11 Father's Education												−0.04	0.12
12 Traditionality of Mother's Career													−0.01
13 Early Family Socialization													

* Significant at the 0.05 level.
** Significant at the 0.01 level.

Preliminary Analyses

Preliminary analyses were conducted to determine if the set of eight psychological variables, including components of achievement motivation, career motivation, and sex-role orientation, and the set of five environmental variables could predict women's career choice. These analyses were used to provide initial information about the multivariate nature of the relations that are assessed among psychological and environmental variables and career choice (traditional or nontraditional). Two discriminant analyses were carried out, one with the psychological variables and one with the environmental variables predicting the participants' membership in the traditional or nontraditional academic group. For the psychological variables, the discriminant function was significant $X^2(N = 208) = 145.95, p < 0.001$. The canonical correlation was 0.72. The group centroids for the traditional and non-traditional academic groups are presented in Table 4 . The discriminant function separates the traditional academic group from the nontraditional academic group. Career aspiration was the only variable that showed a strong positive correlation with the function. It appears that women in the nontraditional academic group expressed higher career aspirations than women in the traditional academic group.

For the environmental variables, the discriminant function was significant $X^2(N = 208) = 19.48$, $p < 0.01$. The canonical correlation was 0.31. The discriminant function separates the traditional academic group from the nontraditional academic group. Traditionality of mother's career, parental support, and mother's education level showed strongest positive correlations with the function. Thus, women in the nontraditional academic group have higher levels of parental support and have mothers with higher education levels than women in the traditional academic group. Unexpectedly, the nontraditional group members' mothers have careers of higher traditionality than the traditional group members.

Table 4. Group Centroids on the Significant Function for Each Set of Variables for the Two Academic Groups.

Academic Group	Centroid	
	Psychological Variables Function 1	Environmental Variables Function 1
Traditional	−1.10	−0.34
Nontraditional	0.99	0.31

Analyses of Research Hypotheses

To answer the first research question, "Do women enrolled in majors leading to a traditionally male-dominated career differ from women pursuing academic majors leading to a traditionally female-dominated career on a set of psychological variables, including components of achievement and career motivation, and sex-role orientation?" MANOVAS were conducted. First, a MANOVA was performed to test the hypothesis that women in nontraditional majors have higher levels of achievement motivation than women in traditional majors. The independent variable was academic group (e.g. traditional or nontraditional), and the dependent variables were the participants' scores on the three achievement motivation variables: competitiveness, mastery, and personal unconcern.

The results showed that the main effect of academic group (traditional and nontraditional) on achievement motivation was significant ($F(3, 203) = 3.69, p < 0.05$). Univariate analysis showed that this significant effect occurred only for competitiveness ($F(1, 205) = 7.97, p < 0.01$). Participants in the nontraditional academic group demonstrated significantly higher levels of competitiveness ($M = 14.73$) than those in the traditional academic group ($M = 13.43$). The effect of academic group on mastery or personal unconcern was not significant.

A second MANOVA was performed to test the hypothesis that women in the nontraditional group have higher levels of career motivation than women in the traditional group. The two components of career motivation, career aspiration and career commitment, were dependent variables, and academic group was the independent variable. The results showed that the main effect of academic group (traditional or nontraditional) on career motivation was significant ($F(2, 200) = 89.77, p < 0.001$). Significant univariate effects occurred for career aspiration ($F(1, 201) = 179.58, p < 0.001$). As seen in Table 2, participants in the nontraditional academic group expressed significantly higher levels of career aspiration ($M = 79.05$) than those in the traditional academic group ($M = 65.12$). The effect of academic group on career commitment was not significant.

A third MANOVA was performed to test the hypothesis that women in the nontraditional academic group have higher levels of masculinity and masculinity-femininity (androgyny) compared to women in the traditional academic group. Academic group was the independent variable with two levels (traditional, nontraditional), and the dependent variables were the three components of sex-role orientation: masculinity, femininity, and masculinity-femininity. The results showed that the main effect of academic group on sex-role orientation was significant ($F(3, 203) = 7.62, p < 0.001$). Univariate analysis indicated a significant effect of academic group for masculinity ($F(1, 205) = 12.17, p < 0.01$), femininity ($F(1, 205) = 6.93, p < 0.05$), and for masculinity-femininity

($F(1, 205) = 4.46$, $p < 0.05$). Participants in the nontraditional academic group expressed significantly higher levels of masculinity ($M = 22.54$), higher levels of masculinity-femininity ($M = 16.89$), and significantly lower levels of femininity ($M = 24.47$) as compared to the traditional group (see Table 2).

To answer the research question, "Do the two groups differ in terms of environmental influences, including early family socialization, role model influences, and parental support for their chosen career path?" MANOVAS were performed. First, to test the hypothesis that women in the nontraditional academic group had more parental support and less gender-congruent sex-role stereotypical early family socialization, a MANOVA was conducted with academic group as the independent variable and parental support and early socialization as the dependent variables. The results showed that the main effect of academic group on parental support and early family socialization was significant ($F(2, 204) = 4.23$, $p < 0.05$). Univariate analyses showed that this significant effect of academic group occurred only for parental support ($F(1, 205) = 8.17$, $p < 0.01$). Participants in the non-traditional academic group reported significantly higher levels of parental support ($M = 48.41$) than those in the traditional academic group ($M = 45.23$). To test the role model influences hypothesis that compared to women in the traditional group, more women in the nontraditional group have mothers in nontraditional careers, and both their mothers and fathers have higher education levels compared to the parents of women in traditional majors, a MANOVA was conducted. The independent variable was academic group and the dependent variables were the traditionality of mother's career, mother's education level, and father's education level. Results indicated a significant main effect occurred for role model influences ($F(3, 197) = 4.49$, $p < 0.05$). Significant univariate effects of academic group were found for mother's education level ($F(1, 199) = 9.34$, $p < 0.05$), but were not revealed for father's educational level or traditionality of mother's career. Participants in the nontraditional academic group had mothers with significantly higher education levels ($M = 4.27$) than the participants in the traditional academic group ($M = 3.48$).

To answer the final research question, "Do women's psychological characteristics directly predict their career choice, and do their environmental characteristics both directly and indirectly predict their career choice?" a series of analyses was performed. These included two discriminant analyses to determine if the psychological and environmental variables could predict academic group membership, and a canonical correlation to see if the set of environmental variables correlated with the set of psychological variables.

As shown in the preliminary analyses section, the two discriminant analyses for the psychological and environmental variables yielded significant functions which were useful in predicting participants' membership in the traditional

Table 5. Academic Group – Logistic Regression Results with All Variables.

Significant Predictors	Dependent Variable Academic Group			
	B	SE	Wald	R
Psychological Variables				
Masculinity	0.15	0.12	1.65	0.00
Masculinity-Femininity	−0.25	0.15	2.88	−0.06
Femininity	−0.17	0.05	13.14*	−0.21
Competitiveness	0.19	0.12	2.62	0.05
Mastery	−0.00	0.15	0.00	0.00
Personal Unconcern	−0.11	0.20	0.30	0.00
Career Commitment	−0.04	0.06	0.49	0.00
Career Aspiration	0.72	0.13	30.19*	0.34
Environmental Variables				
Early Family Socialization	0.11	0.12	0.83	0.00
Father's Education Level	−0.16	0.18	0.80	0.00
Mother's Education Level	0.25	0.24	1.07	0.00
Parental Support	−0.03	0.05	0.29	0.00
Traditionality of Mother's Career	0.67	0.40	2.78	0.06

*Significant at the 0.001 level.

or nontraditional group. In other words, the psychological and environmental variables can predict career choice.

Although not part of the original research questions, the following post hoc questions were addressed. First, when all variables (psychological and environmental) were entered, which variables predict career choice when the other variables are held constant? Second, do the environmental variables increase the predictability of career choice when added to the psychological variables? To test the first post hoc research question, a logistic regression analysis was conducted with academic group regressed on both the environmental and psychological variables. Table 5 presents the results of the effect of all variables on career choice. As shown in the table, only two psychological variables were significant. With all variables entered in the regression analysis, the model correctly classified 95.4% ($p < 0.001$) of the participants in the traditional and nontraditional academic groups.

To test the second post hoc research question, "Do the environmental variables increase the predictability of career choice when added to the psychological variables?" a second logistic regression using a stepwise procedure was performed. On step one of the logistic regression, psychological variables were entered; on step two, the environmental variables were entered. The dichotomous criterion variable was academic group (traditional or nontraditional). The difference between the two models (psychological variables versus both psychological and environmental variables) was not significant. Therefore, adding environmental variables to psychological variables did not improve the prediction of career choice.

DISCUSSION

Discussion of Results

The purpose of this study was to examine the differences between women pursuing traditionally female-dominated career paths and women in nontraditional, male-dominated fields of study on a number of psychological and environmental variables and to investigate the prediction of career choice from a social cognitive perspective using these variables.

As hypothesized, when considering achievement motivation, women in the nontraditional academic group evidenced significantly higher levels of competitiveness than their traditional counterparts. Interestingly, using competitiveness as an indicator of female achievement-motivated behavior is often criticized in the literature based on a view that competitiveness is a trait valued in males but judged harshly in females. Traditional definitions of achievement motivation which have included competitiveness are believed to neglect the importance of the feminine sex-role which discourages competitiveness and emphasized the development of socially desirable, nurturant traits in women (Mednick, Tangri & Hoffman, 1975; Offermann & Beil, 1992; Spence & Helmreich, 1983). This research demonstrates, however, that women in nontraditional fields of study, are competitive – significantly more so than their peers in more traditional fields like elementary education and library science. Undoubtedly, to gain entry and to thrive in a math and science-related field, an individual must strive to perform at a high standard. Perhaps women's social learning experiences are changing as the millennium approaches, and women who grew up in the past two decades have heard messages that do not discourage competition.

Previous research has linked women's achievement motivation with the traditional feminine sex-role (Alper, 1974; Moss & Kagan, 1961), and it is not surprising that women who have learned, through socialization experiences, to value more traditional sex-typed behaviors demonstrate lower levels of achievement motivation. As hypothesized, women in nontraditional academic majors demonstrated higher levels of masculinity and masculinity-femininity than women in traditional academic majors. This result is consistent with previous research which has shown that a masculine and androgynous sex-role orientation is often characteristic of women in male-dominated careers (Betz & Fitzgerald, 1987; Segal, 1980; Stockton, Berry, Shepson & Utz, 1980; Yanico, Hardin &

McLaughlin, 1978). These findings also lend support to the masculine definition of achievement motivation and to the disparity between the traditionally defined feminine sex-role and achievement motivation.

It appears that the link between achievement motivation and sex-role orientation serves to pigeonhole individuals by providing a framework for behavior. This framework, if translated through the socialization process, may limit an individual's career options. Specifically, through socialization, males may be encouraged for individuality, autonomy, and competitive behaviors, while females are often discouraged from having these masculine sex-typed characteristics (Stein & Bailey, 1973). However, these masculine sex-typed characteristics essentially comprise the traditional and accepted definition of achievement motivation. The definition of achievement motivation does not have to be reliant on gender roles – the definition needs to be stretched and broadened to include traits and attitudes that are not sex-role specific. Both women and men can be achievement-motivated without being competitive. For example, if an individual values cooperation and teamwork and works toward that goal, they are demonstrating achievement-motivated behavior. The definitions of achievement motivation and sex-roles appear to neglect individual differences across both genders.

No significant difference was demonstrated for the achievement variable of personal unconcern. Personal unconcern refers to an individual's lack of concern for how others react to their personal achievement (Spence & Helmreich, 1978). The hypothesis that women in the nontraditional academic group would demonstrate higher levels of personal unconcern than their traditional peers was not supported, suggesting that women in divergent fields do not necessarily limit their achievements based on the perceptions of others.

Career motivation has been given little attention as a psychological variable important to an individual's career decision-making, particularly when comparing women in traditional and nontraditional fields of study. In the present study, two aspects of career motivation were examined: career commitment and career aspiration. Only career aspiration was found to significantly differ between the two academic groups. This finding is consistent with prior research which has shown career aspiration to differentiate women in traditional academic fields from women in nontraditional majors (Murrell et al., 1991). Women may seek careers in male-dominated arenas if they hold occupational prestige as a value. Undoubtedly, money is a societal value which is linked to occupational prestige, and careers traditionally held by females, tend to be of lower status and income. Women who have learned that money and prestige are important values may be more likely to pursue male-dominated fields. The role of career commitment in determining career choice remains inconclusive. In other words, the importance of how much one emphasizes planning for a career and viewing career as giving meaning to their life for determining a woman's choice of a male-dominated or female-dominated career path was not illustrated in the present study.

As hypothesized, women in the nontraditional male-dominated academic group reported higher levels of parental support for their career choice than women in the traditional group. This finding is consistent with previous research which has linked parental support with female participation in male-dominated occupational arenas (Haber, 1980; Trigg & Perlman, 1976). Previous research has also suggested that women with a feminine sex-role can overcome their discomfort and participate in traditionally masculine achievement situations if they perceive support from their parents (Farmer & Fyans, 1983).

Mother's education level was also found to be a discriminating environmental variable when comparing women in traditional and nontraditional fields of study. Results of the present study indicated that women in the nontraditional academic group had mothers with significantly higher education levels than the participants in the traditional academic group. This finding is consistent with previous research which has suggested that having a mother who is college-educated is associated with nontraditional career choice in women (Elder & MacInnis, 1983; Tangri, 1972). Surprisingly, father's education level and the traditionality of mother's career were not shown to differ between the two groups.

This study attempted to illustrate a social cognitive process of career choice in which an individual's psychological characteristics and subsequent behaviors (e.g. career choice) are shaped by environmental factors, including family socialization and role model influences. As hypothesized, a set of psychological characteristics directly predicted traditional versus nontraditional career choice. Similarly, as hypothesized, a set of environmental variables directly predicted traditional versus nontraditional career choice. However, the idea that the social cognitive process of environmental variables also indirectly influences career choice through their direct prediction of psychological characteristics was not supported in this study.

Limitations of the Research

Participants in this research were solicited at four Midwestern universities. Although all four schools could be defined as having rigorous admissions requirements, other important differences among the schools exist. Two of the schools have traditional residential campuses, and the majority of their students come from the state in which the university is located. A third school could be described as a commuter campus in an urban setting where the average student age is 28 years, significantly higher than the more traditional universities included in this study. This undoubtedly led to a limitation of the current research in that the participants' mean age was 24.5 years. The fourth school specializes in the education of engineering students. Moreover, the majority of participants were white, creating a sample that was very homogenous in terms of cultural background. These limitations may restrict the generalizability of the results beyond the sample.

In considering the influence of role models in determining women's career choice, a more useful variable to examine may have been the father's specific employment and the influence of other male role models. For example, male teachers and older brothers may be important role models for adolescent females during the time when they are beginning to plan their higher education and to identify potential career paths.

Implications for Library Administrators

This study calls on professionals in traditionally female-dominated careers to reevaluate who is attracted to their field and how their career expectations may or may not be met. For example, the stereotypical view of librarians as possessing characteristics that lead them to enter a traditionally female-dominated field may be considered outdated by some, even library administrators. Specifically, library science is now a very technology-driven field, and traditionally defined female sex role traits, such as personal unconcern, are not perhaps as necessary as they were in the past for successful performance in the field. Instead, flexibility and adaptive behavior in light of continuous change in the field are characteristics leading to increased success and contentment in the field of library science. Interestingly, such skills are probably not far from the traditional female sex role orientation, however, when its definition is considered broadly. For example, women's concern about maintaining and protecting interpersonal relationships is often evidenced by behavior that could be termed flexible, adaptive, and accommodating. In other words, women with traditional sex role orientations work hard to smoothly navigate any change process, often with a positive benefit of easing the transition for others around them. Thus, it is still an aspect of the traditionally defined feminine sex role that enhances one's fit with the field, even as the field evolves with increased technology usage and decreased direct service.

Secondary to the idea that sex role orientation is more or less important than in the past is the probability that many women may still enter library science with an assumption that it is a feminized profession in terms of the expectations such a career includes – expectations that are consistent with a traditionally defined feminine sex role. Therefore, some women may enter the profession and become disappointed very quickly when their expectations do not match the actuality of an evolving field that is relying heavily on technological resources, while moving farther from direct service to patrons. Certainly, the traditional views of library science exist, and some students may seek the opportunities offered by the traditional definition of the field. Then, of course, the difficulty arises when individuals have entered a profession that differs from their expectations. For example, administrators may find themselves in a position of supervising an employee who believes they were misled in their educational development and who is ultimately disappointed with their career choice. Fortunately, library administrators can serve as role models, helping new professionals see the traditional and nontraditional characteristics of the field while coaching them to find their fit within the mix. Role models continue to be an important factor contributing to women's career decision-making.

The challenge for the library administrator becomes one of helping new professionals who have found a gap between their career expectations and the reality of the field. In a supervisory and mentoring role, the administrator is in a unique position however, to help the new professional to understand how her role continues to maintain a connection with traditional definitions of the field. In addition, the supervisor may need to help the new professional understand how technology actually enhances the quality of direct service that can be provided to users. Educating new professionals about how the field has maintained its traditional focus on direct service while increasing its productivity and service capacity is also a new and important role for library administrators who find themselves supervising a new employee who is confused and disappointed about the field. Specifically, the administrator may point out how working in a field that is embracing technology more and more calls for people who are able to adapt and to change without tremendous discomfort.

The original values of the field have certainly not disappeared simply because the field has evolved to include more technology, and, fortunately, women may, in fact, continue to enter library science because they want to play a role in advancing the traditional goals and values of the field. Thus, continuing to attract women who have more traditionally feminine sex role orientations to the field may allow the original values to be perpetuated. It is undoubtedly the human influence that will create congruence between the original goals of the profession and the values and needs of those who choose to pursue a career in library science, regardless of how the mode of service delivery changes. The organizational culture of the profession may actually be enhanced if women continue to enter the field with expectations derived from a traditionally female sex role orientation. Again, the challenge to educate new and continuing professionals about how their original career expectations may be realized even as the field changes lies with library administrators.

Implications for Career Counseling

The results of this study emphasize the importance of career counseling for young women as they begin their career decision-making process. Career counselors must rely not only on the results of interest and ability assessments in helping young women to identify potential career paths, but also must consider the importance of factors such as sex-role beliefs, role model influences, and the support of significant others.

Results also indicated that mother's education level was a discriminating factor when comparing women in traditional and nontraditional career paths. This finding emphasizes the potential importance of a same-sex role model for women in identifying their educational and professional goals. As career counselors develop career exploration activities for adolescent females, the inclusion of female role models from a range of traditional and nontraditional occupations would be very beneficial. Career counselors can develop mentoring and internship programs that offer young women exposure to female role models in various fields. Seeing women actually working in a male-dominated profession such as engineering or architecture may create an option for a young woman that was out of the range of possibilities before, regardless of her previously demonstrated academic strengths in math and science. According to Douvan (1976), the career choices of women are impeded by the lack of women in certain career paths. Therefore, career counselors can recruit the women who are working and thriving in male-dominated fields to be mentors for their clients, and thus, expand their clients' perceived career options.

As the millennium approaches and women continue to behave outside the definition of the traditional feminine sex-role and the traditionally masculine definition of achievement motivation, research examining the usefulness of such definitions will be valuable. The traditional definition of achievement motivation, which includes behaviors that are valued in males but discouraged in females, is inadequate as a framework for discussing women's achievement behaviors. Spence and Helmreich's (1978) inclusion of personal unconcern as a component of women's achievement motivation was a first step in accounting for the differences in how women and men make the decision to pursue achievement behavior. An examination of personal unconcern, not only in women, but also in men, may be a useful research direction as the roles of men and women continue to gain flexibility. The importance men place on their relationship needs when evaluating an opportunity for achievement has been neglected in the literature.

Results of this study have demonstrated that career aspiration and the value an individual places on occupational prestige and money should be considered when examining women's career decision-making. A future investigation could examine the factors related to the development of this value. For example, the role of environmental variables like family socialization and role model influences in the development of career aspiration deserves further inquiry. In other words, how do young girls learn to value money and prestige? Do they hear messages from parents, teachers, siblings, or other role models, which suggest that money and prestige are important factors to weigh when considering their career options? The role of the entertainment industry and the media is also important to consider. Do young girls see messages on television and in the movies that emphasize occupational prestige and money? Furthermore, including both males and females in such a study would be important for illustrating the gender differences in career aspiration and the desire for money and prestige attached to one's occupation.

REFERENCES

Almquist, E. M. (1974). Sex stereotypes in occupational choice: The case for college women. *Journal of Vocational Behavior, 5*, 13–21.

Almquist, E. M., & Angrist, S. S. (1970). Career salience and atypicality of occupational choice among college women. *Journal of Marriage and the Family, 32*, 242–249.

Alper, T. (1974). Achievement motivation in women: Now-you-see-it-now-you-don't. *American Psychologist, 29*, 194–203.

Bailyn, L. (1973). Family constraints on women's work. *Annals of the New York Academy of Sciences, 208*, 82–90.

Bartholomew, C. G., & Schnorr, D. L. (1994). Gender equity: Suggestions for broadening career options of female students. *The School Counselor, 41*, 245–255.

Basow, S. A., & Howe, K. G. (1979). Model influence on career choices of college students. *The Vocational Guidance Quarterly, 27*, 239–243.

Bem, S. L. (1975). The measurement of psychological androgyny. *Journal of Consulting and Clinical Psychology, 42*, 155–162.

Betz, N. E., & Fitzgerald, L. F. (1987). *The career psychology of women.* New York: Academic Press.

Crider, A. B., Goethals, G. R., Kavanaugh, R. D., & Solomon, P. R. (1989). *Psychology* (3rd ed.). Boston: Scott Foresman.

Douvan, E. (1976). The role of models in women's professional development. *Psychology of Women Quarterly, 1*, 5–20.

Eccles, J. S. (1984). Sex differences in achievement patterns. In: T. B. Sonderegger (Ed.), *Nebraska Symposium on Motivation: 1983 Psychology and Gender* (pp. 97–132). Lincoln, NE: University of Nebraska Press.

Eccles, J. S. (1994). Understanding women's educational and occupational choices. *Psychology of Women Quarterly, 18*, 585–609.

Elder, G. H., Jr., & MacInnis, D. J. (1983). Achievement imagery in women's lives from adolescence to adulthood. *Journal of Personality and Social Psychology, 45*, 394–404.

Farmer, H. S. (1980). Environmental, background, and psychological variables related to optimizing achievement and career motivation for high school girls. *Journal of Vocational Behavior, 17*, 58–70.

Farmer, H. S. (1985). Model of career and achievement motivation for women and men. *Journal of Counseling Psychology, 32*, 363–390.

Farmer, H. S., & Fyans, L. J., Jr. (1983). Married women's achievement and career motivation: The influence of some environmental and psychological variables. *Psychology of Women Quarterly, 7*, 358–372.

Farmer, H. S., Wardrop, J. L., Anderson, M. Z., & Risinger, R. (1995). Women's career choices: Focus on science, math, and technology careers. *Journal of Counseling Psychology, 42*, 155–170.

Fyans, L. J., Jr. (1980). *Achievement motivation.* New York: Plenum Press.

Gelso, C., & Fassinger, R. (1992). Personality, development, and counseling psychology: Depth, ambivalence, and actualization. *Journal of Counseling Psychology, 39*, 275–298.

Gilligan, C. (1982). *In a different voice.* Cambridge, MA: Harvard University Press.

Haber, S. (1980). Cognitive support for the career choices of college women. *Sex Roles, 6*, 129–138.

Hackett, G., & Betz, N. E. (1981). A self-efficacy approach to the career development of women. *Journal of Vocational Behavior, 18*, 326–339.

Harmon, L. D. (1972). Variables related to women's persistence in educational plans. *Journal of Vocational Behavior, 2*, 143–153.

Holland, J. (1973). *Making vocational choices: A theory of careers.* New York: Prentice Hall.

Horner, M. (1968). Sex differences in achievement motivation and performance in competitive and non-competitive situations. Unpublished doctoral dissertation. University of Michigan, Ann Arbor.

Hoyt, K. B. (1988). The changing workforce: A review of projections-1986 to 2000. *Career Development Quarterly, 37*, 31–39.

Lemkau, J. P. (1979). Personality and background characteristics of women in male-dominated occupations: A review. *Psychology of Women Quarterly, 4*, 221–240.

Lemkau, J. P. (1983). Women in male-dominated professions: Personality and background characteristics. *Psychology of Women Quarterly, 8*, 144–165.

Long, B. C. (1989). Sex-role orientation, coping strategies, and self-efficacy of women in traditional and nontraditional occupations. *Psychology of Women Quarterly, 13*, 307–324.

Lyson, T. A. (1980). Factors associated with the choice of a typical or atypical curriculum among college women. *Sociology and Social Research, 64*, 559–571.

Mednick, M. T., Tangri, S. S., & Hoffman, L. W. (Eds) (1975). *Women and achievement.* New York: Wiley.

Moss, H., & Kagan, J. (1961). Stability of achievement and recognition seeking behaviors from early childhood through adulthood. *Journal of Abnormal and Social Psychology, 62*, 504–513.

Murrell, A. J., Frieze, I. H., & Frost, J. L. (1991). Aspiring to careers in male- and female-dominated professions: A study of Black and White college women. *Psychology of Women Quarterly, 15*, 103–126.

National Science Foundation. (1990). *Women, minorities, and persons with physical disabilities in science and engineering.* Washington, DC: National Science Foundation.

Offermann, L. R., & Beil, C. (1992). Achievement styles of women leaders and their peers. *Psychology of Women Quarterly, 16*, 37–56.

O'Leary, V. E. (1974). Some attitudinal barriers to occupational aspiration in women. *Psychological Bulletin, 81*, 809–816.

Paludi, M. A. (1990). Sociopsychological and structural factors related to women's vocational development. *Annals of the New York Academy of Sciences, 602*, 157–168.

Penn, J. R., & Gabriel, M. E. (1976). Role constraints influencing the lives of women. *School Counselor, 23*, 252–254.

Rehberg, R. A., & Sinclair, J. (1970). Adolescent achievement behavior, family authority structure, and parental socialization processes. *American Journal of Sociology, 75*, 1012–1034.

Rossi, A. S. (1965). Women in science: Why so few? *Science, 148*, 1196–1202.

Segal, J. (1980). Profiles of successful women working in nontraditional occupations with special reference to their androgynous characteristics. *Dissertation Abstracts International, 41*, 4852.

Spence, J. T., & Helmreich, R. L. (1978). *Masculinity and femininity: The psychological dimensions, correlates, and antecedents*. Austin: University of Texas Press.

Spence, J. T., & Helmreich, R. L. (1983). Achievement-related motives and behaviors. In: J. T. Spence (Ed.), *Achievement and Achievement Motives: Psychological and Sociological Approaches*. San Francisco: Freeman.

Spence, J. T., & Helmreich, R. L. (1986). Personal Attributes Questionnaire. Unpublished Manuscript.

Spenner, K. I., & Featherman, D. L. (1978). Achievement ambitions. In: R. Turner, J. S. Coleman & R. Fox (Eds), *Annual Review of Sociology: Vol. 4* (pp. 373–420). Palo Alto, CA: Annual Review.

Standley, R., & Soule, B. (1974). Women in male-dominated professions: Contrasts in their personal and vocational histories. *Journal of Vocational Behavior, 16*, 360–367.

Stein, A. H., & Bailey, M. M. (1973). The socialization of achievement orientation in females. *Psychological Bulletin, 80*, 345–367.

Stockton, N., Berry, J., Shepson, J., & Utz, P. (1980). Sex-role and innovative major among college students. *Journal of Vocational Behavior, 16*, 360–367.

Super, D. E. (1957). *The psychology of careers*. New York: Harper and Row.

Super, D. E. (1976). Vocational guidance: Emergent decision-making in a changing society. *Bulletin of the International Association for Educational and Vocational Guidance, 29*, 16–23.

Tangri, S. S. (1972). Determinants of occupational role innovation among college women. *Journal of Social Issues, 28*, 177–199.

Trigg, L. J., & Perlman, D. (1976). Social influences of women's pursuit of nontraditional careers. *Psychology of Women Quarterly, 1*, 138–150.

U.S. Department of Labor Women's Bureau (1995). *Nontraditional occupations for women in 1995*. Washington, DC: U.S. Department of Labor, Women's Bureau.

U.S. Department of Labor Women's Bureau (1995). *Twenty leading occupations of employed women*. Washington, DC: U.S. Department of Labor, Women's Bureau.

Williams, E., Radin, N., & Allegro, T. (1992). Sex role attitudes of adolescents reared primarily by their fathers: An 11-year follow-up. *Merrill-Palmer Quarterly, 38*, 457–476.

Yanico, B. J., Hardin, S. I., & McLaughlin, K. B. (1978). Androgyny and traditional versus nontraditional major choice among college freshman. *Journal of Vocational Behavior, 12*, 261–269.

APPENDIX A

Background Information Questionnaire

Please complete the following information:

1. Your age: _____
2. Your year in college __ Freshman__ Sophomore
   __ Junior __ Senior
3. Your Academic Major: _____
   (Be as specific as possible – e.g. electrical engineering instead of engineering.)
4. Your Ethnicity:
   __ African-American __ Asian-American __ Caucasian__ Hispanic
   __ Native American   __ Other
5. While you were growing up, what was your mother's primary occupation?
   _____

6. While you were growing up, what was your father's primary occupation?
   _____

7. What is your mother's highest level of education?
   __ Some high school
   __ High School Diploma
   __ Some College (No degree)
   __ Two-year college degree (Associates degree)
   __ Bachelor's Degree
   __ Some Post-Bachelor's Graduate Work (No degree)
   __ Masters Degree
   __ Doctorate
8. What is your father's highest level of education?
   __ Some high school
   __ High School Diploma
   __ Some College (No degree)
   __ Two-year college degree (Associates degree)
   __ Bachelor's Degree
   __ Some Post-Bachelor's Graduate Work (No degree)
   __ Masters Degree
   __ Doctorate
9. Please indicate your overall ACT score with an "x":
   __ 14–18
   __ 19–23
   __ 24–28
   __ 29 or above   or   above

APPENDIX B

Work and Family Orientation Questionnaire-2

The following statements describe reactions to conditions of work and challenging situations. For each item, indicate how much you *agree* or *disagree* with the statements, as it refers to yourself, by choosing the appropriate letter on the scale, A, B, C, D, or E.

1. I would rather work in a situation where group effort is stressed and more important rather than one in which my individual effort is stressed.

A	B	C	D	E
Strongly agree	Slightly agree	Neither agree nor disagree	Slightly disagree	Strongly disagree

2. I more often attempt difficult tasks that I am not sure I can do than easier tasks I believe I can do.

A	B	C	D	E
Strongly agree	Slightly agree	Neither agree nor disagree	Slightly disagree	Strongly disagree

3. It is important for me to do my work as well as I can even if it isn't popular with my co-workers.

A	B	C	D	E
Strongly agree	Slightly agree	Neither agree nor disagree	Slightly disagree	Strongly disagree

4. I would rather do something at which I feel confident and relaxed than something, which is challenging and difficult.

A	B	C	D	E
Strongly agree	Slightly agree	Neither agree nor disagree	Slightly disagree	Strongly disagree

5. I would rather learn fun games that most people know than a difficult thought game.

A	B	C	D	E
Strongly agree	Slightly agree	Neither agree nor disagree	Slightly disagree	Strongly disagree

6. If I am not good at something I would rather keep struggling to master it than move on to something I may be good at.

A	B	C	D	E
Strongly agree	Slightly agree	Neither agree nor disagree	Slightly disagree	Strongly disagree

7. I really enjoy working in situations involving skill and competition.

A	B	C	D	E
Strongly agree	Slightly agree	Neither agree nor disagree	Slightly disagree	Strongly disagree

8. When a group I belong to plans an activity, I would rather organize it myself than have someone else organize it and just help out.

A	B	C	D	E
Strongly agree	Slightly agree	Neither agree nor disagree	Slightly disagree	Strongly disagree

9. Once I undertake a task, I dislike goofing up and not doing the best job I can.

A	B	C	D	E
Strongly agree	Slightly agree	Neither agree nor disagree	Slightly disagree	Strongly disagree

10. I think more of the future than of the present and past.

A	B	C	D	E
Strongly agree	Slightly agree	Neither agree nor disagree	Slightly disagree	Strongly disagree

11. I hate losing more than I like winning.

A	B	C	D	E
Strongly agree	Slightly agree	Neither agree nor disagree	Slightly disagree	Strongly disagree

12. I worry because my success may cause others to dislike me.

A	B	C	D	E
Strongly agree	Slightly agree	Neither agree nor disagree	Slightly disagree	Strongly disagree

13. It is important to me to perform better than others on a task.

A	B	C	D	E
Strongly agree	Slightly agree	Neither agree nor disagree	Slightly disagree	Strongly disagree

14. I feel that winning is important in both work and games.

A	B	C	D	E
Strongly agree	Slightly agree	Neither agree nor disagree	Slightly disagree	Strongly disagree

APPENDIX C

Career Motivation Measure

People consider work important for a variety of reasons, many of which are described below. Please circle the number that best describes your opinion about each statement below. Although some statements appear to be asking the same thing, they are all different in some important way. There are no right or wrong answers; your opinion is what counts.

	Strongly Disagree	Disagree	Not Sure	Strongly Agree	Agree
1. I enjoy making plans about my future.	1	2	3	4	5
2. I often think about what type of job I'll be in, ten years from now.	1	2	3	4	5
3. To me, a career is a means of expressing myself.	1	2	3	4	5
4. I would like to have a job of which I am really proud.	1	2	3	4	5
5. I like to have a career goal toward which I can work.	1	2	3	4	5
6. My mother was/is a role model for the importance I place on career.	1	2	3	4	5
7. I really don't think too much about whether or not I'll get ahead in my job.	1	2	3	4	5

	Strongly Disagree	Disagree	Not Sure	Strongly Agree	Agree
8. Planning for and succeeding in a career is *not* my main concern.	1	2	3	4	5
9. I could be happy without having a career.	1	2	3	4	5
10. If I hit the jackpot or made it in the lottery I would quit my job.	1	2	3	4	5
11. I would want to move ahead in my occupation, not stand still.	1	2	3	4	5
12. My career will give meaning to my life.	1	2	3	4	5
13. The occupation that interests me most will give me a chance to really be myself.	1	2	3	4	5
14. My father was/is a role model for the importance I place on career.	1	2	3	4	5
15. Planning for a specific career is not worth the effort.	1	2	3	4	5
16. I do not consider myself "career minded."	1	2	3	4	5

17. Please answer the following question:
What occupation do you expect to end up in?

_____

(Be as specific as possible – e.g. electrical engineer instead of engineer or kindergarten teacher instead of teacher)

APPENDIX D

Personal Attributes Questionnaire

The items below inquire about what kind of a person you think you are. Each item consists of a *pair* of characteristics, with the letters A–E in between. For example:

Not at all artistic   A... B... C... D... E   Very artistic

Each pair describes contradictory characteristics – that is, you cannot be both at the same time, such as very artistic and not at all artistic.

The letters form a scale between two extremes. You are to choose a letter which describes where *you* fall on the scale. For example, if you think you have no artistic ability, you would choose A, if you think you are pretty good, you might choose D. If you are only medium, you might choose C, and so forth.

1.	Not at all aggressive	A	B	C	D	E	Very aggressive
2.	Not at all independent	A	B	C	D	E	Very independent
3.	Not at all emotional	A	B	C	D	E	Very emotional
4.	Very submissive	A	B	C	D	E	Very dominant
5.	Not at all excitable in a MAJOR crisis	A	B	C	D	E	Very excitable in MAJOR Crisis
6.	Very passive	A	B	C	D	E	Very active
7.	Not at all able to devote self completely to others	A	B	C	D	E	Able to devote self completely to others
8.	Very rough	A	B	C	D	E	Very gentle
9.	Not at all helpful to others	A	B	C	D	E	Very helpful to others
10.	Not at all competitive	A	B	C	D	E	Very competitive
11.	Very home oriented	A	B	C	D	E	Very worldly
12.	Not at all kind	A	B	C	D	E	Very kind
13.	Indifferent to others' approval	A	B	C	D	E	Highly needful of others' approval
14.	Feelings not easily hurt	A	B	C	D	E	Feelings easily hurt
15.	Not at all aware of others' feelings	A	B	C	D	E	Very aware of others' feelings
16.	Can make decisions easily	A	B	C	D	E	Has difficulty making decisions
17.	Gives up very easily	A	B	C	D	E	Never gives up easily

18. Never cries	A	B	C	D	E	Cries very easily
19. Not at all self-confident	A	B	C	D	E	Very self-confident
20. Feels very inferior	A	B	C	D	E	Feels very superior
21. Not at all understanding of others	A	B	C	D	E	Very understanding of others
22. Very cold in relations with others	A	B	C	D	E	Very warm in relations with others
23. Very little need for security	A	B	C	D	E	Very strong need for security
24. Goes to pieces under pressure	A	B	C	D	E	Stands up well under pressure

APPENDIX E

Early Family Socialization Measure

The questions ask for information about your parents' attitudes and actions. "Parent" includes stepparent, foster parent, or any other adult guardian who has been responsible for you all or most of your life. If a question asks about "parents" and you were brought up by only one, answer for him or her. Answer every item by picking the number on the scale below which best describes how characteristic or uncharacteristic it is as it applies to your experience in your family.

1. My mother didn't mind if I played with toys that were supposed to be for the opposite sex.

1	2	3	4	5
Very Uncharacteristic				Very Characteristic

2. My mother is very sympathetic to "women's lib."

1	2	3	4	5
Very Uncharacteristic				Very Characteristic

3. My father didn't mind if I played with toys that were supposed to be for the opposite sex.

1	2	3	4	5
Very Uncharacteristic				Very Characteristic

4. My father is very sympathetic to "women's lib."

1	2	3	4	5
Very				Very
Uncharacteristic				Characteristic

APPENDIX F

Parental Support Measure

The first seven questions ask for information about your parents' attitudes and actions. "Parent" includes stepparent, foster parent, or any other adult guardian who has been responsible for you all or most of your life. If a question asks about "parents" and you were brought up by only one, answer for him or her. Answer every item by picking the number on the scale below which best describes how characteristic or uncharacteristic it is as it applies to your experience in your family.

1. If I go on after I finish my education and have a very successful career, my parents will be very pleased.

1	2	3	4	5
Very				Very
Uncharacteristic				Characteristic

2. My mother encouraged me to do my best on everything I did.

1	2	3	4	5
Very				Very
Uncharacteristic				Characteristic

3. My mother frequently praised me for doing well.

1	2	3	4	5
Very				Very
Uncharacteristic				Characteristic

4. My mother always took an interest in my activities.

1	2	3	4	5
Very				Very
Uncharacteristic				Characteristic

5. My father encouraged me to do my best on everything I did.

1	2	3	4	5
Very Uncharacteristic				Very Characteristic

6. My father has always set up high standards for me to meet.

1	2	3	4	5
Very Uncharacteristic				Very Characteristic

7. My mother has always set up high standards for me to meet.

1	2	3	4	5
Very Uncharacteristic				Very Characteristic

For questions 8–11, please consider as your mother and father those people with whom you have had a parental relationship. Again, mother and father could include a stepparent, foster parent, or any other adult guardian who has been responsible for you all or most of your life. For these questions, please answer using the following scale:

1	2	3	4	5
Not Supportive at all	Slightly Supportive	Moderately Supportive	Considerably Supportive	Extremely Supportive

8. How supportive do you perceive your mother has been toward your choice of your present college major?

1	2	3	4	5
Not Supportive at all	Slightly Supportive	Moderately Supportive	Considerably Supportive	Extremely Supportive

9. How supportive do you perceive your father has been toward your choice of your present college major?

1	2	3	4	5
Not Supportive at all	Slightly Supportive	Moderately Supportive	Considerably Supportive	Extremely Supportive

10. How supportive do you perceive your mother has been toward your future career goal?

1	2	3	4	5
Not Supportive at all	Slightly Supportive	Moderately Supportive	Considerably Supportive	Extremely Supportive

11. How supportive do you perceive your father has been toward your future career goal?

1	2	3	4	5
Not Supportive at all	Slightly Supportive	Moderately Supportive	Considerably Supportive	Extremely Supportive

E-METRICS: MEASURES FOR ELECTRONIC RESOURCES

Rush Miller and Sherrie Schmidt

The research library today can be described as a "hybrid" library: a library in transition from a focus on print-based collections and services to one that emphasizes electronic, or digital information resources and services. The quickening pace of change in this field is evident in the supplemental statistics data gathered by the Association of Research Libraries. The percentage of acquisitions dollars that ARL member libraries devote to electronic resources has risen from 3.6% in 1992–1993 to 12.9% in 1999–2000. Nine libraries spent more than 20% of their materials budget on electronic or digital materials, and five libraries spent more than $2 million on such resources in 1999–2000, with the University of Pittsburgh being at the top of the list spending $2,163,220. One hundred and five ARL libraries reported spending a total of almost $100 million on electronic resources out of their materials expenditures budget. The cost of mounting digital information resources is far higher when infrastructure and personnel costs are factored into the picture (ARL, 2001). Clearly, the total expenditures related to electronic resources and services within ARL libraries would be measured in the hundreds of millions of dollars if it could be counted accurately and consistently.

That, of course, is the problem. While libraries, particularly ARL libraries, have 60 years of consistently defined and collected statistics related to budgets, collections, services, and personnel (Kyrillidou, 2000, 2001), no such data is available for the electronic resources that are becoming ever more important. Problems and challenges in collecting and analyzing such data are many and obvious, including: there is a lack of clear and consistent definition of data elements; vendors do not

Advances in Library Administration and Organization
Advances in Library Administration and Organization, Volume 20, 203–212
© 2003 Published by Elsevier Science Ltd.
ISSN: 0732-0671/PII: S0732067102200097

"count" things in the same manner as one another; membership in a consortium can skew the statistics of the individual libraries in that consortium; libraries structure themselves differently in regard to electronic resources, making data gathering difficult; libraries do not control access to and use of important data about vendor-supplied resources; and the nature of electronic resources is changing rapidly and, therefore, data elements are shifting. Even as libraries are increasing their invest-ment in electronic resources and the opportunities for information management are growing dramatically with the advent of the World Wide Web as a delivery vehicle, we know much less about this aspect of our collections and services than the traditional ones.

Questions related to the measurement of digital resources and services must be answered if libraries are to be accountable to their constituents and funders alike. Questions such as, "Who uses these resources?" or "Are these huge outlays of funds justified in terms of use, or value derived from use?" or "What difference do all of these resources make to students and faculty in universities?" must be answered if university administrators, trustees, students, and faculty are expected to support ever-increasing levels of funding for the acquisition and development of these resources and services. Just as important is the need for reliable mea-sures in order to make sound decisions about the acquisition or de-acquisition of electronic resources, selection of what to digitize, and development of criteria and benchmarks that can be communicated to stakeholders.

ARL has been concerned with performance measurement issues since the 1990s (Kyrillidou, 2001a). The ARL Statistics and Measurement Committee and the ARL Leadership and Management Committee launched the New Measures Initiative in January 1999, following a retreat held in Tucson. The New Measures Initiative arises from two challenges facing research libraries: (1) the need to demonstrate the impact research libraries have on areas of interest to their host institutions, and (2) the need to respond to pressure to maximize resources through cost containment and reallocation, which in turn requires the identification of "best practices." Coming out of the Tucson retreat, several representatives wrote white papers in areas of acknowledged interest (Baker, 1999; Deiss, 1999; Franklin, 1999; Haka, 1999; Kobulnicky, 1999; Presser, 1999). Those attending the retreat addressed a set of questions regarding the data needed to describe research libraries in today's environment, the need for new measures, and the means by which useful data and measurement tools could be developed. The retreat participants recognized that "any new measures must: (a) be consistent with organizational missions, goals, and objective; (b) be integrated with an institution's program review; (c) balance customer, stakeholder, and employee interests and needs; (d) establish accountability; and (e) include the collection and use of reliable and valid data" (Blixrud, 2001).

During 1999, the library leaders engaged in this set of activities decided that it was not enough to simply frame the issues – research libraries needed to move into testing new methods and experimenting with specific projects. With limited resources and many ideas to test and implement, a variety of projects have emerged as outlined in the annual *ARL Activities Report* (ARL, 2001a). There are five major projects that are being pursued within the Association under the aegis of New Measures. These are: (1) an investigation into higher education outcomes assessment, with an examination of both learning outcomes (Smith, 2000) and research outcomes; (2) measurement of library service quality (Heath et al., 2002); (3) cost studies; (4) interlibrary loan and document delivery investigation; and (5) an examination of measures for networked statistics and electronic resources (ARL, 2002a).

The examination of measures for networked statistics and electronic resources has evolved into the ARL E-Metrics Project. The E-Metrics Project began in February 2000 at a retreat in Scottsdale, Arizona, attended by representatives from 36 ARL libraries. This retreat focused on the challenges involved in measuring the commitment to and impact of electronic resources and services in ARL libraries. Due to his extensive funded research in this area (McClure, 2000), ARL employed a consultant for the meeting – Dr. Charles McClure, Francis Eppes Professor and Director of the Information Management Use and Policy Institute at the School of Information Studies at Florida State University. Rush Miller, Hillman University Librarian at the University of Pittsburgh, and Sherrie Schmidt, Dean of Libraries at Arizona State University, agreed to serve as project co-chairs. Martha Kyrillidou, Senior Program Officer for Statistics and Measurement, staffs the project for ARL. Susan Jurrow served as facilitator for the retreat.

The Scottsdale retreat was essential for defining the scope of a project to be undertaken, since the project was to be self-funded as well as self-managed by libraries willing to put forth a significant commitment of money and staff time. Prior to the meeting, attendees were asked to submit answers to questions about their efforts to measure the impact of electronic services and resources and their decision-making process related to these materials. Also, some attendees provided examples of the statistics they were collecting; these examples reflected the lack of consistency in current practices, as well as the lack of adequate data provided by vendors. After a full day of intensive discussions, a project began to take shape. The group identified four major areas that should be explored in the project:

(1) Study of users and uses.
(2) Cost and benefit analysis.
(3) Study of staff impact and needs.
(4) Engagement with information providers and their usage data services.

The project co-chairs worked with McClure and his staff to develop a project prospectus (McClure, 2000b). In the meantime, the level of commitment in terms of the number of ARL libraries electing to participate in this project doubled initial expectations, for a total of 24 libraries agreeing to support and participate in the project:

- University of Alberta
- Arizona State University
- Auburn University
- University of Chicago
- University of Connecticut
- Cornell University

- University of Illinois – Chicago
- University of Manitoba
- University of Maryland – College Park
- University of Massachusetts
- University of Nebraska – Lincoln

- University of Notre Dame
- University of Pennsylvania

- Pennsylvania State University
- University of Pittsburgh
- Purdue University
- University of Southern California
- Texas A&M University
- Virginia Polytechnic Institute & State University (Virginia Tech)
- University of Western Ontario
- University of Wisconsin – Madison
- Yale University

- Library of Congress
- The New York Public Library, Research Libraries

The project was formalized as the E-Metrics Project and a formal contract was negotiated with the Information Use Management and Policy Institute at Florida State University to accomplish the three phases of deliverables outlined below:

Phase One: A knowledge inventory of ARL libraries and the organization of a Working Group on Database Vendor Statistics.

Phase Two: Statistics and performance measures to collect and analyze data collected within libraries or provided by vendors.

Phase Three: An outline of a proposal for measuring outcomes of electronic resources, to be funded separately.

The Phase One Report (Shim et al., 2000) was submitted to ARL on 7 November 2000. In this report, McClure and the Institute staff report the findings from their collection of data related to the current state-of-the-art within ARL libraries in measuring electronic information resources and services. Their data was gathered using survey questionnaires as well as site visits to several libraries that were considered advanced in this area after an analysis of the surveys.

The survey responses revealed a wide range of data collection and use activities among the 24 project participants. The most consistently collected and used data related to patron-accessible resources and costs. Data related to use and users was collected less often since much of the data collected was provided by vendors and was not kept in-house. Collected data was used primarily when making acquisitions decisions. Not surprisingly, the largest impediment to survey respondents lay in the lack of consistent and comparable statistics from database vendors.

Site visits were conducted at Virginia Tech, the University of Pennsylvania, Yale University, and the New York Public Library. These visits documented current practices and clarified survey responses. Again it was clear that a lack of standardized reporting practices makes it difficult to collect and analyze data.

Another aspect of Phase One was the organization of a working group to deal with vendor-supplied statistics. This working group met with 12 major vendors for ARL libraries in order to explore issues related to the perceived lack of consistency in vendor statistics and to solicit vendors' assistance in developing and field-testing standard data elements. The vendors who accepted the invitation to participate in the meeting include:

Academic Press/IDEAL	Bell & Howell	EBSCO
Elsevier/ScienceDirect	Gale Group	JSTOR
Lexis-Nexis	netLibrary	OCLC/FirstSearch
Ovid	SilverPlatter	

As the project entered Phase Two, the focus shifted to the definition and testing of data elements. Without solid and comparable data, measurement would be less helpful and meaningful in the long run. It was becoming clear that the project framers had underestimated the complexity of the issues and challenges. It also became clear that this project was one of many being undertaken in the United States and in other countries to accomplish similar, if not the same, goals.

A number of projects designed to improve the availability of consistent and comparable statistical data about electronic resources and services have been undertaken over the past several years. All of these projects are related, in one way or another, to the E-Metrics Project. However, none of them duplicated the ARL effort in terms of goals and timeframes. Close communication links and collaboration with the projects was undertaken by project co-chairs. These projects are:

- European Commission EQUINOX Project (European Commission, 2002).
- Publishing and Library Solutions Committee (PALS) Working Group on Online Vendor Usage Statistics (UK).
- International Coalition of Library Consortia (ICOLC) review of ICOLC *Guidelines for Statistical Measures of Usage of Web-based Indexed, Abstracted, and Full-Text Resources.*

- National Commission on Libraries and Information Science (NCLIS) project to standardize online database usage statistics and reporting mechanisms (public libraries).
- Institute of Museum and Library Services (IMLS) project to develop national network online statistics and performance measures for public libraries.
- Council on Library and Information Resources (CLIR) report by consultant Judy Luther related to network statistics (Luther, 2000).
- NISO Forum on Performance Measures and Statistics (NISO, nd).

During Phase Two of the project, statistical data elements were discussed within the Vendor Statistics Working Group and with participants at various meetings held at CNI, ALA, and other meeting opportunities. The consultants worked with participants to develop a set of measures to be tested in the field. These included statistical elements from vendors – worked out as a separate trial with 12 vendors – and internal library statistics to be collected by library staff.

A total of 18 measures were agreed upon to be adopted for a field test. These elements were grouped into categories and included:

(1) *Information Content.* This category includes elements such as the number of electronic full-text journals or reference sources to which a library subscribes. It also includes virtual "visits" to the library's electronic resources and the percentage of all monographs represented by electronic books, among other elements.
(2) *Information Services.* These elements measure usage of library digital collections as well as the percentage of reference and other transactions that are digitally based.
(3) *Technical Infrastructure.* Technical infrastructure is measured in terms of the cost of digital collections along with support costs and management information, such as the expenditures for electronic journals and books and other components.

An effort to field test vendor statistics in selected libraries was also underway. This effort was designed not only to collect and analyze data elements that are agreed upon and consistent with the ICOLC Guidelines (Guidelines, 1998), but to gather information related to the vendor's definition and compilation of these data. Judging from the work so far, vendors have varying methodologies and internal processes, which affect the consistency and standardization of the data provided. Each vendor defines a search and retrieval set differently, which dramatically affects the statistics provided. It is safe to say that, until now, comparing the data from one vendor with that of a second vendor was unreliable and misleading.

One benefit of this project will be to assist vendors and libraries alike in standardizing data element definitions to gain more consistency across the data.

Internal data elements were field tested in 13 libraries (including the University of Texas, which is not a participant in the project, but agreed to assist with the field testing, because Sue Phillips, a member of their staff, was serving in a liaison role between the ARL project and the ICOLC group that was revising the related guideline). Along with the data itself, these libraries were asked to track the amount of effort expended in providing the data. There was little consistency in the number of staff hours reported – it ranged from 3 to 167 hours. Much of the variance can be explained by the variability of infrastructure and experience within ARL libraries in maintaining data such as these. Libraries that are already engaged in collecting and analyzing usage and management data related to electronic resources found it easier to adapt to this field-test; those with little history or experience found it much more difficult to comply. Libraries in the field test were also asked to analyze how useful they felt the collected data would be to them. Overall, libraries clearly saw these measures as good things to have in the absence of more detailed data.

The field-testing of these data elements was critical to a better understanding of the challenges and issues facing research libraries in systematizing e-metrics. This kind of data collection does not derive from traditional library structures, such as acquisitions, accounting, and cataloging, or from other information systems in place in libraries. Few ARL libraries have a system in place for managing electronic resources, although the number is growing. Additionally, many of the definitions and procedures for collecting this data during the field test varied from current practices within the participating libraries, although one major outcome of the project will be to develop a more standardized mechanism for gathering data. Defining changing concepts such as electronic books or full-text retrievals is painfully difficult, and the distinctions among various resource types can often be arbitrary and fluid. And, of course, in ARL libraries, electronic resources are often dispersed throughout a large institution and are not centrally managed, making data difficult to collect centrally. The field test allowed the project managers and consultants to refine the data elements further. The Phase Two report proposes a refined set of measures for implementation on an ongoing basis (Shim et al., 2001). These elements include measures of the nature and size of the digital resources available within an institution, the cost of providing these resources by category, and the amount of activity documenting the use of these resources. The report from Phase Two is available on the Web and has been distributed to all ARL member libraries. It includes a procedures manual that provides ARL libraries with definitions and techniques for collecting standardized data related to electronic resources; these definitions and techniques will guide ARL libraries in the implementation of ongoing data collection relating to electronic resources measures. It is anticipated that these data elements will not be static – as the traditional ones have tended to be – but subject to continuous change. This is, after all, the nature of the networked environment.

From the outset of the E-Metrics Project, libraries looked beyond the development of metrics to the development of outcomes measures. Simple data is not sufficient to answer the question, "What difference does this tremendous outlay of resources make to the users of libraries?" Phase Three of the project is envisioned to study and recommend strategies and a framework for measuring outcomes, i.e. assessing the impact and value of electronic resources on user behavior and effectiveness. We all want to know what difference electronic resources make, not in terms of inputs, but in terms of outputs. Some people are asking, "Are we determined to get it right this time in terms of measuring important things rather than just convenient things?" The answer is probably that we always wanted to get it right, and we always did what we thought was the right thing; yet, what is right may differ from context to context. There is often a scientific positivism associated with statistics and measures that sometimes blinds us to the emerging context and uniqueness of specific environments. Vice versa, one could argue that too much emphasis on the uniqueness of a local context fosters an isolationist attitude that may not be appropriate for a highly interconnected information environment with global dimensions that are changing, shifting, and affecting all libraries in similar ways.

The consultants working on this project have presented the results of Phase Two with some analysis of the strategy ARL might follow to achieve this higher level of institutional outcomes investigation. However, outcomes assessment is viewed as being a separate project, for which additional funding and time will be required.

CONCLUSION

The ARL E-Metrics Project is a key development in the ongoing effort to quantify and better understand the impact of emerging information technologies on library collections and services. It has provided the Association with a new measurement model – to which individual libraries have committed significant resources and effort beyond the Association structure and budget – to further develop and test in Phase Three of the project.

It is difficult to overstate the hurdles encountered in carrying out what appeared at the outset to be a rather simple idea – collecting statistics on the effort that ARL libraries are making to mount electronic resources and services. The problems of definition, reliability, and consistency of data provided by the vendor community alone are daunting. But, they are matched equally by librarians' lack of agreement on what is important to collect, how to collect it, and how to use what is collected. Most libraries lack experience with the collection and analysis of data related to their investment in electronic resources. This is a new, emerging, and changing field, and these issues are very complex and difficult to get a handle on.

However, in less than the two years to which participants committed their funds and support, the project is producing a viable and implementable program of data collection related to electronic networked resources in ARL libraries. This accomplishment is to the credit of the directors and staff of these 24 libraries; it is also largely due to the expertise and hard work of the director and staff of the Information Use Management and Policy Institute at Florida State University.

In developing e-metrics, libraries are only part of a larger networked community concerned with similar issues. Some libraries are concerned with the competition presented by Internet search engines, gateways, and portals. Some libraries feel the need to demonstrate large numbers of web hits and other e-metrics to justify their investment in electronic resources. Yet, no matter how large an electronic library is, it is doubtful that it will ever receive more web hits than popular search engines, gateways, and portals such as Yahoo and Google. Libraries, though, have much more valuable resources to offer than do any Internet search engine – it is our challenge to try to measure these contributions.

REFERENCES

Association of Research Libraries (2001). *ARL Supplementary Statistics 1999–2000.* Washington, DC: Association of Research Libraries, 2001. Also available at: http://www.arl.org/stats/arlstat/#sup

Association of Research Libraries (2001a). *ARL Activities Report 2001.* Washington, DC: Association of Research Libraries, 2001; also, see *ARL Activities Report 2000* and *ARL Activities Report 1999.*

Association for Research Libraries (2002a). Measures for electronic resources (E-Metrics) homepage. Retrieved August 26, 2002 from http://www.arl.org/stats/newmeas/emetrics/index.html

Baker, S. (1999). ARL new measures: Ease and breadth of access. Retrieved August 26, 2002 from http://www.arl.org/stats/program/Access.pdf

Blixrud, J. (2001). The association of research libraries statistics and measurement program: From descriptive data to performance measures. 67th IFLA Council and General Conference, August 16–25, 2001. Retrieved from http://www.ifla.org/IV/ifla67/papers/034–135e.pdf

Deiss, K. J. (1999). Organizational capacity white paper. Available at: http://www.arl.org/stats/program/capacity.pdf

European Commission. Telematics for Libraries Programme (2002). EQUINOX: Library performance measurement and quality management systems homepage. Retrieved August 26, 2002 from http://equinox.dcu.ie/index.html

Heath, F., Cook, C., Kyrillidou, M., & Webster, D. (2002). The forging of consensus: A methodological approach to service quality assessment in research libraries – the LibQUAL+™ experience.

International Coalition of Library Consortia (ICOLC) (1998). Guidelines for statistical measures of usage of web-based indexed, abstracted, and full-text resources prepared by the International Coalition of Library Consortia. (ICOLC), November 1998.

Kyrillidou, M. (2000). Research library trends: ARL statistics. *Journal of Academic Librarianship, 26*, 236–427.

Kyrillidou, M. (2001). To describe and measure the performance of North American research libraries. *IFLA Journal, 27*(4), 257–263.

Luther, J. (2000). *White paper on electronic journal usage statistics*. Washington, DC: Council on Library and Information Resources.

McClure, C. R. (2000). Study proposal: Developing statistics and performance measures to describe electronic information services and resources in ARL libraries. Tallahassee: School of Information Studies, Florida State University. Retrieved August 26, 2002 from http://www.arl.org/stats/newmeas/emetrics/phase twoappendix.pdf

McClure, C. R. (2000b). Developing statistics and performance measures to describe electronic information services and resources in ARL libraries. Retrieved from http://arl.org/stats/newmeas/emetrics/phasetwoappendix.pdf

National Information Standards Organization <http://www.niso.org/stats-rpt.html>

Presser, C. Library impact on research: A preliminary sketch. Available at: http://www.arl.org/stats/program/presser.pdf

Shim, W., McClure, C. R., & Bertot, J. C. (2000). *ARL E-Metrics project: Developing statistics and performance measures to describe electronic information services and resources in ARL libraries: Phase One report*. Tallahassee, FL: Information Use Management and Policy Institute. Retrieved August 26, 2002 from http://www.arl.org/stats/newmeas/emetrics/phaseone.pdf

Shim, W., McClure, C. R., Fraser, B. T., Bertot, J. C., Dagli, A., & Leahy, E. H. (2001). *Measures and statistics for research library networked services: Procedures and issues: ARL E-Metrics Phase II report*. Washington, DC: Association of Research Libraries. Retrieved August 26, 2002 from http://www.arl.org/stats/newmeas/emetrics/phsetwopreface.pdf

Smith, K. (2000). *New roles and responsibilities for the University Library: Advancing student learning through outcomes assessment*. Washington, DC: Association of Research Libraries.

MANAGING SERVICE QUALITY WITH THE BALANCED SCORECARD

Roswitha Poll

THE DATA IN THE CONTROLLING SYSTEM

Traditionally, libraries have collected statistical data about their collections, acquisitions, lending, and inter-lending activities. In time, the number of statistics was enlarged and differentiated, and in many cases, it now comprises several hundred data points. These range from the number of incunabula or microforms in the collection, the expenditure on preservation or buildings to the number of issues made, claims and reservations placed or visits made to exhibitions and special events. These statistics are, for the most part, collected nationally, but libraries also tend to collect additional statistics, (e.g. for special tasks and activities like legal deposit right, special collections, or services for special user groups).

All those statistical data could be used as steering instruments for library management. But such use is more often accidental than systematic, and many data are collected laboriously without ever being evaluated or used. For several decades libraries have tried to assess, not only the quantity of their resources and activities, but also the quality – the "goodness" of a library's services and products. Performance measures for libraries have been developed and tested in national and international projects and standardized in an international standard (ISO 11620, 1998). Though there are lists of recognized and established performance indicators, such indicators have not been collected and used systematically, like in the national collection of statistics, but rather in the evaluation process of a single library.

Advances in Library Administration and Organization
Advances in Library Administration and Organization, Volume 20, 213–227
Copyright © 2003 by Elsevier Science Ltd.
ISSN: 0732-0671/PII: S0732067102200103

Statistics, as well as performance indicators, were developed for use in the traditional library that has print collections, reading rooms and lending services. The growing importance of electronic services in libraries has led to a revision of both statistics and performance indicators. The international standard of library statistics has been revised and enlarged to include the data of the "digital library" (ISO 2789, 2003), and a working group of ISO (the International Organization of Standardization) has edited a Technical Report about performance indicators for electronic library services. (ISO TR 20983, 2003)

Another sector of management data has evolved over the last few years: cost data. Libraries have always registered data relating to their income and expenditure. But the general demand for transparency of costs has led to questions like:

- What are the costs of each single service or product of a library (e.g. one issue, one reference question answered)?
- How do the costs of a service or product split up as to staff costs, administrative costs, equipment etc.?

More and more libraries are involved in cost analysis projects of programs within their institutions, or are trying to analyze their costs in order to present reliable data when applying for funds or allocating resources. Models for cost analysis in libraries have been developed and tested (Ceynowa & Coners, 2003; Poll, 2000) and will probably be used widely in the future.

Nowadays, there is an immense pool of management data available in libraries, to include statistics on resources, services, use, and cost data and combined data like performance indicators for the quality of library services. The quantity, diversity and complexity of the data stress the need for an integrated system designed to make this management data useful for evaluating programs, developing strategy, and initiating action.

THE BALANCED SCORECARD MODEL

A German project, sponsored by the German Research Council (DFG), has developed an integrated quality management system for academic libraries. The project was chaired by the University and Regional Library of Münster and included as partners the Bavarian State Library in Munich and the State and University Library in Bremen. The three libraries are among the largest in Germany, each with special tasks, activities, and operating conditions. Thus, the project could rely on a broad and differentiated view of management issues in academic libraries. The project started in June 1999 and finished in the autumn of 2001. The results have been published in a handbook, with a software package designed to facilitate

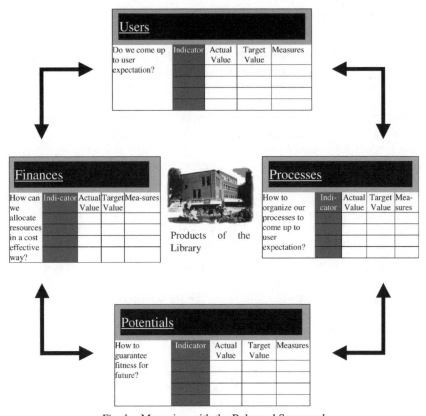

Fig. 1. Managing with the Balanced Scorecard.

the collection of data and the management process (Ceynowa & Coners, 2002). The project partners decided to use the Balanced Scorecard (Kaplan & Norton, 1992, 1996) as a tool in developing this management system. This concept was originally developed for the commercial sector. It "translates" the planning perspective of an institution (mission, strategic vision and goals) into a system of performance indicators that covers all important perspectives of performance: finances, users, internal processes and improvement activities (Fig. 1).

The system thus integrates:

- financial and non-financial data;
- input and output data;
- the external perspective (funding institutions, users) and the internal perspective (processes, staff);

- goals and measures taken;
- causes and results.

The basic model of the Balanced Scorecard, adapted to the conditions of academic libraries, deviates from the original model in placing the user perspective rather than the financial perspective foremost, because libraries do not strive for maximum financial gain, but for best service.

The following sections show the different performance perspectives of the Balanced Scorecard Model, the respective indicators for each perspective, and the actual values found in the project libraries. Performance indicators have not yet been used systematically in German academic libraries, and a broad comparison of output measures is not feasible at this time. Therefore, the project libraries decided to publish their own data, collected during the course of the project (the year 2000), in order to help libraries using the Balanced Scorecard Model estimate the position of their own data collection efforts. The three project libraries vary greatly as to mission, structure and clientele:

- The State and University Library (SuUB) Bremen has a one-tier library system on a campus.
- The University and Regional Library (ULB) Münster has a two-tier library system with 159 institute libraries.
- The Bavarian State Library (BSB) München does not serve a university, but the general academic community in a broad frame.

As a result, a large number of the indicators are not applicable for comparison between the three libraries. The indicator "market penetration," for instance, shows lower values for the two-tiered system in Münster than for Bremen, since the central library shares this task in Münster with the institute libraries. It does not apply at all to the Bavarian State Library because that library does not serve a clearly defined population. Libraries testing the performance indicators of the model for their own use will have to decide which of the three library types considered is best comparable with their own mission, structure and clientele.

The User Perspective

The indicators chosen for the *user perspective* correspond to the fundamental goals of reaching as large a part of the population as possible and of satisfying their informational needs with the services offered.

- *Market penetration* = Percent of the population registered as actual users.
  For an academic library, the population to be served will probably consist of the members of the institution (university, scientific institute etc.) it is set up

to serve. Actual users are those that have transacted at least one loan during a specified time period (usually one year). It would, of course, be even more interesting to assess the proportion of the population who made use of other library services during a specified time, including electronic services and remote use. But, for many libraries, this is still difficult to measure. Market penetration for the test libraries was:

SuUB Bremen	74.5%
ULB Münster	71.2%
BSB München	not applicable

The project libraries chose to assess "actual users" instead of "registered users" for this indicator, since in many libraries students' enrollment automatically includes registration for library services and market penetration could not be measured.

- *User satisfaction rate*
  This indicator is assessed using satisfaction surveys on a 5-point-scale. Overall satisfaction with the library is generally assessed in a broader survey that asks for satisfaction with different library services and for frequency of use of those services. The data showed that the average user satisfaction rating was:

SuUB Bremen	2.39
ULB Münster	2.40

The BSB München restricted its satisfaction survey to the users of the reading rooms and did not produce comparable data.

- *User satisfaction with opening times*
  Open times of libraries have always been regarded as an important quality indicator. But the library's location and surroundings, mission and population may influence the need for a certain set of operating hours. Therefore user satisfaction with the opening hours of the library was chosen as the more relevant indicator. Satisfaction ratings for the hours of operation of the libraries were:

SuUB Bremen	1.59
ULB Münster	2.15

The BSB München restricted the survey to the users of its reading rooms.

- *Library visits per member of the population*
  The visits to the library premises (counted by turnstile, electronic counter etc.) per year are compared to the number of members of the population. "Virtual visits" (cases of remote use) by the population should also be counted and evaluated separately, as activities and length of time differ too much from those of traditional visits. As yet, however, most libraries are not able to differentiate

exactly between remote use coming from members of the population and other use, making comparison difficult. The number of visits per year per member of the population was:

SuUB Bremen	13.2 visits
ULB Münster	22.0 visits
BSB München	not applicable

- *Immediate availability*
This indicator is measured based on the percent of immediate loans among the total number of loans made (including reservations and ILL)

$$\text{The indicator is } \frac{A}{B} \times 100\%,$$

where

A = number of loans minus those made by reservation

B = number of all loans from the library collections

$\times$ (including those by reservation) + ILL − loans

The indicator shows whether the collection covers all topics asked for by users and whether there are sufficient copies of specific titles required. By this measure, immediate availability rates were:

SuUB Bremen	92.6%
ULB Münster	84.8%
BSB München	95.0% (data from 1999)

The results clearly showed a high number of books on loan when requested in the Münster library, a library serving a university that has one of the largest populations among German universities (45,000 students).

Two indicators assess the use of electronic services offered by the library and the growing portion of that use that is coming from outside the library building:

- *Percent of the population using the electronic library services*
This indicator is assessed using a survey. Electronic services include the OPAC, the library's website, electronic databases, journals, and other electronic documents, and electronic document delivery. For the libraries studied, the percentage of patrons using these services were:

SuUB Bremen	94.2%
ULB Münster	94.5%
BSB München	between 46.3–64.0%

Bremen assessed the data in a general satisfaction survey that queried only users coming into the library. Münster assessed the data in a special telephone survey, choosing a relevant sample of its population. München assessed the data in its survey of reading-room users. All libraries included more detailed questions as to the use of certain services (e.g. electronic journals).

- *Percent of remote accesses to electronic library services of all accesses*
  This indicator assesses what percentage of electronic services use was from outside the library. One access (or session) is defined as one established connection to an electronic library service. Data collection in the project was restricted to the OPAC and the website and was developed by evaluating the log files of the web server. Remote use of the OPAC and website was as follows:

SuUB Bremen	OPAC	49.9%
	Website	52.3%
ULB Münster	OPAC	62.3%
	Website	40.1%
BSB München	OPAC	40.4%
	Website	46.7%

The data of München refer to the year 1999, the other data to the year 2000.

The Financial Perspective

The indicators for the *financial perspective* answer the question as to whether the library is operating in a cost-effective way. The goals comprise low costs per instance of use or per product and a high proportion of the total budget spent on the print and electronic collection.

- *Total costs of the library per active user*
  The total costs comprise staff costs, collection building and maintenance, administrative costs, operating costs, depreciation and rent. If the library has no cost accounting procedure, the total expenditure could be used as a substitute. "Active users" were chosen for this indicator instead of "members of the population" in order to show the library's options for optimizing cost data. If market penetration rises and there are more active users, costs per user will automatically go down. Costs calculated using this measure were:

SuUB Bremen	322.83 €
ULB Münster	313.14 €
BSB München	350.37 €

München used the expenditure data of 1999 instead of cost data. Bremen and Münster apply cost accounting procedures and used data for the year 2000.

- *Total costs of the library per library visit*
  The costs of individual library visits were:

SuUB Bremen	27.03 €
ULB Münster	11.22 €

For Münster, only the visits in the central library were counted and compared with the central library's costs. In München, only the visits to the reading-rooms were counted. Thus, the data could not be compared to the overall costs there.

- *Acquisitions expenditure compared to the total costs of the library*
  Acquisitions expenditure comprises expenditure for print, electronic, and other media (including licenses and cost-per-view, if paid by the library), but excludes expenditures for preservation. The percentages of the entire library budget at individual institutions were:

SuUB Bremen	40%
ULB Münster	20%
BSB München	33.4% (data from 1999)

Bremen's high percentage of acquisition expenditure shows the possibilities provided within the library's global budget to shift resources between staff and other budget items.

- *Percent of staff costs per library service/product to total staff costs*
  The model differentiates as to the following services/products:
  - collection building (including cataloguing);
  - information services;
  - user services 1: loans/reading-rooms;
  - user services 2: document delivery/ILL;
  - preservation;
  - administration/IT-services;
  - special services/projects.

Staff costs were counted in standardized average rates. Staff members were classified as to their assignment to departments/working groups, not as to specified activities. As a result, short time work in other departments is not represented. The percentage of staff time in each library assigned to each activity was:

• collection building	SuUB Bremen	30.3%
	ULB Münster	27.2%
	BSB München	44.8%
• information services	SuUB Bremen	27.6%
	ULB Münster	8.3%
	BSB München	(all user services): 43.9%
• user services 1	SuUB Bremen	13.0%
	ULB Münster	16.6%
	BSB München	(all user services): 43.9%
• user services 2	SuUB Bremen	7.4%
	ULB Münster	10.2%
	BSB München	(all user services): 43.9%
• preservation	SuUB Bremen	1.3%
	ULB Münster	2.2%
	BSB München	4.9%
• administration/IT-services	SuUB Bremen	13.6%
	ULB Münster	15.8%
	BSB München	6.4%
• special services/projects	SuUB Bremen	6.8%
	ULB Münster	19.7%
	BSB München	not assessed

The results show, for instance, the high percentage of time devoted to collection building in the BSB München with its large special collections, and a high percentage for special services/projects in Münster with special collection tasks and cost-intensive services for the institute libraries in the system.

A last indicator shows the allocation of resources to the electronic library:

• *Percent of acquisitions expenditure spent on electronic media*
Acquisitions expenditure for electronic media includes licenses, the library's own expenditure in consortia, and pay-per-view costs paid by the library. These constitute the following percentages of the acquisitions budget:

SuUB Bremen	7.2%
ULB Münster	3.8%
BSB München	3.3% (data from the year 1999)

The Perspective of Processes

For the *perspective of processes*, the underlying goals are to organize all processes
in such a way that, despite budget restrictions, space for investment into new
developments and improvement of service is allowed. The indicators pick out
background activities as examples of process organization.

* *Acquired media per staff year*
  The processing department comprises all activities from acquisition and
  cataloguing to binding and shelving the new media. Book processing is seen
  here as a typical example for the effectiveness of background processes.
  Staff members in the processing department are counted in FTE (full time
  equivalent). Electronic media are not included in this indicator. The number of
  items processed per person were:

SuUB Bremen	3,748 media
ULB Münster	3,057 media
BSB München	2,797 media (data from the year 1999)

  While Bremen und Münster have integrated acquisition and cataloguing in a
  processing department, München still had two separate departments in 1999.
* *Average media processing time*
  Processing time is seen as the time between the day a document arrives in the
  library and the day it becomes accessible for users. In the project, measuring was
  restricted to purchased print monographs, and the average processing times were:

SuUB Bremen	25.1 days
ULB Münster	17.5 days
BSB München	40.1 days

  The libraries measured processing time as to the separate stages of processing
  (e.g. inventory, cataloguing, subject cataloguing, technical treatment, shelving).
  Books given to commercial firms for binding were excluded. In all libraries,
  subject cataloguing proved to be the most time-consuming part of the process.
* *Number of stages involved in providing a product/service* (for every library
  service/product)
  This indicator tries to determine how well processes are organized and
  streamlined. Processing print monographs and document delivery services were
  evaluated as typical examples. One person performing several activities in a
  sequence for the same product was seen as one stage, but a different person

taking over or the same person taking over again after somebody else was seen as different stages. The number of stages involved in various processes were:

Processing print monographs (purchased monographs only)	
SuUB Bremen	15
ULB Münster	13
BSB München	19
Electronic document delivery	
SuUB Bremen	7
ULB Münster	4–6
BSB München	5–7

Again, one indicator was chosen to show the allocation of resources to the electronic services:

• *Percent of all staff costs spent on electronic services*
Library staff involved in planning, maintaining, providing, and developing electronic services is calculated in FTE (full time equivalent). The definition does not include staff in user services (e.g. reference and training services, staff cataloguing electronic media, and the staff involved in developing the contents of the library website). Only regular staff was counted, not persons working on projects or student assistants. The percentage of staff costs devoted to this area were:

SuUB Bremen	3.9%
ULB Münster	7.5%
BSB München	6.7% (data from 1999)

The Perspective of Potentials

The last perspective, named "potentials," describes the capability of the library to cope with future challenges and addresses its ability to change and improve. The institution's engagement for the library is indicated by the budget it allocates to the library; staff as the main factor for all development, is represented by two indicators for learning and engagement.

• *Library budget as percent of the institution's budget*
Project funding is excluded.
The indicator measures the budget as a percentage of the university budget, not the specific amount.

The percentage for these institutions is:

SuUB Bremen	5.9%
ULB Münster	4.5%
BSB München	not applicable

- *Percent of the library's expenditure from project funding (special grants) or income generation*
  "Special grants" comprise all funding the library gets by special claims, outside of the "normal" budget; funding for staff is included. This indicator assesses whether the library is successful in claiming additional funding or in generating income and is expressed as a percentage of library expenditures.

  For these institutions, the percentages are:

SuUB Bremen	4.5%
ULB Münster	7.4%
BSB München	15.9% (data from 1999)

- *Number of training lessons per staff member*
  This indicator assesses the average number of times each staff member has participated in training lessons. In the project, the data were also assessed per service area (collection building, user services, ...)

SuUB Bremen	0.36 lessons
ULB Münster	1.08 lessons
BSB München	0.69 lessons (data from 1999)

Only external training (not in-house) was considered for the indicator. For in-house training there is often no exact boundary between formal and informal training lessons, so it was excluded.

- *Number of short-time illnesses per staff member*
  A short-time illness is an absence from one to three days. In German public service, such short-time absence need not be accounted for by a medical certificate. Short-time absence is here seen as an indicator of motivation. Data collection in this case must be discussed with staff representatives and must be strictly anonymous. As one of the project libraries did not agree with this indicator and another could not get permission for publishing the data, no data are mentioned here.

  An alternative indicator for staff motivation might be the fluctuation rate. The best indicator – staff satisfaction rate, assessed by a survey – was regarded as too time-consuming for the project.

STRATEGY WITH THE BALANCED SCORECARD

One great advantage of the Balanced Scorecard is its ability to visualize relationships of cause and effect between target values, evaluation data and actions taken.

The following example shows the planning process from the definition of goals and target values and the choice of adequate indicators to the actions that the library takes to achieve the target value (Fig. 2).

As the mission of academic libraries is identical in many aspects, the indicator system within the project might be used as a reference model for benchmarking purposes. Individual differences between libraries can be expressed by different target values and operational actions. Thus, a library whose main task is to provide basic information for students will establish the use of electronic media by offering multimedia-learning material. A special research library, on the other hand, would perhaps offer its scientific journals in electronic form to achieve the same result. Despite such differences, benchmarking is possible. The implementation and continuous use of the Balanced Scorecard demands a large set of data. In the project, a special tool called *Library Audit* was developed that is based on a system of data analysis (OLAP) and that allows for the multidimensional and flexible analysis of data collections. The library in Münster has already filed the *Library Audit* with several thousand bits of data, classified as to the library's products and services. Benchmarking data of other libraries are added continuously. Many of these data will not be used in the strategic evaluation of the Balanced Scorecard, but the large data pool can be useful in addressing many operational problems.

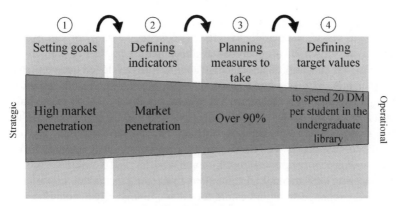

Fig. 2. The Balanced Scorecard.

The number of indicators for the Balanced Scorecard has been purposely kept small in order to avoid a flood of data without direct relevance for strategic management. When choosing the indicators for the Balanced Scorecard, the project libraries oriented themselves using the concept of the hybrid library that combines electronic and traditional library services in a comprehensive function.

Structuring and implementing a scorecard model for a library demands a clear formulation of mission and strategic goals – a duty that has not yet been performed by every academic library. The most important issue in the integrated controlling concept is not to look at different quality aspects separately, but to keep them all in view. An example shows the steps of measuring quality in collection building:

(1) The costs per document processed are low. Does that mean that there are backlogs?
(2) Processing time proves quick and adequate. Processes are well organized. But perhaps there is no time for claiming overdue orders?
(3) Claiming is done regularly and in good time. Maybe staff is overworked, and absence rates due to illness are rising?
(4) Illness rates are quite normal, and a staff satisfaction survey shows high satisfaction with the job.
(5) Everything looks fine. But collection use is going down, and a user survey shows dissatisfaction with the collection: Apparently, much well organized labor has been spent on the wrong material.

Service quality has many aspects – the Balanced Scorecard integrates them, providing a tool for the assessment of programs.

CONCLUSION

Libraries as yet are comparatively free to choose their own models of evaluation, though evaluation and cost analysis have been made compulsory in many institutions of higher education. The scorecard architecture developed in our project is an attempt to connect vision and mission statement, strategy and goals, programs for action, and indicators for results in a consistent management model. The Balanced Scorecard focuses exclusively on indicators with strategic relevance. Thus the model compels library managers to restrict themselves to measures of the critical issues of service quality. The choice of certain indicators and the priority for certain aspects will probably be questioned by some libraries, and the workload connected with assessing the data might detain others from using the model. Libraries could, of course, exchange some indicators for others, though effort would be required to insure that relevant data for controlling the chosen variables are available.

The scorecard developed in this project has already influenced management issues in German academic libraries. The university libraries in North Rhine-Westphalia have agreed on collecting ten "core data" sets that rely very much on the scorecard indicators. The scorecard will probably also be taken into consideration when building up a benchmarking-system for German academic libraries. The Bertelsmann Foundation has for several years been sponsoring a benchmarking project for public libraries with 18 indicators (Bertelsmann-Stiftung). The foundation is now starting a new project for academic libraries together with the German Library Association (Deutscher Bibliotheksverband). The goal is to define a concise set of indicators for controlling and benchmarking and to initiate evaluation and benchmarking procedures on a national scale.

REFERENCES

Bertelsmann-Stiftung, Bereich Öffentliche Bibliotheken: Bibliotheksindex (http://www.bix-bibliotheksindex.de).

Ceynowa, K., & Coners, A. (2003). Cost management for university libraries. Frankfurt a. M.: Klostermann.

Ceynowa, K., & Coners, A. (2002). *Balanced scorecard fur wissenschaftliche Bibliotheken* (Balanced Scorecard for Academic Libraries) Frankfurt a. M.: Klostermann (Zeitschrift fur Bibliothekswesen und Bibliographie. Sonderheft 82).

Kaplan, R. S., & Norton, D. P. (1992). The balanced scorecard – measures that drive performance. *Harvard Business Review, 70*, 71–79.

Kaplan, R. S., & Norton, D. P. (1996). *The balanced scorecard: Translating strategy into action.* Boston: Harvard Business School.

ISO 11620 (1998). *Information and documentation – performance indicators for libraries.*

ISO 2789 (2003). *Information and documentation – international library statistics.*

ISO TR 20983 (2003). *Information and documentation – performance indicators for electronic library services – technical report.*

Poll, R. (2000). The costs of quality: Cost analysis and cost management as counterpart to performance measurement. In: *Proceedings of the 3rd Northumbria international conference on performance measusrement in libraries and information services* (pp. 43–52). Newcastle upon Tyne: Information North.

PERFORMANCE MEASURES OF QUALITY FOR ACADEMIC LIBRARIES IMPLEMENTING CONTINUOUS IMPROVEMENT PROJECTS: A DELPHI STUDY

John B. Harer

INTRODUCTION

Academic libraries have endured rapid change in the past two decades that has had repercussions on how they manage their organization and deliver library services. Skyrocketing costs, especially for journals, explosive growth in new technologies, fiscal exigencies caused by a tightening of public financing of most academic institutions, demands for greater accountability, and the onslaught of electronic delivery of networked information, are just some of the major obstacles libraries are encountering (Lubans, 1996; Riggs, 1993; Shaughnessy, 1987). Customers of academic libraries are increasingly less satisfied because of limited resources and the difficulties they encounter in accessing printed material in a traditional library facility (Doughtery, 1992). The emergence of textual materials in electronic form has added a new dimension to this discontent. While such resources have the potential for meeting the information needs more dynamically, the costs for information have been exorbitant, particularly since full electronic texts have not been sufficient in coverage to supplant printed resources (Tenopir,

Advances in Library Administration and Organization
Advances in Library Administration and Organization, Volume 20, 229–296
ISSN: 0732-0671/PII: S0732067102200115

1993). These phenomena require academic libraries to use a more integrated and flexible approach to problem solving (Gapen, Hampton & Schmitt, 1993).

Because Continuous Quality Improvement (CQI) has had celebrated successes in recognizing industries for developing higher quality operations and for finding effective responses to adversity, some academic libraries are adopting this management strategy, at least in some form, as a means for creating a flexible organization able to respond to change and capable of adapting existing structures and processes for library management and service delivery to meet these challenges (Boelke, 1995). Libraries do not possess their own, unique management science and often adopt management models from other sources. There has been a natural progression from for-profit paradigms to non-profit organizational approaches, beginning with traditional management models and migrating to continuous improvement and learning organizations (Jurow & Barnard, 1993). Just as other popular management theories such as scientific management and management by objectives gained the attention of library managers who adapted them for use in our community, it is only natural that the success of Continuous Quality Improvement in the private sector has lead libraries to look seriously at this management system.

Continuous Quality Improvement (CQI) has its roots in the work of Walter Shewhart, a quality engineer who worked for Bell Labs beginning in the 1920s (Garvin, 1998). Shewhart is known for the development of statistical tools such as the control chart and for the development of an efficient American telephone system. Juran (1991) considers the control chart, along with utilization of sampling techniques, to be the watershed developments in the history of quality control. In the 1950s, two pioneer quality consultants, W. Edwards Deming and Joseph Juran, were asked by the Japanese to teach them the principles of quality control (Ishikawa, 1985). Though Deming and Juran had promoted their views on quality within American industry, they found U.S. manufacturers more interested in high levels of production than in quality control (Ishikawa, 1985). With their industries devastated by the war, Japan faced a monumental task rebuilding their economy and was not helped by a reputation for poor quality in manufactured goods. Thus, Deming and Juran found a more receptive audience for their ideas on quality assurance.

By the 1970s, Japanese products were synonymous with high quality. Gradually, American industry realized that this was due to the implementation of Continuous Quality Improvement programs utilizing Deming's and Juran's ideas and began to adopt CQI for use in the manufacturing and service industries. While private industry made strides in the production of quality goods and services in the 1980s, the assumptions of the traditional approach to library management were questioned by innovators in the profession (Stuart & Drake, 1993). Financial pressures and service demands increased the pressure on libraries to assess their programs and demonstrate their ability to deliver better services (Shaughnessy, 1987). Many librarians are now realizing that models of service must also be able to manage knowledge that is driven by user needs, a prime tenet of Continuous Quality Improvement. The digitizing of materials, coupled with a burgeoning growth in the use of information technology, is causing library leaders to view strategic planning as an absolute necessity as well (Gapen, Hampton & Scmidt, 1993). These phenomena encouraged managers to adapt CQI for academic libraries.

Continuous Quality Improvement (CQI) emphasizes continuous, incremental improvement of critical processes in an organization. Jurow and Barnard (1993) explain that there are some essential elements to any continuous improvement program. They include a focus on employee training, the breakdown of internal barriers between units and/or functional areas, development of strong relationships with external groups, especially stakeholders and suppliers, the elimination of fears of reprisal, the use of problem solving teams, long-range planning, and decision making based on data and statistics gathered for use in improving processes. While the implementation of CQI in academic libraries has barriers to overcome, continuous improvement processes are suitable for libraries in many ways. Libraries are complex, highly structured and hierarchical organizations which operate within functional silos, (like the division between public and technical services), and conflict often results (Jurow & Barnard, 1993). Continuous Quality Improvement breaks down these interdepartmental barriers by teaching employees to work together on problem-solving teams that use a shared knowledge of problem-solving tools and techniques. Miller and Stearns (1994) cite four key principles of CQI and how they differ from traditional library management. First, a library that has implemented CQI focuses resources on customer needs, not on the needs of the organization. Second, major innovations and change for change sake are replaced with a continual process designed to improve quality and service. Third, decisions are made on data and objective fact using standard tools to get at root causes. Fourth, team empowerment creates a collaborative working environment, rather than competition between individuals.

Statement of the Problem

University libraries have found that the implementation of Continuous Quality Improvement presents them with many of the same obstacles that have been encountered by the TQM movement within education in general (Boelke, 1995). The applicability of continuous improvement has been challenged by some professionals because the private sector model for meeting customer needs is not seen as relevant for publicly supported organizations (Doughtery, 1992). Stuart and Drake (1993) also found that, within the profession, there was a fear of loss of control, and employees were reluctant to suggest changes out of fear of management repercussions.

But the experiences of libraries that have implemented Continuous Quality Improvement programs indicate that many of the same factors demonstrating a need for quality improvement in private sector industries are applicable to library organizations (Brockman, 1999). Lubans (1996) reports that his institution was driven to a continuous improvement approach by the rising costs of library materials, fiscal pressures from funding sources, newer technologies for information delivery, and the expectations of library support staff for a reasonable career ladder. There have been two published surveys that reported on libraries that are in various stages of implementing CQI (ARL, 1993). They made it clear that the societal forces Lubans reports are driving more libraries to at least consider continuous improvement. It has become clear that there is a need for systematic, qualitative and quantitative measures of quality programs if CQI is to be applied more widely (Boelke, 1995). Penniman (1993) has suggested that an award similar to the Malcolm Baldrige National Quality Award is needed for library institutions so that libraries will change the way they measure success. An assessment of existing programs is required as we begin to develop these measures.

Purpose of the Study

The purpose of this study was to identify critical processes and performance measures of quality that can serve as a framework for academic libraries that intend to implement continuous improvement programs. It was also designed to forecast significant trends in academic libraries that represent serious challenges to the organization or substantial changes that were taking place in the way libraries conduct their business. The study began by asking three research questions:

(1) What are the critical processes that are fundamental to academic library operations within each of the seven Malcolm Baldrige National Quality Award's Education Criteria for Performance Excellence categories?
(2) What are the performance measures that can serve as indicators of quality for these critical processes?
(3) What will be the most important processes for developing quality academic library operations in the future?

Some operational definitions were important to aid in the design and understanding of the study. These included, but were not limited to:

- Critical processes – That method or strategy by which a library addresses a specific function and has been found to produce results that are replicable over time.
- Performance measures – Numerical information on the results of processes, production and services that quantifies input, output and factors influencing those processes, production and services for the purpose of rating or evaluating them for quality.
- Continuous Quality Improvement – Any strategy that incorporates the principles of W. Edwards Deming for developing work processes that focus on customers and emphasize improving the process on a continual basis.
- Quality – A state of excellence as measured or assessed by a known instrument for measuring quality or by wide-spread acceptance and praise by customers who use products or services deemed to be excellent or considered of an acceptable level of quality.

Significance of the Study

A growing number of educational leaders view higher education institutions, including libraries, as "professional bureaucracies" that are experiencing a paradigm shift from organizations in which professional standards and the operation of the organization are controlled exclusively by the members of the profession working within them to a model best described by the criteria for the Malcolm Baldrige National Quality Award's Education Criteria for Performance Excellence (MBNQA) (Seymour, 1996). These critical processes and performance measures will be useful for academic libraries seeking to develop high quality programs, processes and services, whether any or all aspects of CQI are undertaken. The identification of these critical processes can also assist libraries in understanding the role processes play in improving services and achieving results. It assists libraries in moving from a function-based to a process-based management paradigm, i.e. one where each work process, such as the flow of work in and out of a unit, is the focus of continuous improvement strategies. At the same time, these measures serve as a means of evaluating existing programs or guiding the planning of new processes and services and assist libraries that wish to use the MBNQA's Education Criteria for Performance Excellence for self-assessment and improvement.

LITERATURE REVIEW

Organizations in both the public and private sector share the common experience of coping with changes in organizational dynamics that stem from significant paradigm shifts that threaten the foundational purpose of their organization. These include societal changes influenced by generational differences, the economy, innovations in technology, and demands for operating organizations more effectively, often in the form of new theories of organizational management. When everything is considered, the one thing that has remained constant is that organizations continuously change (Barker, 1993; Conger, 1992; Drucker, 1997). All organizations, public or private, are being challenged to sustain their viability, and change threatens this goal. Paradigm shifts can destroy large sectors of industry (Barker, 1993). The way organizations view their means for remaining effective has also shifted over the years as new theories of how one manages organizations have been promulgated, tried and played out (Cole, 1995; Drucker, 1997; Drummond, 1992).

Continuous Quality Improvement

Continuous Quality Improvement was born out of crisis. The antecedents to the CQI philosophy come from Shewart, Deming, Juran, Crosby and others, but quality as a strategic initiative required more than the advocacy of quality control engineers. Industry leaders had to be shocked into introducing this kind of preventive quality control throughout their organizations by foreign competition that gained market advantage by emphasizing products of the highest quality (Oakland, 1993). By the late 1970s, the Japanese began to seriously cut into the American share of the world markets (Schmidt & Finnigan, 1992). While this was happening, the American economy suffered some serious blows, to include a major gasoline crisis and rising inflation, and all of this combined to make it difficult for industry to be productive and profitable, and changes were in order (Hart & Bogan, 1992). In this climate, CQI succeeded in gaining industry-wide acceptance.

There is a faddish nature to the nomenclature surrounding the Continuous Quality Improvement approach. Total Quality Management is a more well known term for this kind of program, but it has developed a negative connotation in recent years (Cole, 1995). Japanese writers, such as Ishikawa, harken to Feigenbaum's work and refer to the process as "Total Quality Control" (Ishikawa, 1985). Japanese industry also uses the term, "Company-Wide Quality Control (CWQC)." Whether the term used is "Total Quality Management" or "Continuous Quality Improvement," the quality improvement process has had, and continues to have, a significant impact on American industrial competitiveness. Schmidt and Finnigan (1992) suggest this process comes from the following roots:

- Scientific management: Finding the best way to do a job.
- Employee involvement: Workers have influence in the organization.

- Socio-technical systems: Organizations operate as open systems.
- Organizational development (OD): Help to learn and change.
- The New leadership theory: Inspiring and empowering others to act.
- The Linking-pin concept: Creating cross-functional teams.
- Strategic planning: Determining where to take the organization, and how and when to get there.

The Malcolm Baldrige National Quality Award

Events in post-war industrial production in America, as discussed, led some American corporate leaders and prominent authors on American culture to believe there was a crisis of quality in the manufacturing and delivery of American goods and services. The defining moment has often been seen as the 1980 airing of the NBC-TV documentary "If Japan Can, Why Can't We?" After that event, many large corporations sought out W. Edwards Deming, the quality engineer responsible for introducing Continuous Quality Improvement to Japanese industry (Dobyns & Crawford-Mason, 1991). Later, in 1981, William Ouchi wrote a powerful book entitled *Theory Z: How American Business Can Meet the Japanese Challenge* that questioned the prevailing views on managing organizations and introduced Americans to some concepts used in Japanese business management, especially quality circles (Ouchi, 1981). Tom Peters followed this in 1982 with *In Search for Excellence*, discussing at length the crisis in quality in American business practices (Peters, 1982).

By 1982, two forces from the public sector and the private sector converged to promote a national award as a means for energizing American industry by building productivity and competitiveness through quality standards and improvement (Bell & Keys, 1998). In the private sector, the American Society for Quality Control (ASQC), a professional society for quality engineers, and the American Productivity Center (APC), now known as the American Productivity and Quality Center (APQC), a professional association concerned with increasing industrial productivity, began to promote just such an award (Bell & Keys, 1998). In the public sector, the Federal government formed the White House Conference on Productivity that, in turn, created the Committee to Establish a National Quality Award. When the award was created in 1987, it was named for Malcolm Baldrige, Ronald Reagan's Secretary of Commerce and a major proponent of the award.

The Baldrige Award System

This study utilized the MBNQA's Education Criteria for Performance Excellence, first established in 1999 and built on the original award criteria. It consists of seven categories, and within these categories there are at least eight specific criteria items (Baldrige National Quality Program, 1993). (See Appendix 1.) Of the seven categories, the "Leadership" category is the driver of the system. (Brown, 1993). Any plan for organizational quality and quality processes requires a strong and supportive leadership. Without this, there can be a lack of the kind of direction and commitment that is needed to maintain the functionality of the organization and the quality system. Data gathering (Information and Analysis, Category 4) is a key element in the system. Strategic planning (Category 2) is integral to the directions the organization will take over the short and long terms. Human resources issues are addressed in Category 5, Faculty and Staff Focus, and the design and delivery of services is covered in Category 6. Two other categories focus on the School Performance Results. Category 7 focuses on evidence that shows that the organization has achieved the products of the system, and Category 3, Student and Stakeholder Focus, represents the ultimate goal of quality programs (Brown, 1993).

Continuous Quality Improvement in Libraries

Libraries are not immune to the influences of change, the demands of those they serve, or the concerns about quality services or programs (Boelke, 1995; Riggs, 1993; Shaughnessy, 1987). Change has always been a factor in libraries, as they have at various times had to deal with rapid growth after a long period of dormancy. Technological changes have always been a catalyst for change, beginning with the invention of the card catalog and moving to the introduction of the OPAC (Boelke, 1995). Likewise, quality services and programs are not new concepts for libraries and those who manage them (O'Neil, 1994) because there has always been a strong commitment to service and quality within the library profession.

In recent years, libraries have been willing to utilize Continuous Quality Improvement as a means to organize themselves to provide better quality programs and services. O'Neil (1994) indicates that the possible reasons for this are:

- Times are getting tougher and there is a need to prove the worth of libraries more than ever before.
- Libraries have seen successes in business and industry and see the parallels.
- A realization exists that knowledge, and the potential for acquisition and access is so dramatic, that there is a need for customer input.
- CQI/TQM is seen as a useful and effective vehicle for change (1994, p. xi).

Benefits of Implementing Continuous Quality Improvement in Libraries

Gapen, Hampton and Schmitt (1993) report that, "Librarians are rich in their tradition of service. The services which librarians have historically provided have evolved from a tradition of trying to present the most effective library programs, for the largest number of library users, within the limitations of the available tools, while considering the nature of the materials" (p. 18). The movement to utilize CQI in libraries enhances the improvement efforts of the past by providing a systematic, formalized process for improving library programs and services. While improving performance is an ideal no matter what management method is used, Continuous Quality Improvement is beneficial for libraries in several ways, including:

- Management by fact: use of data is feedback for improvement.
- Eliminating rework: because much of the work in a library is labor-intensive, there is a need to simplify the work and make sure it is done right the first time.
- Respecting people and ideas: Team work and an emphasis on ideas from people at the user's level serves libraries as a service organization.
- Empowering people: the process develops the ability of staff to use authority to make decisions at the lowest possible level (Riggs, 1993).

Barriers to Implementing Continuous Quality Improvement in Libraries

There are many proponents of applying CQI/TQM in libraries, but the movement is not without its detractors in the profession. Libraries potentially present many barriers that have to be overcome as one implements Continuous Improvement, particularly the belief that it's just another management fad (Lubans, 1996). Jurow and Barnard (1993) find four primary barriers to implementing CQI/TQM in libraries:

- The vocabulary barrier: a specialized vocabulary from the business sector.
- The commitment barrier: many articles indicate CQI is not a quick fix, and that it requires a significant commitment from the organization.
- The process barrier: individuals in organizations have been taught to solve a problem quickly, then to move on, creating impatience with process.
- The professionalization barrier: some professionals resist CQI/TQM, objecting to the concept that the library user will be viewed as a "customer" (Jurow & Barnard, 1993, pp. 5–6).

Veaner (1994) has been the most vocal opponent based on his views regarding the issue of the professional nature of librarianship. He stresses the intellectual character and leadership functions of librarians and feels that this is at odds with CQI concepts (Veaner, 1994).

Performance Measures for Libraries

In a recent issue of *American Libraries*, in their article "Lies, damn lies and indexes," Lance and Cox (2000) criticize a statistical study of public libraries. The study, authored by Thomas Hennen used numerical measures to rank public libraries, in much the same manner as the Association of Research Libraries (ARL) ranks academic and other research libraries. The Hennen study used data from public libraries that included:

- Circulation per capita;
- Expenditures per capita;
- Periodicals per 1000 residents;
- Staff FTE per 1000 population;
- Cost per circulation (Lance & Cox, 2000, p. 83).

Lance and Cox (2000) find fault with this study based on the poor statistical method, but they also acknowledge the concerns of many in the profession about the use of numerical measures. They argue that the public library is unique in the community it serves, that measures should be defined in the terms of that community, and that the body of statistical data used in this study does not capture this local uniqueness. This is further evidence of an ongoing debate in the library profession on the nature of appropriate performance measures. Blixrud (1998) explains that, within the history of libraries, building, housing, and making collections available have been our prime functions and that quantitative and extensiveness measures were the means for measuring library effectiveness. As a result, comparisons were based on five data categories:

- Volumes held;
- Volumes added, gross
- Current serials;
- Total library expenditures;
- Total professional plus support staff (Kyrillidou & Crowe, 1998, p. 9).

The Movement from Quantitative to Qualitative Measures

As the profession debates the efficacy of using quantitative data as a measurement, the need to develop better output and performance measures and different types of measures continue to emerge (Kyrillidou, 1998). The call for new measures rises, in part, out of a call for accountability and an increase in quality assessment in higher education. Recently, a Pew Higher Education Roundtable, sponsored by ARL and the Association of American Universities, concluded that there was a need to move away from statistical comparisons in libraries based on the "tonnage model" (for example, the number of volumes and serial subscriptions owned) (Blixrud, 1998). Pritchard (1992), ARL's Associate Executive Director in the early 1990s, is generally seen as having begun the initiative for new measures in an article for the ARL newsletter. Pritchard believed that "ARL's active program for statistical analysis, research and management development must center on maintaining the useful approaches of the past and exploring responses to the challenges of the present and future" (1992, p. 2).

There have been two important international efforts to develop indicators of effectiveness or quality. First, there has been considerable work done toward the development of ISO 11620, an approved standard on Library Performance Indicators (Kyrillidou, 1998). The ISO 11620 standard includes twenty-nine indicators grouped into: (1) user satisfaction; (2) public services, including indicators on the delivery of services; and (3) technical services. For Kyrillidou (1998), this standard is notable because of the emphasis it places on user satisfaction, and because of its inclusion of cost-effectiveness indicators. Second, the International Federation of Library Associations (IFLA) has developed international guidelines for performance measurement in academic libraries (Poll & te Boekhorst, 1996). In the United States, the National Association of College and University Business Officers (NACUBO) has also developed benchmarks for the performance of academic departments for thirty-nine functional areas of universities and colleges, including libraries. The data collected by NACUBO has been criticized because it has been used in some quarters as indicators of efficiency or best practices, or even quality despite ARL's repeated warnings that such data should not be interpreted in this way (Kyrillidou, 1998). Additionally, John Minter and Associates has been developing performance measurement initiatives. This work is based on the Integrated Post-Secondary Education Data System (IPEDS) and is regularly published as *Academic Library Statistical Norms*. Minter and Associates report ratios for different types of libraries based on categories from the Carnegie Classification System.

Performance Measures for Libraries Related to the Malcolm Baldrige National Quality Award Criteria
Recent discussions within the profession have suggested that the criteria used for the Malcolm Baldrige National Quality Award provides a base upon which we can develop a means for the assessment of libraries. The expansion of the award into education, and subsequently libraries, is important because it advances institutional commitment to the core values of the organization (Mullen, 1993). Ashar and Geiger (1998) state that libraries must join the national quality movement because the Internet, among other sources of online information, have changed the position

of libraries as the main source of information for research and study, and the quality movement offers the opportunity for libraries to compete with these other sources.

Performance measures of a qualitative nature have not been reported in the literature to the extent that quantitative measures have. As Lubans (1992) has noted, it is not that performance or productivity is not a concern, but that it is not often discussed by library managers in specific contexts. Townley (1989) argues that libraries are labor intensive, but more importantly, that they are made up of a labor force that is highly intelligent, motivated, and skilled. This poses special challenges for library leaders. Townley offers at least four performance measures for leadership that are qualitative in nature:

- Activities that encourage personnel development.
- Actions that point out organizational goals, indicate how these can relate to an individual's goals, and identify possible development activities.
- Support for values that encourage development activities.
- Actions taken to evaluate the results, reward performance, and identify new goals.

The challenge for leaders is to create an organization that has an effective process for employee development. To establish development processes and requirements for employees but not for leaders would be counter-productive.

The decision-making process presents other qualitative measures. Though control of processes is understood as necessary for achieving outcomes, some researchers argue that control of behavior is a prime goal of traditional organizational structures (Ouchi, 1978). Martel (1987) theorizes that power and self-interest project negative connotations. He describes two elements for a new model: formal participation and self-regulation (Martel, 1987). Self-regulation can be defined as control by the employee over those decisions that directly effect the work to be performed (Martel, 1987). Self-regulation occurs best in a team environment, or, at least, in a group setting.

Employee satisfaction is another category of activities where qualitative performance measures can be employed. Locke (1976) reminds us that there is a distinction between "job satisfaction" and "staff morale." Job satisfaction is "an emotional reaction that results from the perception that one's job fulfills or allows the fulfillment of one's important job values" (1976, p. 1307). Morale differs from this in that it often applies to the attitude of a working group, not an individual. When an organization uses teams to achieve goals or to conduct a process, qualitative measures of success are important. Lubans (1998) praises the use of teams, not only for their ability to achieve great success and quality, but also for higher values, including: (1) a sense of decency in the organization; and (2) the respectful and honest exchange of ideas (1998, p. 146). Russell (1998) suggests that, in order to create a successful team environment, there also must be a means for evaluating the effectiveness of the teams, as opposed to just evaluating individuals.

Conclusion of the Review of Literature

Libraries face new challenges under conditions of constant change. Traditional structures of library management are not flexible enough to meet those challenges and still maintain quality (Gapen, Hampton & Schmitt, 1993). Defining and measuring quality are challenges in and of themselves, but transforming library organizations into structures that can build quality into their processes, programs and services to anticipate and address the impact of these changes is a greater challenge. Furthermore, a strong customer focus and the use of customer data for improving library services have in the past been lacking (Riggs, 1993).

During the past decade, librarians looked to the value and benefits of implementing Continuous Quality Improvement to begin the development of library organizations that could respond to the changes being experienced and to anticipate future change. The more recent literature has suggested that there is less emphasis on implementing Continuous Quality Improvement. Some professionals argue that CQI/TQM threatens the professional nature of librarians because it tends to flatten the organization and thereby diminish the status of professionals, and because the emphasis on data gathering is more oriented toward factory-like organizations than it is to knowledge based ones (O'Neil, Harwood & Osif, 1993; Veaner, 1994).

Despite this decline in interest in Continuous Quality Improvement, there is a growing discussion of performance measures that fit within the rubric of CQI/TQM. The profession is working towards evaluative programs combining a qualitative approach with the use of quantitative measures (Kyrillidou & Crowe, 1998). Many of the new measures spring from the principles of CQI. When applying these new measures, data gathering is still a key concept, but the emphasis is on using tools that gather data that are based on service quality indicators, benchmarking, and other qualitative measures (Lakos, 1998). Other performance measures concentrate on customer data and many professionals are making a case for gathering data from key stakeholders using customer data gathering tools, such as the LIBQUAL+ instrument (Lakos, 1998). There is significant concern for using a more comprehensive approach to performance measurement. That movement is calling for the use of qualitative measures based on many of the principles of CQI.

RESEARCH METHODOLOGY

The purpose of this study was to identify the most important critical processes and performance measures of quality in academic libraries implementing Continuous Quality Improvement programs and to forecast the most significant changes that will affect the ability of academic libraries to deliver quality programs and services. The Delphi technique for forecasting future issues of the future and for gaining consensus from a group of experts was used to survey professional librarians who had significant knowledge of Continuous Quality Improvement applications in libraries, either as students of library management or as practitioners who had implemented some significant aspect of Continuous Quality Improvement in a library.

The Delphi Technique

Scientific research seeks to answer questions on topics of importance to at least one sector of society. There are a number of ways to gather information that will answer questions in a scientific manner. Dalkey (1969) describes a continuum of information from "knowledge" to "speculation." Knowledge is data or information that is common to empirical scientific research, often gathered by a carefully planned research methodologies that build in validity and reliability into the data gathering. Speculation, on the other side of the continuum, is information based on very little factual evidence. Dalkey (1969) argues that, in between knowledge and speculation, there is a vast gray area, which is often called "wisdom," "insight," and "informed judgment." At the heart of the Delphi technique is a mechanism for determining informed judgment. The argument made by those who use the Delphi method is that everything that is not knowledge cannot be assumed to be speculation. The Delphi technique is a systematic, scientific means for determining information as informed judgment (Ziglio & Ziglio, 1996).

Linstone and Turoff (1975) have identified three prime reasons for considering the use of the Delphi process:

- The problem does not lend itself to precise analytical techniques.
- The problem at hand has no monitored history or adequate information on its present and future development.
- Addressing the problem requires the exploration and assessment of numerous issues connected with various policy options where the need to pool judgment can be facilitated by judgmental techniques (Linstone & Turoff, 1975).

Often, organizations or scholars must work on problems under conditions of uncertainty where there is insufficient data, and where a theory of the phenomena under study has not been completely formulated. Ziglio and Ziglio (1996) notes that there are two approaches that can be taken in these cases. First, the scholar can wait until there is a nearly complete theory and sufficient data. Second, the scholar can gather the relevant, intuitive insights of experts, creating an informed judgment, as a means for developing the theory and/or data needed to proceed. The second approach is the heart of the Delphi technique.

The Delphi technique was chosen here because the identification of critical processes and performance measures does not lend itself to precise measurement and the theory on the processes and measures for libraries is in a state of fluidity and, therefore, incomplete. A panel was chosen to develop an initial set of qualitative performance measures that could be validated through consensus as the most likely to be considered important for academic libraries to assess quality, especially in institutions implementing Continuous Quality Improvement. The criteria for panel membership emphasized the individual's knowledge and/or experience with the implementation of Continuous Quality Improvement in libraries, especially academic libraries. At the time of this study, all panel members either are currently or were on the faculty and staff of a research library that is a member of the Association of Research Libraries.

Population

The population of this study consisted of professional librarians working in four-year colleges or universities, either as practitioners in academic libraries or as professors of library science, who were identified by an extensive set of criteria as knowledgeable about the theory and implementation of Continuous Quality Improvement/Total Quality Management in an academic library setting. The group consisted of twelve individuals from a cross section of institutions in the United States, including six deans of university research libraries, three assistant or associate deans of university research libraries, and three practitioner librarians who had developed and implemented Continuous Quality Improvement programs.

The participants were identified by using a carefully constructed set of criteria developed by the author with the assistance of the staff of the Association of Research Libraries' Office of Leadership and Management Services. The most important criteria was substantial evidence of knowledge of Continuous Quality Improvement (CQI) in academic libraries, determined by a search of the literature for publications on this topic. A second criteria was membership or involvement in programs that emphasize Continuous Quality Improvement (CQI), such as quality award examiners, including some for the Malcolm Baldrige National Quality Award. A third criteria involved evidence that the potential panelist had implemented a CQI/TQM program or service within an academic library setting.

Instrumentation

There were two phases in the creation and dissemination of the instruments for this study. The first instrument for the study was created to test an initial set of critical processes and performance measures and to refine and revise that list utilizing the advice of experts on an instrument review panel. Prior to the creation of the first instrument, the 1999 Malcolm Baldrige National Quality Award's Education Criteria for Performance Excellence was reviewed by the author. Upon review, the language of the criteria was examined and revised to reflect terminology more appropriate for the library profession and libraries as institutions. It was then reviewed by two other colleagues of the author, including a certified Baldrige examiner for 1996, 1997, 1998, and 1999 – and a judge for the Texas Quality Award (2000). A structure for the first instrument was created using the exact structure of the Malcolm Baldrige National Quality Award's Education Criteria for Performance Excellence. The structure consisted of the seven categories of the award and the items listed within each category. Within this structure, a series of critical processes and performance measures were devised for each of the eighteen items linked to the seven categories used in the award structure. The critical processes were created from a review of the Malcolm Baldrige National Quality Award's Education Criteria for Performance Excellence. The MBNQA criteria listed specific critical processes in the wording of the explanation of each item and within the subsequent text of the booklet in which the categories and items were published. The critical processes for libraries were formulated from the language of the publication on the education criteria and reflected the terminology most appropriate for libraries.

Performance measures were then sought for each item listed in the first instrument. An extensive search of the literature was made to determine the state of research on performance measures for academic libraries and to formulate appropriate measures. Performance measures were sought in known texts on performance measurement in libraries, especially works by Lancaster (1977), Kantor (1984), Riggs (1984), and Hernon (1990). Publications of the Association of Research Libraries (ARL) were then examined for performance measures, because ARL has provided the most recent forum for the discussion of both quantitative and qualitative measures. Publications that have analyzed and interpreted the Malcolm Baldrige National Quality Award criteria for the annual MBNQA awards were also consulted, especially Brown (1993). Furthermore, numerous professional articles in library journals discussing a specific topic or performance measures in general were also reviewed, and measures were culled and revised from them for this study (Ashar and Geiger, 1998; Martel, 1987; Russell, 1998; Townley, 1989).

For the first instrument, the participants in the instrument review panel were asked to list the critical processes and performance measures they deemed useful in priority order. For the second instrument, however, four-point, Likert-type scales were provided for use with each critical process and performance measure to enable each participant to score each item on the instrument according to its perceived importance. The most common form of the Likert-type scale consists of five points, however, other scale ranges are permitted (Anderson, 1988). The use of the four-point scale is recommended by Anderson (1988) and others, along with other even number scales, to avoid an option that permits a "not sure" response.

In this first phase, a panel of experts was formed from a list of potential panelists that met the criteria for selecting panelists as a whole. These panelists consisted of a university library dean who had been a member of the Pennsylvania Quality Award's Board of Examiners, a former dean of a graduate school of library science who published several articles on Continuous Quality Improvement, and two members of the Association of Research Libraries' Office of Leadership and Management Services' executive staff who were the authors of several articles on performance measures. The initial instrument was sent to this panel to review for face validity and clarity and to make recommendations on the critical processes and performance measures to be included. The wording of the critical processes and performance measures was revised based on recommendations of this panel. Furthermore, each panelist provided a prioritized list of critical processes and performance measures. These processes and performance measures were compiled so that the top two critical processes for each item and top two performance measures remained on the compiled list. Where there were discrepancies among the panelists, electronic messages were sent to solicit agreement to secure only two critical processes for each item and two performance measures for each critical process.

The second instrument was structured in the same manner as the first, using the exact structure of the Malcolm Baldrige National Quality Award's Education Criteria for Performance Excellence, including the seven categories and eighteen items of the criteria. (See Appendix 1 for a final list.) The critical processes and performance measures identified through the process of reviewing and revising the first instrument were also included so that each critical process and performance measure corresponded with the appropriate MBNQA category and item. The instrument was designed so that for each MBNQA item, the corresponding critical processes and performance measures were set in tabular form with the item, all assigned critical processes, and all assigned performance measures within the table. (See Appendix 1.) Space was also provided to add an additional critical process and an additional performance measure in each table. The instrument also included an open-ended question that asked the participants to forecast a significant change that will affect academic libraries within the next twenty years. There were nineteen tables in the second instrument, including the tables for each of the eighteen items and one table for the open-ended forecast. Two sets of instructions were provided with the instrument: (1) a cover sheet with detailed instructions on how to score the critical processes and performance measures included in the instrument, how to include any additional critical process or performance measurement, how to score the open-ended question on the forecast of significant changes, and how to return the completed instrument and (2) brief instructions on the first page of the instrument for scoring the critical processes and performance measures, and including additional processes and measures and brief instructions on scoring the open-ended question on the last page.

A third instrument was created with the same structure as the second, including each of the MBNQA's seven categories, eighteen items, and the critical processes and performance measures of the second instrument. Any critical process or performance measure provided by a participant during the completion of the second instrument was added in the appropriate table and linked to the appropriate MBNQA item and critical process, respectively. The first responses from each participant to the open-ended question were included in the final table. The third instrument was then formulated so that the distribution of the scores of each participant for each critical process and each performance measure was linked in a column immediately next to the corresponding process or measure, the participants own score given on the second instrument listed in a column next to the column with the distribution scores of all participants, and a final column to record their revisions, if any for the final phase. Ziglio and Ziglio (1996) describes the use of the distribution of scores as appropriate for Delphi studies utilizing a panel with few members (10–15). To complete the process of a Delphi review of the open-ended forecast (question eight on the second and third instruments) a brief and final instrument was sent to the participants that included only the responses to the open-ended question with the format for reviewing all of the scores of the participants, including the distribution of the scores for each response, their score for each forecast, and a column to record any changes in their score from instrument to instrument.

The first phase began by contacting the instrument review panel. The two professional librarians were mailed a cover letter thanking them for agreeing to participate and providing them with instructions for completing the review along with: (1) the first instrument which included all of the critical processes and performance measures discovered during the literature review process; (2) an unedited copy of the Malcolm Baldrige National Quality Award's Education Criteria for Performance Excellence; and (3) a copy of the edited MBNQA's Education Criteria for Performance Excellence that reflected the terminology more appropriate for libraries. In September 1999, the author met with the two senior officers of the ARL Office of the Leadership and Management Services over a three-day period. During these meetings, the language of the edited version of the MBNQA's Education Criteria for Performance Excellence was discussed, and minor changes were suggested. The first instrument was also reviewed with suggestions made as to which critical processes and performance measures should be included. Responses were then gathered from all of the participants of the instrument review panel and incorporated into the second and complete instrument for the Delphi panel.

A list of potential Delphi panelists was made up by the author prior to the onsite visit to the Association of Research Libraries. Nine professional librarians and library scholars were identified through this process. Discussions with the senior staff of the ARL Office for Leadership and Management Services on possible participants generated the names of three more librarians. A letter was prepared and sent to each of the twelve selected individuals describing the study and soliciting their participation. Ten invitees agreed to participate, one declined due to pressing commitments, and one professional librarian suggested a colleague within her institution. That colleague was queried about her qualifications and then included in the panel.

In late February 2000, each panelist was sent a packet consisting of: (1) a cover letter thanking them for their agreement to participate and a brief explanation of the steps in the process, (2) the second instrument, including the complete instructions on a separate sheet, (3) an unedited copy of the Malcolm Baldrige National Quality Award's Education Criteria for Performance Excellence, (4) an edited copy of the MBNQA's Educational Criteria for Performance Excellence reflecting the changes made to more appropriate library terminology, (5) two copies of the "Informed Consent Document" to comply with the regulations for research on human subjects protocol, and (6) a self-addressed, stamped envelope for ease of return of the completed instrument. The instructions for returning the completed instrument asked the participants to send their response and one copy of the signed "Informed Consent Document" to the author by March 31, 2000.

Responses were received from eight of the eleven participants on time. Follow up calls were made to the remaining participants, and these secured two more responses. Repeated calls to the final participant did not yield any response. One participant included responses that were not part of the instructions. Instead of using the four-point Likert-type scale as described, this participant used half-points on seventeen items. An e-mail message clarified this by agreement to drop the half-point from each of these responses.

The responses to the critical processes and performance measures were compiled on an Excel spreadsheet, and the open-ended responses to the forecast question were collected. These were then added to the third instrument, with the distribution of the scores for each critical process and performance measure in one column and the participant's own score in the adjacent column. The open-ended responses were also included in a table for question 8, with instructions to provide two separate scores: (1) rank in order of importance and (2) rank the probability that the prediction would occur.

The Delphi panel was then sent a second packet that included the third instrument and a cover sheet with the detailed instructions. The packets were sent mid-June and included instructions to return the completed instrument by July 7, 2000. Seven responses were completed on time, while the remaining responses were received after follow-up calls were made. As a result of the first two rounds with the Delphi panel, responses were overwhelmingly ranked as: (1) very important, and (2) somewhat important. A third round was not conducted because the rankings had resulted in consensus.

Data Analysis

To analyze the data, the responses for each critical process, performance measure, and prediction of the future were entered on several spreadsheets. A spreadsheet was created for the data as a whole while other spreadsheets were created for each subset of data. The data was analyzed by calculating descriptive statistics primarily, including mean and standard deviation. Rosenberg (1968) states that much can be learned from simply examining the contents of a contingency table. The set of data was very small, and descriptive statistics explained a lot of what the data projects. A four-point Likert-type scale was used which did not allow for any ambiguous responses. The results were clustered around a small range of means and deviations, with very little variation in scores. Furthermore, Rosenberg (1968) has shown that the cross-tabulation or contingency table permits a very sophisticated analysis of quantitative survey data.

Changes by Panelists in the Number of Questionnaire Responses Between Rounds
The first iteration of the questionnaire consisted of forty critical processes identified by an examination of the 1999 Malcolm Baldrige National Quality Award's Education Criteria for Performance Excellence through a process that revised the language of the Education Criteria to reflect library terminology. The critical processes were structured and linked by the seven categories of the Malcolm Baldrige National Quality Award. The first questionnaire also included

seventy-six performance measures that were identified through an extensive literature search and linked to a critical process.

During the first iteration, the panel was given the opportunity to add critical processes and performance measures they believed were significant but not included in the questionnaire. The panelists added two critical processes to the Leadership category in the first round. Five performance measures were also added to critical processes in the instrument, two for the two critical processes suggested during this round, two in the Strategic Planning category and one in the Library Performance Results category. This brought the total number of critical processes for the second round to forty-two and the total number of performance measures to eighty-one.

Changes in Ratings Between Rounds

A descriptive analysis of the data shows that slightly more than 8% of all the scores made were changed from Round One to Round 2. With forty critical processes and seventy-six performance measures, the panelists that completed both Round 1 and Round 2 scoring had a potential total of one-thousand-forty-four changes in scoring. A total of eighty-six items were changed at least one rank, plus or minus, from Round 1 to Round 2 scores, yielding a quotient of 0.082 or 8.2%.

A further descriptive analysis shows that the panel as a whole changed 7.8% of the scores made on critical processes between Round 1 and Round 2 scores. With forty critical processes, potentially three-hundred-sixty score changes on critical processes could have been made. The panel made a total of twenty-eight score changes at least one rank, plus or minus, between the two rounds. As for performance measures, potentially six hundred eighty-four score changes on performance measures could have been made at least one rank, plus or minus. The panel as a whole made fifty-eight changes in performance measure scores between Round 1 and Round 2.

Research Question One

This study first asked: What are the critical processes that are fundamental to academic library operations within each of the seven Malcolm Baldrige National Quality Award's Education Criteria for Performance Excellence categories? Virtually every critical process in both Round 1 and in Round 2 had a preponderance of scores of either very important or somewhat important. More specifically, critical process number 3.1.1, "How the Library determines the needs and expectations of its current and future students and stakeholders to maintain a climate conducive to learning and inquiry for all students and stakeholders,"

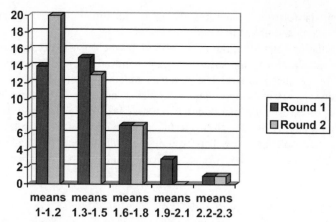

Fig. 1. Distribution of the Means of Critical Processes: Round 1 and Round 2.

received a unanimous response of very important. A total of thirty-two critical processes out of a possible forty, or 80%, in the first round had an overwhelming response from the panel as "important." This factor improved in Round 2. While there was one critical process with a unanimous response of very important in Round 1, there were nine unanimous responses of very important in Round 2, fully 21.4% of all the critical processes. A total of thirty-five of forty-two, or 83.3%, critical processes were seen by the panel as a whole as important.

An examination of the means in a distribution of the responses for each critical process also bears out the view that the Delphi panel saw the identified critical processes as important. Figure 1 compares the distribution of the means of Round 1 with Round 2 for the critical processes.

This figure demonstrates that the mean scores cluster closest to a response of very important. There is no mean above two point three. Fully 50% of the means lie below one point five.

Analysis by Category: Category One: Leadership
The Malcolm Baldrige National Quality Award criteria publications define the leadership category as how the school's senior leaders guide the school in setting directions, seeking future opportunities, and building and sustaining a learning environment and how senior leaders address values, focus on student learning, and provide for performance excellence. For the purposes of this study, the language of the award criteria for each category, including *Category 1: Leadership*, was altered to reflect the terminology of librarianship and academic libraries. For example, "school" was changed to "library" and additional terms for stakeholders

were added to the concept of "customer," not just "students." The Malcolm Baldrige National Quality Award further divides the leadership category into two distinct sub-categories: (1) Leadership System and (2) Public Responsibility and Citizenship.

Five critical processes form the major items for assessing the Leadership System (1.1.1 through 1.1.5) and are critical processes leading to quality in how library leaders set directions and sustain a system of leadership capable of high performance, individual development, initiative, and innovation. Two critical processes were added by the experts. (1.1.6 and 1.1.7). There are also two critical processes for sub-category two, Public Responsibility and Citizenship. (See Appendix 1 for a list of all critical processes.)

In examining the individual critical processes in the sub-category "Leadership System," the critical processes that emphasize communication by leaders gathered a unanimous response from the panel with a score of very important from each member in the second round. Furthermore, processes that address how values and expectations and shared values and directions are communicated were seen by the panel of experts as the most crucial processes required as senior leaders work to make an effective and viable leadership system.

Two critical processes were identified as methods for building an organization's public responsibility and citizenship. The Delphi panel had less to say about this sub-category. Clearly, the panel saw the critical process, "How leaders communicate and promote opportunities for practicing good citizenship . . ." only as somewhat important, yielding a mean of 2.0 (s.d., 71). As for the other critical process, that concerning reducing risk factors, the panel had less agreement as to its importance.

Category 2: Strategic Planning
Strategic planning, as defined by the Malcolm Baldrige National Quality Award's criteria, is how the library sets strategic directions, and how it develops key action plans to support the directions, how plans are deployed, and how performance is tracked. The MBNQA criteria publication divides this category into two sub-categories: (1) strategic development process, and (2) library organizational strategy. (See Appendix 1 for a list of all critical processes.)

The first sub-category "Strategic development process" is known in the language of the MBNQA criteria as an "approach" sub-category. The critical processes in this sub-category address how an organization goes about beginning the strategic planning process. The expert panel views the approach to strategic planning as very important. The panel sustained this agreement from Round 1 to Round 2 because there were no ratings changes between rounds, except that due to a lower response in Round 2. Both the means and standard deviation bear out this scoring (second round means 1.11 [s.d., 0.33] and 1.22 [s.d., 0.66] respectively).

The second sub-category, library organizational strategy, is considered by the MBNQA criteria to be the "deployment" sub-category. The critical processes in this sub-category address how an organization takes the strategic planning developed in the approach and implements it within the organization. In this sub-category, three of the critical processes have been noted as at least somewhat important.

Category Three: Student, Faculty and Stakeholder Focus

Student, faculty and stakeholder focus is defined by the Malcolm Baldrige National Quality Award criteria publications as how the library determines requirements, expectations, and preferences of its external customers, (primarily students, but also other significant stakeholders such as the faculty and administrators of the college or university). The MBNQA publications also emphasize questions relating to how the library builds relationships with students, faculty and stakeholders and how it determines their satisfaction. As with other categories, there are two sub-categories here: (1) Knowledge of student and faculty needs and expectations, and (2) Student, faculty and stakeholder satisfaction and relationship enhancement. (See Appendix 1 for a list of all the critical processes).

Category 3: Student, faculty and stakeholder focus has the greatest degree of agreement and the least deviation in scores of any of the categories. The first sub-category relates to how the library approaches determining student, faculty and stakeholder needs and expectations. In this subcategory, critical process number 3.1.1, which deals with basic data gathering methods used in determining student, faculty and stakeholder needs and expectations, was ranked as being very important by every panelist in both rounds. The other critical processes achieved a unanimous score of very important by Round 2.

Category 4: Information and Analysis

Category 4: Information and analysis is defined by the Malcolm Baldrige National Quality Award criteria publications as the selection, management, and effectiveness in the use of information to support key library processes and action plans, as well as the library's performance management system. There are three sub-categories in this category: (1) Selection and use of information and data, (2) Selection and use of comparative information and data, and (3) Analysis of library performance. (See Appendix 1 for a list of all of the critical processes.)

In the Malcolm Baldrige National Quality Award prescription for assessing an organization's effectiveness, the use of data to make decisions is extremely important. The first two sub-categories address approaches to data gathering and delineate a difference between data on the organization itself and comparable data from other similar institutions. The third sub-category concerns use of the data for improving performance.

Some distinct and different patterns emerge when the critical processes are examined in this category. For the deployment sub-category, "analysis and review of library performance," the experts scored the critical processes, on the average, as very important. For example, in considering critical process number 4.3.1, "how data is analyzed to assess performance," a large majority of panelists scored this as being very important in both rounds. Inter-round changes in the mean and standard deviation show that the panelists made several changes in rating this item, however. At the same time, the critical processes for comparative data gathering were seen as less important. In fact, when the data on the critical processes in this sub-category are compared to the data on the processes in the other two sub-categories, it appears that the experts believe that comparisons are not as important as institutional data.

Category 5: Faculty and Staff Focus
The Malcolm Baldrige National Quality Award criteria publications define faculty and staff focus as how the library enables faculty and staff to develop their full potential and use that potential to improve their performance. This category has three sub-categories, including: (1) Work systems, (2) Faculty and staff education, training, and development, and (3) Faculty and staff well-being and satisfaction. (See Appendix 1 for a complete list of all of the critical processes.)

In *Category 3: Student, faculty and stakeholder focus*, the critical processes addressed the means for assessing the external customer's needs and expectations. In *Category 5: Faculty and staff focus*, the critical processes are related to measurements of the internal customer's needs and expectations. In public institutions such as libraries, the concept of the internal customer is not as common as the external customer. Nevertheless, Continuous Quality Improvement tenets stress the important role played by the internal customer in building quality into programs, services, and processes. The first sub-category deals with the way that an organization uses job design, compensation, and recognition to encourage faculty and staff to be effective employees. The other two sub-categories measure the systems that effect faculty and staff in a direct way. The issues of education and training have been promoted heavily by experts in organizational development, such as Tom Peters and Peter Senge. Education and training are crucial to building a work force that can keep current and effective. Additionally, many publications on employee effectiveness discuss morale issues such as health and safety and general satisfaction with the job.

The critical processes for "work systems" were rated by the panel, on the whole, as very important. All three processes garnered a score of very important from at least 60% of the panelists in both rounds. The process on consistency between the library's compensation and recognition system and work structures, number 5.1.2, was the only critical process among the three in this sub-category that received any score below somewhat important.

Two critical processes were identified that address faculty and staff education and training. The scores indicate that these processes are also very important to the panel. Both critical processes received a score of very important from at least 70% of the experts in both rounds. Four critical processes were identified that address the concerns of faculty and staff morale, well-being and satisfaction. A look at the scores in this sub-category shows less of a concern by the experts for faculty and staff well-being and satisfaction, or at the very least, more deviation in opinion as to the importance of these critical processes. Of the four processes, the means in Round 2 range a low of 1.55 (s.d., 0.71) to a high of 1.88 (s.d., 1.39). Processes concerning faculty and staff health and safety, as well as measurement of faculty and staff well-being and satisfaction, received a score of very important from at least 50% of the experts. However, there was less consensus in this area from the rest of the panel.

Category 6: Library Program and Service Delivery and Support Management
The Malcolm Baldrige National Quality Award's criteria publications terminology for this category has been adapted from the education criteria to more accurately reflect the missions of libraries and address key aspects of process management. The critical processes and performance measures are designed to examine how key processes are designed, implemented, managed, and improved to enhance performance. For libraries, performance is measured within a context of program and service delivery, especially information delivery.

There are two sub-categories in Category 6: (1) Library program and service delivery design and delivery, and (2) Library support processes. The first addresses the production and service driven processes of the library. The second sub-category is concerned with specialized units or services that have a support function for administrative, technical, or operational missions. (See Appendix 1 for a list of all of the critical processes.)

Organizations ultimately seek to get good results, that is, products or services that are characterized by a high degree of quality. This category is followed by the last category, Library Performance Results, because the processes in this category are directly tied to the results sought. The purpose of the critical processes in this category is to achieve the management of processes that get the desired results, including aspects of design, implementation, management, and improvement of those processes.

Three critical processes cover the facets of actual program and service design and delivery. Overall, the experts view these processes as important. Two of these three processes garnered a score of very important from at least 60% of the panel. Critical process number 6.1.2, how the library delivers its educational and information offerings, was rated as being very important by 80% of the experts, for example.

The second sub-category describes the critical process identified for support program management. The panel regards the one critical process in this category as very important. Fully 80% of the experts rated this process very important. The mean for this critical process in Round 1 and Round 2 is 1.3 (s.d., 0.67) and 1.33 (s.d., 0.71).

Category 7: Library Performance Results
The Malcolm Baldrige National Quality Award criteria publications describe the elements of this category in terms of school performance in general and, specifically, in terms of student performance. Libraries are a service-type organization, but they serve to build the success of students in conducting and producing research. This category has four sub-categories: (1) Student performance results, (2) Student and stakeholder satisfaction, (3) Faculty and staff results, and (4) Library specific results. (See Appendix 1 for a list of all of the critical processes.)

Organizations need a results-oriented focus to meet the challenges that face them today and in the future. This category is made up of the major ingredients from *Sub-category 4.3: Analysis and Review of Library Performance*. The award criteria in these sub-categories are intended to identify causal connections to primarily support improvement activities, as well as activities relating to planning and change management.

There is one critical process identified for each sub-category. The panel of experts views these processes as important, on the whole. All of the critical processes were rated as very important by at least 50% of the panel. Three of the four processes were rated as very important in 70% of the responses in the second round. The critical process number 7.2.1, "how the library uses student and stakeholder satisfaction data," received a unanimous rating of very important.

There were forty critical processes in Round 1 and forty-two in Round 2. Every critical process in both rounds received scores of either very important, somewhat important, or a combination of the two from a majority of the experts. Only five critical processes were scored unimportant by any expert, and each received this rating only once for each process. This data has indicated an overwhelming sense that each of these critical processes is important to the measurement of effectiveness.

Research Question Two

This study also asked: What are the performance measures that can serve as indicators of quality for these critical processes? Performance measurement is represented by the output results that an organization would use to determine the effectiveness of its programs and services. Performance measures are linked to the critical processes and are a means for measuring the output of the respective critical process. A precursory examination of the data in both the first and second rounds shows that most of the performance measures were considered to have been rated on a scale from somewhat important to very important. For example, in the first round, three performance measures, numbers 2.1.2.1, 3.1.2.1, and 3.1.3.1, (see Appendix 1) were ranked as very important by the entire panel. Furthermore, thirteen performance measures in Round 1 received scores from the experts of only very important and somewhat important. All total in Round 1, fifty of the seventy-six performance measures, or 65.8% of the total, can be categorized as important.

An examination of the distribution of the means of the responses for each performance measure also bears out the conclusion that the Delphi panel viewed the identified performance measures as important. Figure 2 compares the distribution of the means of Round 1 with those of Round 2 for the performance measures. The bar chart shows that the means are clustered near the score of very important.

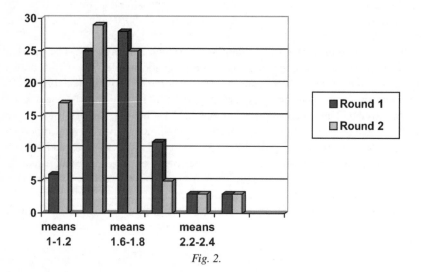

Fig. 2.

Category 1: Leadership

The Malcolm Baldrige National Quality Award criteria for leadership is included in Category 1. The category contains two sub-categories: (1) Leadership system and (2) Public responsibility and citizenship. A total of nine performance measures were identified for the original five critical processes of this sub-category through a literature search. The panelists also suggested one performance measure for each of the new critical processes. In the second sub-category, two critical processes were identified from the MBNQA publications and four performance measures for these original critical processes were formulated from a review of the literature. An expert suggested one more performance measure during his review of the first questionnaire. (See Appendix 1 for a list of all of the performance measures.)

Leadership is not a characteristic that can be easily quantified. Performance measures of leadership emphasize subjective qualities such as what student, stakeholders and employees say about the leaders' visibility or the existence of systems, plans, or mechanisms for leadership activities. One performance measure uses a standard job evaluation, which can provide quantitative data.

In sub-category 1, a scan of the score distribution for these performance measures shows that five of the measures received a score of very important from a majority of the panelists in the first round and all nine had at least 80% of the scores in the distribution listed as either very important or somewhat important in both rounds. Of the nine performance measures, measures relating to the communication of values, directions and expectations (1.1.2.1) and those that account for needs and expectations (1.1.1.1 and 1.1.2.2) were rated as very important by most of the experts.

The experts did not treat the issue of "promoting an environment conducive to learning" as well. Two performance measures were listed for this critical process (number 1.1.3), and neither received a majority of ratings of very important. "How leaders review the leadership system" was also viewed as important in the eyes of the experts. The two performance measures for this critical process have a substantial number of scores of importance, with seven panel members rating "administrator evaluations" as very important.

Sub-category 2: Public responsibility and citizenship has two performance measures for each of two critical processes. The ratings for these performance measures reflect the de-emphasis placed on the critical processes for the sub-category. For example, while critical process number 1.2.1, making risk factors and legal and ethical requirements an integral part of improvement, had a mean of 1.6 (s.d., 0.71) in the second round, the two performance measures had several panel members who scored these as somewhat unimportant and garnered a mean of 1.9 (s.d., 0.92) in the first round. Educating employees on good citizenship was seen as more important by the panel.

Category 2: Strategic Planning
The Malcolm Baldrige National Quality Award Education Criteria for Performance Excellence for strategic planning is included in Category 2. This category
contains two sub-categories: (1) Strategic development process and (2) Library
organizational strategy. Six critical processes were identified from the MBNQA
publications that address strategic planning, two in sub-category 1 and four in
sub-category 2. Eleven performance measures were discovered from a literature
review, with two linked to each critical process except number 2.2.3, "what faculty
and staff resource plans are in place." Two additional performance measures in
this category were added by the panel of experts to critical process number 2.1.1,
"how the library develops its view of the future." (See Appendix 1 for a list of all
of the performance measures.)

Strategic planning is becoming increasingly important for the success of
organizations. This aspect goes beyond setting goals and objectives and now
includes efforts to examine the direction of the organization for the short-term and
long-term future and to anticipate trends that may impact the organization. This
questionnaire identified several performance measures that were thought to be very
important.

The Delphi panel has demonstrated a strong preference for student and
stakeholder information in the analysis of the performance measures. Clearly,
performance measure number 2.1.2.1, "evidence that student and other user
requirements are used in developing goals and plans," has been viewed as very
important to strategic planning. The panel rated this measure a unanimous score
of one (1) in both rounds. As for developing a view of the future, evidence of
a systematic process is seen as more important than evidence that process and
technology capabilities/limitations are considered in developing goals.

Some contrasting performance measures exist in sub-category 2, library organizational strategy. The Delphi panel viewed performance measure 2.2.2.2, "extent
that deployment of plans is part of evaluation," as more important than the optional
measure, number 2.2.2.1, "evidence that key learning strategies are linked to past
learning strategies." Performance measure 2.2.4.1, "proving the integrity of data
from past performances and comparable institutions to support projected performance," had one of the highest means of all the performance measures. However,
the optional measure for this critical process, "comparisons of projections with
performance levels attained by the organization," is also highly regarded.

Category 3: Student, Faculty and Stakeholder Focus
The Malcolm Baldrige National Quality Award criteria for student, faculty and
stakeholder focus is included in Category 3. The category has two sub-categories:
(1) Knowledge of student and faculty needs and expectations, and (2) Student,

faculty and stakeholder satisfaction and relationship management. When the questionnaire for this study was formulated, five critical processes were identified. Ten performance measures were also identified through a literature search, two for each critical process. (See Appendix 1 for a list of all of the performance measures.)

One of the prime tenets of Continuous Quality Improvement is a strong customer orientation. This category addresses the concept of the external customer, the clientele to whom an organization offers goods and services. There is much agreement by the Delphi panel that is evident in the scores assigned to the performance measures. Two measures, number 3.1.2.1, "evidence that satisfaction data is used to design and enhance operations," and number 3.1.3.1, "use of a systematic process to evaluate the importance of trends in student data," were unanimously scored very important in both rounds. A third, "a comprehensive system for tracking student data," achieved a unanimous score of very important, in the second round. Performance measure means in this category ranged from a high of 2.1 (s.d., 0.87) to a low of 1.0 (s.d., 0) in Round 1, and a high of 2.0 (s.d., 0.71) to a low of 1.0 (s.d., 0) in Round 2.

"How data is used" appears to be the most important type of performance measures for this category. The two performance measures achieving a unanimous score of very important in both rounds emphasize use of the data. In measure 3.1.2.1, for example, data on satisfaction and dissatisfaction is to be used to design and enhance operations. "Use of a systematic process" to evaluate trends in student requirements is another performance measure with a unanimous score of very important. In yet a third measure with a full consensus, "use of student comments and complaints" is emphasized as very important. "Use of a systematic process based on student requirements" (measure number 3.1.2.2), had a mean of 1.3 (s.d., 0.67), nearly that of its optional measure of use of student satisfaction data, while performance measure number 3.2.2.2, "extent to which student categories are included in customer satisfaction data," had an average of 1.2 (s.d., 0.42).

Category 4: Information and Analysis

The Malcolm Baldrige National Quality Award criteria for information and analysis is included in Category 4. The category contains three sub-categories: (1) Selection and use of information and data, (2) Selection and use of comparative information and data, and (3) Analysis and review of library performance. Five critical processes were identified from a review of the MNBQA publications, one for sub-category 1 and two each for sub-categories 2 and 3. The questionnaire design identified two performance measures for each of the critical processes. (See Appendix 1 for a list of all of the performance measures.)

One of the most important principles of Continuous Quality Improvement is that decision making should be based on facts and data. In order to build quality into a process, the interrelated components of the process-output, and feedback from customers must be measured to locate the root cause of problems in order to improve the system. This category emphasizes critical processes and performance measures for gathering and using data for measuring performance of operations and services.

Generally, the performance measures identified for this category are considered by the Delphi panel as important, but the scoring does not indicate a very strong propensity towards a score of very important. Seven of the measures attained a score of very important from 50% or less by the panel. Four of these measures were rated very important by less than 50% of the experts. No performance measure in this category achieved a unanimous rating of very important in either round.

Category 5: Faculty and Staff Focus

Category 5 contains three sub-categories: (1) Work systems, (2) Faculty and staff education, training and development, and (3) Faculty and staff well-being and satisfaction. As the questionnaire was designed, nine critical processes were identified through the MBNQA publications. Two performance measures for each critical process, eighteen in total, were also identified by a review of the literature. (See Appendix 1 for a list of all of the performance measures.)

In *Category 5: Faculty and staff focus*, the critical processes and performance measures describe the means for achieving effective internal customer service. The internal customer concept, as an integral part of a quality organization, is a unique aspect of Continuous Quality Improvement. Quality is built into work processes by attending to both external and internal customer needs and expectations.

An overall review of the performance measures in this category shows that almost all of the measures are seen as important, though there is a difference of opinion on the degree of importance. All but one of the measures has a majority of scores of very important or somewhat important, or a combination of the two. Only the performance measure number 5.3.2.2, on "turn over rates" as a measure of faculty and staff well-being and satisfaction, does not have a clear majority of importance scores. No performance measure in this category mustered a unanimous rating, as have other measures in other categories.

Performance measures for critical processes of faculty and staff education, training, and development had the strongest importance scores. Of the four performance measures in this sub-category, each one was assigned scores of a combination of very important and somewhat important by at least 90% of the experts in the first round. One of these measures, "evidence that supervisors include education and training needs suggestions in their employee evaluations," was the only measure in the category that had scores of only one (1) or two (2). The other measures in this sub-category had means ranging from 1.4 (s.d., 0.51) to 1.7 (s.d., 0.94) in Round 1 and a range of 1.22 (s.d., 0.44) to 2.11 (s.d., 1.16) in Round 2.

Several performance measures in this category had sharply different scores than the trend for most of the performance measures in the study. Three performance measures in this category received relatively few ratings of very important or somewhat important. When asked to rate the measures of faculty and staff well-being, two optional measures were listed. As noted, the panel as a whole did not prefer the performance measure "turn-over rates," which may be considered a traditional measure of staff morale. The mean score in the second round was 2.66 (s.d., 0.5). Though this measure was not rated highly, the optional measure for this critical process, a generically written measure requiring some form of mechanism for measuring faculty and staff well being, did not fair much better. It was rated as somewhat important, with a mean of 1.88 (s.d., 0.6).

The work systems' performance measures addressed such issues as the existence of a performance measurement and feedback mechanisms, the use or measurement of compensation and recognition to support performance measurement, and the evaluation of team effort as well as individual effort. Half of the scores for both performance measures on maintaining a safe and healthy work environment were scored as very important, but the other half fluctuated between somewhat important and somewhat unimportant. These diverse scores were true of all six performance measures for the sub-category "work systems."

Category 6: Library Program and Service Delivery and Support Management
The Malcolm Baldrige National Quality Award criteria are included in *Category 6: Library program and service delivery and support management*. This category consists of two sub-categories: (1) Library program and service delivery design and delivery, and (2) Library support processes. As this study was designed, four critical processes were identified through a search of the MBNQA publications, three for the first sub-category and one for the second sub-category. There were two performance measures identified through a review of the literature for each of these four critical processes. Generally, scores of very important were assigned to these performance measures. There appears to be the overall sense that the items in this category are compatible with the Malcolm Baldrige National Quality Award's Education Criteria. (See Appendix 1 for a list of all of the performance measures.)

Ultimately, organizations want to achieve quality results. The last two categories of the Malcolm Baldrige National Quality Award flow one from the other toward this objective. It is difficult to achieve quality results without processes and measures for design, implementation, management and improvement of those processes. Issues such as the design of programs and services as well as those relating to the delivery of those programs and services are crucial to achieving quality results. All organizations have functions that are directly involved with the production of goods and services or the delivery of services to external customers, as well as with functions such as personnel or accounting services, that support the organization in achieving the production or service aspects. This category looks at production and service functions as well as support functions.

Of the eight performance measures in this category, the two on the design of educational and information delivery programs and services (6.1.1.1 and 6.1.1.2), and the two on support process management (6.2.1.1 and 6.2.1.2), were viewed by most of the panel as very important. As for design, one measure, number 6.1.1.1, seeks evidence that program and service design is based on student and stakeholder requirements. The other performance measure for this critical process is a generic statement on using a systematic method to translate these requirements into services and programs. By the second round, all but one panel member scored these as very important. This scoring distribution was similar for the two performance measures concerning support process measurement (critical process number 6.2.1), with an average score of 1.3 (s.d., 0.71) each. However, a split decision was apparent in the case of two other critical processes. As for the two measures for the delivery of educational and information delivery offerings (6.1.2), one measure, "the use of procedures to verify corrective measures to produce desired results," was seen as important, while the other was less so. Performance measure number 6.1.2.2, on "corrective measures for desired results," had nine panel members assign a score of very important or somewhat important. Lastly, there were two performance measures for the critical process that addressed the use of information during the design stage and how that information is used to improve performance (6.1.3). These measures were also viewed as important but not to the degree of many other performance measures.

Category 7: Library Performance Results
The Malcolm Baldrige National Quality Award's criteria on performance results are included in *Category 7: Library performance results*. This category is divided into four sub-categories: (1) Student and clientele performance results, (2) Student and stakeholder satisfaction results, (3) Faculty and staff results, and (4) Library specific results. Four critical processes were identified, one for each sub-category. Six performance measures were also identified, two for each of sub-categories one and four, and one for each of sub-categories two and three. A seventh performance measure, assigned to the critical process for library specific results, was suggested by one of the experts. In all, these critical processes encompass a significant number of processes needed to measure library performance results. Organizations need

to emphasize performance results, making measures in this category extremely important to the entire Malcolm Baldrige award process. (See Appendix 1 for a list of all of the performance measures.)

Quality results are achieved through a leadership system that uses strategic planning and decision making with data and information and that attends to external and internal customer needs and expectations, essentially the first six categories of the MBNQA award assessment process. Most importantly, quality is achieved in results by continually seeking ways to improve the processes of achieving results. The critical processes and performance measures of category seven ask organizational leaders to demonstrate the results of the CQI process, especially that the organization has achieved quality by using data to improve program and service processes.

Above all else, the panel has consistently viewed student and stakeholder satisfaction as extremely important. The performance measure on student and stakeholder satisfaction for this category was accorded the same importance as those in category three. On the opposite end of the scale, purchasing ratios such as volumes added per faculty or student (7.1.1.2), was a performance measure of how performance is improved that was included in the first critical process. No expert rated this as very important. The mean for this measure stayed almost the same, (3.11 with a standard deviation of 0.78) in both rounds. The performance measure, added by the panel after the first iteration, on "evidence of increased usage of library gateways" that was added by the panel after the first iteration, was scored as very important by all but one panelist in the second round.

Research Question Three

This study also asked: What are the most important processes for quality academic library operations in the future? The panelists were asked to predict trends or processes that will be important to academic libraries to meet standards of quality that would most likely occur over the next twenty years. During the first round of the study, twelve separate predictions were made by the nine panelists who responded (Appendix 2). During the second round, the experts were asked to rate these predictions on two scales. The first scale asked them to assign a score of importance to each prediction, using a four-point Likert-type scale. The second scale asked them to predict the likelihood that each forecast would actually occur, also using a four-point Likert-type scale, with one being either most important or most likely to occur. (See Appendix 2 for a list of all of the predictions and the scores on importance and likelihood of occurrence.)

The most important prediction made by those participating in this study is the changing nature of scholarly communication and its impact on the role of libraries, the second forecast in the list. Through two scoring rounds, this prediction held a near perfect score of importance. Only one out of the nine experts scored this item as anything other than very important. This forecast predicts a change in the way library work is performed due to technological change. This forecast stresses the idea that libraries need to be publishers of information as the central theme of the prediction. It was considered highly important, having garnered a mean of 1.44 (s.d., 0.88) in the first scoring and improved to a mean of 1.33 in the follow-up.

Other predictions with a high degree of importance include: (h) commercialization of information and privatization of knowledge, (i) customization and personalization of resources and services for a diverse and dispersed clientele, and (k) an increased need for marketing and promotion of library services. These three items have means ranging from 1.33 (s.d., 0.5) to 1.44 (s.d., 0.88) in the first round and all have a mean of 1.16 in the follow-up.

The second scoring request asked the panel to predict the likelihood that their forecasts would actually occur. According to these experts, the most likely changes will be in any item in which the Internet serves as a central theme. Two of the predictions use the Internet as the central message of the forecast. In the first round, item (c) predicting the impact of the Internet in 1–15 years had a forecast mean of 1.33 (s.d., 0.5) as compared to item (l) a more general treatise on the Internet, which had a forecast mean of 1.11 (s.d., 0.33). Two other predictions are seen as nearly as likely to occur. The impact of the changes in scholarly communication, which was seen as the most important prediction, was rated very likely to occur, with a first round mean of 1.22 (s.d., 0.44) and a follow-up mean of 1.0 (s.d., 0). Furthermore, the concept of new acquisitions coming in electronic form was seen by the experts as very likely to occur, with a first round mean of 1.33 (s.d., 0.5) and follow-up mean of 1.0 (s.d., 0) as well. The least likely prediction to occur, based on the ratings of this set of experts, is changes in the concept of marketing and promotion of library services. This prediction had the highest mean in both the first round and in the follow-up, 2.11 (s.d., 0.6) and 2.17, respectively.

SUMMARY OF THE ANALYSIS OF RESULTS

Results of the final, second round of this study indicate that virtually all of the original and additional critical processes and performance measures are considered important by this panel of experts. Clearly, all critical processes and most performance measures that emphasize a student and stakeholder focus are viewed by the experts as the most important processes and measures. Leadership processes and performance measures also are considered very important in most cases. Though there are mixed results for processes and performance measures concerning faculty and staff focus, faculty and staff education, training and development is seen as very important as well. Most of the remaining categories have varied results in the different critical processes and performance measures. There is a view expressed in the data that the more qualitative measures are more highly regarded by the panel than the quantitative ones. However, there were not enough quantitative measures included in the instrument to make a clear distinction in this regard. Furthermore, all of the predictions of the panel are seen as important and likely to occur, though there are varying degrees of importance and likelihood of occurrence indicated in the data.

STUDY CONCLUSION

This study began with the hypothesis that the framework of the Malcolm Baldrige National Quality Award's (MBNQA) Education Criteria for Performance Excellence, adapted to the language, functions and processes used within libraries, would lead to the identification of useful and effective performance measures of quality for libraries, in general, and for academic libraries in particular. An important aspect of the hypothesis that must be understood first is that these performance measures needed to be linked to critical processes to be valuable. Therefore, the study also hypothesized that the framework of the MBNQA's Education Criteria could identify critical processes as well. After adapting the criteria and conducting an extensive search of the literature, the study was successful in identifying both critical processes and performance measures of quality for libraries. The study identified 42 critical processes through this process and 82 performance measures linked to at least one of these critical processes. (Appendix 1)

This study also sought to assess these critical processes and performance measures of quality for their utility as effective tools for measuring the quality of library services, functions, and processes. By subjecting the identified critical processes and performance measures to a Delphi method of review, the study took the inquiry from one of identifying measures to an inquiry into the level of usefulness of these measures. The study provided a ranked list of importance of the final set of critical processes and performance measures from a review by a panel of experts employing the Delphi method. (See Appendix 1 for a complete list with the panel results.)

This study also sought to assess future trends in libraries that would impact services, functions and processes that would need to be understood for assessing quality and utilizing the performance measures. The study successfully identified 12 predictions of future trends (Appendix 2) that raise concern or will have an impact on how well libraries perform. These predictions were also ranked as to their importance to quality library services and functions, and the Delphi panel rated the likelihood that each prediction would occur.

Key Findings Regarding the Critical Processes

Because there was little variation in the ratings made by the Delphi panel in their findings regarding the identified critical processes, the results of this study show that the experts consider most of the critical processes as "important" at the very least, and many rated them as very important. Only one of the forty-two critical processes had a mean score of more than 2 on a rating scale of 1 to 4, with 1 being "very important." Ten critical processes, or nearly 25%, were unanimously rated "very important." Another 10% had only one expert rating those critical processes as only "important" compared to the rating of "very important" by all the other experts. These results indicate that the experts view most, if not all, of the identified critical processes as significant to the performance measurement process and that these critical processes are highly important to libraries in assessing for quality in the results of their programs, services, and functions.

Within the Malcolm Baldrige Award criteria's seven specific categories, the experts were unanimous in their assessment that the critical processes related to a customer focus, that is the student, faculty and stakeholder focus category, were the most important. No other category had this level of unanimity. Clearly, this study shows that libraries should assess the needs and expectations of students, faculty and other stakeholders in order to plan for quality programs, services and functions. The preponderance of critical processes with a unanimous rating by the panel is not replicated in the other categories. Gauging the needs and expectations of the library's customers is the most important aspect for determining quality programs, services and functions.

In the results found in the other categories, critical processes in the leadership category also were considered very important by the panel. Though all of the critical processes did not receive unanimous ratings, as was true in the stakeholder category, one-third of the nine processes were unanimously rated "very important" by the entire panel, and a fourth was rated "very important" by all but one panel expert. The results in the remaining categories are less clear. Though the critical processes in these categories have low mean scores with small standard deviations for the most part, indicating little variation, there is less agreement among the panel as to their importance. The results of this study indicate that the critical processes for gauging student, faculty and stakeholder needs and expectations, as well as many of those for leadership, methods for gathering information and analysis, and for performance results are regarded as very important to developing, maintaining and assessing quality library programs, services and functions. Within the remaining categories, the study has shown several individual critical processes to also be very important to quality library programs, though the study is less clear as to the categories as a whole.

Key Findings Regarding the Performance Measures

When it comes to an assessment of the identified performance measures, virtually the same pattern of ratings for them as had developed for that of the critical processes was found. The performance measures brought out more overall disagreement amongst the panel of experts, but there is no doubt that the performance measures for *Category 3: Student, faculty and stakeholder focus* (i.e. a customer focus), also received the highest ratings and that there was near unanimous agreement for most of the performance measures in the category. Furthermore, no other category had as many performance measures with this level of agreement amongst the panel of experts.

When the other categories of performance measures are examined, the pattern of ratings of importance for the critical processes holds true, for the most part, in the categories of performance measures. Performance measures in the category for a customer focus are clearly regarded by the panel as more important than any other category, but the categories for leadership, methods of gathering information and analysis, and performance results, follow in the number of measures rated highly by the panel. That is not to say that the experts do not view performance measures for the categories of strategic planning, faculty and staff focus, and program and service delivery as unimportant, but rather that there was more variation in the experts' ratings for the identified measures of these categories. In reality, the panel viewed at least some of the identified performance measures in every category as very important to quality library services, programs and functions. This study shows that when examining this set of performance measures, the experts were in more agreement on performance measures for the categories on a customer focus (student, faculty, stakeholders), leadership, gathering of information and analysis, and performance results, generally in that order, but rated performance measures in all the categories highly. Appendix 1 presents a complete picture of all the performance measures and how these have been rated by the Delphi panel.

Within the categories, there are performance measures that are qualitative and quantitative in nature. Some measures ask for a specific numeric measurement, while others describe a process of measurement. For example, in the customer focus category, a highly rated performance measure is "A comprehensive system or process exists for tracking student and faculty comments and complaints and what is done to address them" and for the leadership category, a highly rated performance measure is "Existence of systems which reinforce the value of continual learning." In more quantitative measures, such performance measures as "turn over rates" in the faculty and staff category, and "purchasing ratios" in the performance results category were included. Measures that were more quantitative in nature were regarded less well, as a whole, than were more qualitative ones. In their responses, some panel members added comments that indicated that quantitative measures were of less value in measuring quality than qualitative measures for now and were likely to remain so in the future.

The study also identified trends and other phenomena that would impact on how well libraries perform in the future. The experts clearly believe that technology will be the most significant change and cause the greatest challenges for library performance. The Internet's proliferation within society, in general, and as a library resource in particular is believed to have the greatest impact on our programs now and in the near future. Some of the technological innovations were perceived as a threat to libraries, and how well institutions approach these innovations will make a difference in the quality of programs, services and functions. The commercialization of information and privatization of knowledge is seen as placing libraries in competition with other information providers, for example. Digitization of information is also seen as a significant impact and may transform the physical state of library organizations from places where people come to visit in person to places visited only electronically.

This study has identified a large body of critical processes and performance measures that can be useful to libraries in the assessment of quality in their programs, services, and functions. By utilizing the Malcolm Baldrige National Quality Award's Education Criteria, these processes and measures also provide libraries with the opportunity to develop quality focused programs, services and functions, and they can contribute to the development of Continuous Quality Improvement for use as a management tool. This body of processes and measures may also contribute to aiding the library profession into developing it's own MBNQA criteria.

The results of this study also show the Delphi panel's opinion about the usefulness of all of the critical processes and performance measures, as well as the most important predictions about future events in libraries. This review provides a window on what processes and measures are important for libraries as they seek to build effective programs, services, and functions. The study shows that, in the judgment of this Delphi panel, libraries must gauge the needs and expectations of their customers and must strive to develop and maintain a strong customer focus in planning for services in order to ensure quality in their efforts. The panel members also noted that processes and measures in the areas of leadership, methods of gathering and analyzing information, and what results libraries actually achieve, must also play a significant role in measuring quality within libraries. This Delphi panel believed that qualitative measures should constitute greater focus in the measurement of quality than quantitative measures and identified specific processes and measures in every category that the panel members saw as very useful or important. The appendix included with this paper should be consulted for a full list of the critical processes and performance measures. Lastly, the Delphi panel identified some important trends that will have an impact on libraries as they plan for, develop and measure quality in offerings. The participants see the ongoing changes in technology as having the most significant impact on libraries.

REFERENCES

Anderson, L. W. (1988). Attitude measurement. In: J. P. Keeves, (Ed.), *Educational Research, Methodology, and Measurement: An International Handbook* (pp. 471–483). New York: Pergamon Press.

Ashar, H., & Geiger, S. (1998). Using the Baldrige criteria to assess quality in libraries. *Library Administration and Management, 12*(3), 147–155.

Association of Research Libraries (ARL) (1993). *Quality improvement programs in ARL libraries: A SPEC kit*. Washington, DC: Association of Research Libraries.

Baldrige National Quality Program (1993). *Education criteria for performance excellence*. Gaithersburg, MD: United States Department of Commerce. Technology Administration. National Institute of Standards and Technology.

Barker, J. (1993). *Paradigms: The business of discovering the future*. New York: Harper Business.

Bell, R., & Keys, B. (1998). A conversation with Curt W. Reiman on the background and future of the Baldrige Award. *Organizational Dynamics, 26*(4), 51–61.

Blixrud, J. C. (1998). Special issue: Issues in research library measurement. *ARL: A Bimonthly Newsletter of Research Library Issues and Actions, 197*(April), 1–2.

Boelke, J. H. (1995). Quality improvement in libraries: Total Quality Management and related approaches. *Advances in Librarianship, 19*, 43–87.

Brockman, F. B. (1999). *Output measures for school library media programs*. New York: Neal Schuman Publishers, Inc.

Brown, M. G. (1993). *Baldrige Award winning quality: How to interpret the Malcolm Baldrige Award Criteria* (3rd ed.). White Plains, NY: Quality Resources.

Cole, R. E. (Ed.) (1995). *The death and life of the American quality movement*. New York: Oxford University Press.

Conger, J. A. (1992). *Learning to lead: The art of transforming managers into leaders*. San Francisco: Jossey-Bass.

Dalkey, N. C. (1969). *The Delphi Method: An experimental study of group opinion*. Santa Monica, CA: The RAND Corporation.

Dobyns, L., & Crawford-Mason, C. (1991). *Quality or else: The revolution in world business*. Boston: Houghton-Mifflin.

Doughtery, R. M. (1992). TQM: Is it the real thing? *Journal of Academic Librarianship, 18*(1/2), 3–4.

Drucker, P. (1997). Introduction: Toward the new organization. In: F. Hesselbein, M. Goldsmith & R. Beckhard (Eds), *The Organization of the Future* (pp. 1–5). San Francisco: Jossey-Bass Publishers.

Drummond, H. (1992). *The quality movement: What Total Quality Management is really about*. East Brunswick, NJ: Nichols.

Gapen, D. K., Hampton, Q., & Schmitt, S. (1993). TQM: The director's perspective. In: S. Jurow & S. B. Barnard (Eds), *Integrating Total Quality Management in a Library Setting* (pp. 15–28). New York: Haworth Press, Inc.

Garvin, D. A. (1998). *Managing quality: The strategic and competitive edge*. New York: The Free Press.

Hart, C. W. L., & Bogan, C. E. (1992). *The Baldrige: What it is, how it's won, how to use it to improve quality in your company*. New York: McGraw-Hill, Inc.

Hernon, P. (1990). *Statistics for library decision making: A handbook*. Norwood, NJ: Ablex Publishing Corp.

Ishikawa, K. (1985). *What is Total Quality Control? The Japanese way*. Englewood Cliffs, NJ: Prentice-Hall.

Juran, J. M. (1991). World War II and the quality movement. *Quality Progress, 24*(12), 19–24.

Jurow, S., & Barnard, S. B. (1993). Introduction: TQM fundamentals and overview of contents. In: S. Jurow & S. B. Barnard (Eds), *Integrating Total Quality Management in a Library Setting* (pp. 1–14). New York: Haworth Press, Inc.

Kantor, P. B. (1984). *Objective performance measures for academic and research libraries*. Washington, D.C.: Association of Research Libraries.

Kyrillidou, M. (1998). An overview of performance measures in higher education and libraries. *ARL: A Bimonthly Newsletter of Research Library Issues and Actions, 197*(April), 3–7.

Kyrillidou, M., & Crowe, W. (1998). In search of new measures. *ARL: A Bimonthly Newsletter of Research Library Issues and Actions, 197*(April), 8–10.

Lakos, A. (1998). The state of performance measurement in libraries: A report from the 2nd Northumbria international conference. *ARL: A Bimonthly Newsletter of Research Library Issues and Actions, 197*(April), 16–19.

Lancaster, F. W. (1977). *The measurement and evaluation of library services*. Washington, DC: Information Resources Press.

Lance, K. C., & Cox, M. A. (2000). Lies, damn lies, and indexes. *American Libraries, 31*(6), 82–87.

Linstone, H. L., & Turoff, M. (Eds) (1975). *The Delphi method: Techniques and applications*. Reading, MA: Addison-Wesley.

Locke, E. A. (1976). The nature and causes of job satisfaction. In: M. D. Dunnette (Ed.), *Handbook of Industrial and Organizational Psychology* (pp. 1297–1349). Chicago, IL: Rand McNally College Publishing Company.

Lubans, J., Jr. (1992). Productivity in libraries? Managers step aside!. *Journal of Library Administration, 17*(3), 23–42.

Lubans, J., Jr. (1996). 'I ain't no cowboy, I just found this hat': Confessions of an administrator in an organization of self-managing teams. *Library Administration and Management, 10*(1), 20–28.

Lubans, J., Jr. (1998). Lessons for libraries from a self-managing team: The Orpheus Chamber Orchestra experience. *Library Administration and Management, 12*(3), 142–146.

Martel, C. (1987). The nature of authority and employee participation in the management of academic libraries. *College and Research Libraries, 47*(March), 110–122.

Miller, R. G., & Stearns, B. (1994). Quality management for today's academic library. *College and Research Libraries News, 55*(7), 406–409.

Mullen, J. A. (1993). Total Quality Management: A mindset and method to stimulate change in higher education institutions. *Journal of Library Administration, 18*(3/4), 91–108.

Oakland, J. S. (1993). *Total Quality Management: The route to improving performance* (2nd ed.). East Brunswick, NJ: Nichols.

O'Neil, R. M. (1994). *Total Quality Management in libraries: A sourcebook.* Englewood, CO: Libraries Unlimited, Inc.

O'Neil, R. M., Harwood, R. L., & Osif, B. A. (1993). A total look at Total Quality Management: A TQM perspective from the literature of business, industry, higher education, and librarianship. *Library Administration and Management, 7*(4), 244–254.

Ouchi, W. (1978). The transmission of control through organizational hierarchy. *Academy of Management Journal, 21*(June), 173–192.

Ouchi, W. G. (1981). *Theory Z: How American business can meet the Japanese challenge.* Reading, MA: Addison-Wesley.

Penniman, W. D. (1993). Quality rewards and awards: Quality has its own reward, but an award helps speed the process. *Journal of Library Administration, 18*(1/2), 127–136.

Peters, T. (1982). *In search of excellence: Lessons from America's best-run companies.* New York: Warner.

Poll, R., & te Boekhorst, P. (1996). *Measuring Quality: International guidelines for performance measurement in academic libraries.* Munich, Germany: K. G. Sauer.

Pritchard, S. M. (1992). New directions for ARL statistics. *ARL: A Bi-monthly Newsletter of Research Library Issues and Actions, 161*(March 2), 1–4.

Riggs, D. E. (1984). *Strategic planning for library managers.* Phoenix, AZ: Oryx Press.

Riggs, D. E. (1993). Managing quality: TQM in libraries. *Library Administration and Management, 7*(2), 73–78.

Russell, C. (1998). Using performance measurement to evaluate teams and organizational effectiveness. *Library Administration and Management, 12*(3), 159–165.

Schmidt, W. H., & Finnigan, J. P. (1992). *The race without a finish line: America's quest for total quality.* San Francisco: Jossey-Bass Publishers.

Seymour, D. (Ed.) (1996). *High performing colleges: The Malcolm Baldrige National Quality Award as a framework for improving higher education.* Maryville, MO: Prescott.

Shaughnessy, T. W. (1987). The search for quality. *Journal of Library Administration, 8*(1), 5–10.

Stuart, C., & Drake, M. A. (1993). TQM in research libraries. *Special Libraries, 84*(3), 131–136.

Tenopir, C. (1993). Forces shaping electronic access. *Library Journal, 118*(September), 154–156.

Townley, C. T. (1989). Nurturing library effectiveness: Leadership for personnel development. *Library Administration and Management, 3*(1), 16–20.

Veaner, A. (1994). Paradigm lost, paradigm regained? A persistent personnel issue in academic librarianship, II. *College and Research Libraries, 55*, 389–402.

Ziglio, M. A., & Ziglio, E. (1996). *Gazing into the oracle: The Delphi method and its applications to social policy and public health.* London: Jessica Kingsley.

APPENDIX 1
CRITICAL PROCESSES AND PERFORMANCE
MEASURES WITH MEANS AND STANDARD
DEVIATIONS FOR BOTH DELPHI ROUNDS

	Round 1 mean	Round 1 s.d.	Round 2 mean	Round 2 s.d.
Category 1: Leadership				
Sub-Category 1: Leadership system				
Critical Process 1.1.1: How leaders account for the needs and expectations of all key stakeholders	1.4	0.96	1.44	1.01
1.1.1.1: What key stakeholders say about the degree to which senior leaders are in touch with the stakeholders' needs and expectations	1.4	0.72	1.22	0.66
Critical Process 1.1.2: How leaders communicate values and expectations and set directions	1.1	0.33	1.0	0
1.1.2.1: What faculty, staff and key stakeholders say about visibility of senior leaders in communicating values, expectations, and in setting directions	1.5	0.52	1.44	0.52
1.1.2.2: What employees say about visibility of senior leaders and the degree to which they are in touch with values	1.3	0.5	1.11	0.33
Critical Process 1.1.3: How leaders promote an environment conducive to learning	1.3	0.5	1.11	0.33

APPENDIX 1 (*Continued*)

	Round 1 mean	Round 1 s.d.	Round 2 mean	Round 2 s.d.
1.1.3.1: Existence of a clear plan for encouraging innovation and creativity	1.9	0.78	1.88	0.78
1.1.3.2: Existence of a method or system of obtaining improvement ideas from employees	1.7	0.66	1.77	0.66
Critical Process 1.1.4: How leaders communicate shared values, directions, and expectations	1.2	0.33	1.0	0
1.1.4.1: Extent to which strategies exist for rewarding all categories and functions of employees for behavior consistent with values	1.4	0.52	1.33	0.5
1.1.4.2: Use of a variety of media to communicate quality values to faculty and staff	1.7	0.52	1.55	0.52
Critical Process 1.1.5: How leaders review the leadership system	1.3	0.5	1.22	0.44
1.1.5.1: Existence of a systematic process for evaluating the integration of quality values into the management approach	1.5	0.72	1.44	0.72
1.1.5.2: Administrator evaluations and feedback mechanisms exist for all key administrators	1.3	0.5	1.22	0.44
Critical Process 1.1.6: How senior leaders share the leadership functions	1.66	1.32	1.66	1.63
1.1.6.1: Extent to which leadership opportunities are afforded other staff	1.11	0.33	1.0	0

APPENDIX 1 (*Continued*)

	Round 1 mean	Round 1 s.d.	Round 2 mean	Round 2 s.d.
Critical Process 1.1.7: How leaders develop leadership throughout the organization	1.22	0.44	1.0	0
1.1.7.1: Existence of systems which reinforce the value of continual learning; for example, reward systems, learning plans	1.22	0.44	1.0	0
Sub-category 2: Public responsibility and citizenship				
Critical Process 1.2.1: How the library makes risk factors and legal and ethical requirements an integral part of performance improvement	1.6	0.71	1.66	0.71
1.2.1.1: A systematic process exists to define standards and goals related to matters of organizational citizenship and public responsibility	1.9	0.92	1.77	0.83
1.2.1.2: Evidence that demonstrates how key goals and standards for public responsibility and organizational citizenship are translated into operational policies	1.9	0.92	1.88	0.78
Critical Process 1.2.2: How leaders communicate and promote opportunities for practicing good citizenship such as strengthening community services, the environment, professional associations, etc.	2.0	0.71	1.88	0.33

APPENDIX 1 (*Continued*)

	Round 1 mean	Round 1 s.d.	Round 2 mean	Round 2 s.d.
1.2.2.1: Existence of a system for monitoring the extent to which employee behavior is consistent with legal/ethical guidelines	2.1	1.05	2.0	1.0
1.2.2.2: Existence of a systematic approach to educate employees regarding legal and ethical behavior	1.7	0.97	1.55	1.01
1.2.2.3: Evidence of involvement in service to key communities and professional associations	1.77	0.66	1.77	0.66

Category 2: Strategic planning

Sub-category 1: Strategic development process

Critical Process 2.1.1: How the library develops its view of the future, sets directions, and translates these directions into a clear basis for communicating, deploying and aligning critical requirements	1.1	0.33	1.11	0.33
2.1.1.1: Evidence that process and technology capabilities/ limitations are taken into consideration when developing long-and short-term plans and goals	1.7	0.71	1.66	0.71

APPENDIX 1 (*Continued*)

	Round 1 mean	Round 1 s.d.	Round 2 mean	Round 2 s.d.
2.1.1.2: Evidence of a systematic process being used to develop the library's view of the future, set directions, and translate these directions into a clear basis for communicating, deploying, and aligning critical requirements	1.3	0.66	1.33	0.71
2.1.1.3: Evidence that faculty and staff capabilities/needs are identified for the strategic plan to be actualized	1.66	0.86	1.33	0.51
2.1.1.4: Evidence that the Library begins planning with a view of where it wants to be and works back to what has to be done today to develop the strategic plan	1.55	0.72	1.5	0.83
Critical Process 2.1.2: How the library gather input for strategic planning, including how key stakeholder needs and expectations and external and internal factors affecting the library are measured	1.2	0.63	1.22	0.66
2.1.2.1: Evidence that student and other user requirements are thoroughly identified and that this information is used in developing goals and plans for the library	1.0	0	1.0	0
2.1.2.2: Inputs are obtained from all appropriate levels and functions in the organization prior to developing operational performance improvement goals and plans	1.4	0.69	1.44	0.72

APPENDIX 1 (*Continued*)

	Round 1 mean	Round 1 s.d.	Round 2 mean	Round 2 s.d.
Sub-category 2: Library organizational strategy				
Critical Process 2.2.1: How the critical action plan requirements, such as faculty and staff development plans and needs, use learning technologies, key measures and indicators, and resources are spelled out and deployed	1.5	0.71	1.44	0.72
2.2.1.1: Evidence of a well-defined and workable process for approach and deployment of long- and short-term plans in the organization to address quality and customer satisfaction are consistent with goals, objectives and programs and services	1.6	0.96	1.66	1.0
2.2.1.2: Evidence that the manner of assigning and deploying resources is consistent with long- and short-term goals and quality services	1.7	1.25	1.33	0.5
Critical Process 2.2.2: How leaders achieve alignment and consistency in key learning strategies and key measures	1.5	0.52	1.55	0.52
2.2.2.1: Evidence that key learning strategies and key measures in the strategic planning process are linked to past learning strategies and measures and classified in the strategic plan	2.3	1.05	2.44	1.01

APPENDIX 1 (*Continued*)

	Round 1 mean	Round 1 s.d.	Round 2 mean	Round 2 s.d.
2.2.2.2: Extent that deployment of plans throughout the organization is part of evaluation	1.8	0.91	1.77	0.97
Critical Process 2.2.3: What faculty and staff resource plans exist to support the overall strategy	1.4	0.96	1.44	1.01
2.2.3.1: Amount of faculty and staff resource plans that support the overall strategic plan	1.5	0.97	1.55	1.01
Critical Process 2.2.4: How projected performance relative to past performance and relative to comparable library organizations and benchmark processes are achieved	2.2	0.91	2.33	0.86
2.2.4.1: Evidence to support the extent to which projections of performance relative to past performance, as well as compared to comparable library organizations, have been accurate	2.5	0.97	2.77	1.09
2.2.4.2: Comparisons of projections with performance levels attained by the organization(s) against which the library benchmarks.	1.5	0.84	1.44	0.88

Category 3: Student, Faculty and Stakeholder Focus

Sub-category 1: Knowledge of student and faculty needs and expectations

APPENDIX 1 (*Continued*)

	Round 1 mean	Round 1 s.d.	Round 2 mean	Round 2 s.d.
Critical Process 3.1.1: How the library determines the needs and expectations of its current and future students, faculty and stakeholders to maintain a climate conducive to learning and inquiry for all students, faculty and stakeholders	1.0	0	1.0	0
3.1.1.1: Identification of the common and unique requirements and expectations for each student and faculty member	1.3	0.48	1.33	0.5
3.1.1.2: Number of contacts with students, faculty and stakeholders that discuss needs and expectations	1.9	0.73	1.77	0.66
Critical Process 3.1.2: How the library maintains awareness of key general and special needs and expectations of current students, faculty and stakeholders	1.1	0.31	1.0	0
3.1.2.1: Evidence that data from satisfied and dissatisfied students, faculty and key stakeholders is used to design, enhance, or change operations and/or services	1.0	0	1.0	0
3.1.2.2: Use of a systematic process to design operational and/or service features based upon student, faculty and stakeholder requirements	1.3	0.67	1.22	0.66

APPENDIX 1 (*Continued*)

	Round 1 mean	Round 1 s.d.	Round 2 mean	Round 2 s.d.
Critical Process 3.1.3: How the library determines and anticipates changing needs and expectations of future students, faculty and stakeholders	1.1	0.31	1.0	0
3.1.3.1: Use of a systematic process to evaluate the importance of trends in student, faculty and stakeholder requirements	1.0	0	1.0	0
3.1.3.2: Evidence exists on the amount of contacts made with future students, faculty and stakeholders that discuss needs and expectations	2.1	0.87	2.0	0.71
Sub-Category 2: Student, faculty and stakeholder satisfaction and relationship enhancement				
Critical Process 3.2.1: How the library provides for effective relationships with key stakeholders to enhance its ability to improve information delivery	1.1	0.31	1.0	0
3.2.1.1: Use of a planned and systematic approach to evaluate and improve service to students, faculty and stakeholders for customer relationship management	1.3	0.48	1.22	0.44

APPENDIX 1 (*Continued*)

	Round 1 mean	Round 1 s.d.	Round 2 mean	Round 2 s.d.
3.2.1.2: Performance evaluation of all functions in the organization is partially based upon the degree to which these functions assist student, faculty and key stakeholder contacts in meeting the identified standards	1.8	1.03	1.66	1.0
Critical Process 3.2.2: How student, faculty and stakeholder satisfaction and dissatisfaction is determined for use in improving the library's ability to improve information delivery and support services	1.1	0.31	1.0	0
3.2.2.1: Comprehensive system or process exists for tracking student and faculty comments and complaints and what is done to address them	1.3	0.67	1.0	0
3.2.2.2: Extent to which students, faculty and key stakeholders in all categories are included in customer satisfaction data	1.2	0.67	1.11	0.33
Category 4: Information and Analysis				
Sub-category 1: Selection and use of information and data				
Critical Process 4.1.1: How information and data are selected and managed for use in support of overall library goals, emphasizing action plans and performance measurement	1.3	0.48	1.11	0.33

APPENDIX 1 (*Continued*)

	Round 1 mean	Round 1 s.d.	Round 2 mean	Round 2 s.d.
4.1.1.1: Existence of specific criteria for selecting measurement indices for programs and services produced for internal and external stakeholders	1.7	0.67	1.55	0.53
4.1.1.2: Existence of a structure/mechanism for collecting information and data for strategic planning	1.3	0.67	1.33	0.71
Sub-category 2: Selection and use of comparative information and data				
Critical Process 4.2.1: How key factors in the selection and use of comparative information and data are selected for use in improving performance relating	1.7	0.82	1.66	0.87
4.2.1.1: Evidence that a systematic process is used to review and follow-up comparable comparisons and benchmark studies that are done	1.7	0.82	1.66	0.87
4.2.1.2: Evidence that a systematic process is used to evaluate processes for gathering comparable and benchmark data	1.8	0.92	1.77	0.97

APPENDIX 1 (*Continued*)

	Round 1 mean	Round 1 s.d.	Round 2 mean	Round 2 s.d.
Critical Process 4.2.2: How the library measures where it stands relative to other library organizations, compares information and compares understanding of their own processes and processes of comparable library organizations	1.8	0.78	1.88	0.78
4.2.2.1: Evidence that a systematic process for selecting comparable institutions for comparison purposes	1.7	0.67	1.66	0.71
4.2.2.2: Scope and breadth of data collected on comparable institutions and benchmark processes	2.1	0.88	2.11	0.93
Sub-category 3: Analysis and review of library performance				
Critical Process 4.3.1: How information and data from all parts of the library are integrated and analyzed to assess performance	1.4	0.69	1.22	0.66
4.3.1.1: Evidence that a systematic process is used to review and follow-up on comparable institutional and benchmark studies	1.8	0.63	1.66	0.5

APPENDIX 1 (*Continued*)

	Round 1 mean	Round 1 s.d.	Round 2 mean	Round 2 s.d.
4.3.1.2: Evaluation measurement indices include measures of internal customer satisfaction, process and output quality	1.2	0.42	1.11	0.33
Critical Process 4.3.2: How the library reviews performance and capabilities, and uses the review findings to improve performance and capabilities relative to goals and plans	1.2	0.42	1.0	0
4.3.2.1: Evidence that analysis data have resulted in changes and improvements in types of data collected and reliability of data	1.4	0.52	1.33	0.5
4.3.2.2: Existence of a structure or mechanism for review of performance of data gathering methods and practices	1.8	0.71	1.77	0.83
Category 5: Faculty and Staff Focus				
Sub-category 1: Work systems				
Critical Process 5.1.1: How faculty and staff compensation and recognition reinforces student achievement and library improvement	1.4	0.51	1.33	0.5
5.1.1.1: Existence of a performance measurement and feedback system for all levels of employees, from senior leaders to individual contributors	1.5	0.71	1.33	0.71

APPENDIX 1 (*Continued*)

	Round 1 mean	Round 1 s.d.	Round 2 mean	Round 2 s.d.
5.1.1.2: Extent to which compensation and recognition is based upon the achievement of quality goals	1.9	0.99	1.77	0.83
Critical Process 5.1.2: How consistency between the library's compensation and recognition system and work structures and processes is defined	1.6	0.96	1.55	1.01
5.1.2.1: Evidence that a systematic, data based approach is used to evaluate the effectiveness of the performance measurement, recognition, and any quality-based compensation systems	1.7	0.67	1.66	0.71
5.1.2.2: Existence of data that indicate levels of employee satisfaction with feedback, recognition, and performance based compensation plans	1.8	0.78	1.77	0.83
Critical Process 5.1.3: How work processes focus on student achievement and needs, and on communication, cooperation, knowledge and skill sharing	1.4	0.51	1.22	0.44
5.1.3.1: Trends showing compensation and recognition being based upon quality/customer satisfaction and operational results, rather than exclusively on financial results and seniority	1.6	0.69	1.55	0.72

APPENDIX 1 (*Continued*)

	Round 1 mean	Round 1 s.d.	Round 2 mean	Round 2 s.d.
5.1.3.2: Trends showing proportional mix of rewards and recognition given out to both teams and individual employees	1.6	0.84	1.44	0.72
Sub-category 2: Faculty and staff education, training and development				
Critical Process 5.2.1: How the library structures and encourages an effective education and training approach for faculty and staff	1.2	0.42	1.11	0.33
5.2.1.1: Existence of a structure or mechanism for determining individual training needs	1.6	0.69	1.55	0.52
5.2.1.2: Evidence that supervisors include education and training needs and suggestions in evaluations	1.4	0.51	1.22	0.44
Critical Process 5.2.2: How the library evaluates the effectiveness of educational and training programs and approaches	1.4	0.69	1.33	0.71
5.2.2.1: Existence of a feedback mechanism for measuring training effectiveness	1.4	0.69	1.33	0.71
5.2.2.2: Amount and objectivity of data collected that indicates the degree to which employees apply knowledge and skills learned in educational courses and training	1.7	0.94	2.11	0.116

APPENDIX 1 (*Continued*)

	Round 1 mean	Round 1 s.d.	Round 2 mean	Round 2 s.d.
Sub-category 3: Faculty and staff well-being and satisfaction				
Critical Process 5.3.1: How the library maintains a safe and healthy work environment	1.7	1.39	1.7	1.39
5.3.1.1: How employees feel about the work environment in terms of health and safety	1.6	0.69	1.44	0.52
5.3.1.2: Extent to which goals and objectives on health and safety are integrated into work functions	1.6	0.69	1.55	0.72
Critical Process 5.3.2: How the library measures well-being, satisfaction, and motivation of all library and staff	1.6	0.69	1.55	0.72
5.3.2.1: Existence of a structure or mechanism for measuring faculty and staff well-being and satisfaction	1.8	0.63	1.88	0.6
5.3.2.2: Turn-over rates	2.6	1.07	2.66	0.5
Critical Process 5.3.3: How the library uses information gathered on the work climate, including faculty and staff well-being, satisfaction, and motivation, to improve the work climate	1.7	0.67	1.66	0.71
5.3.3.1: Amount of information on faculty and staff well-being and satisfaction used in performance improvement	1.9	0.99	1.77	0.83

APPENDIX 1 (*Continued*)

	Round 1 mean	Round 1 s.d.	Round 2 mean	Round 2 s.d.
5.3.3.2: Evidence that employee satisfaction problems are analyzed to determine their root cause	1.7	0.67	1.68	0.71
Critical Process 5.3.4: How the library uses information on the work climate to measure the inter-relatedness of work climate and library organizational results	1.9	0.99	1.88	1.05
5.3.4.1: How data for employee satisfaction indices compare with employee satisfaction data from a parent institution (if any) and/or with comparable libraries	2.2	0.78	2.22	0.83
5.3.4.2: Existence of a structure or mechanism for use of work climate data tied to results	2.2	0.91	2.22	0.83
Category 6: Library Program and Service Delivery and Support Management				
Sub-category 1: Library program and service delivery design and delivery				
Critical Process 6.1.1: How the educational and information delivery programs and offerings are designed, including formative and summative assessments	1.6	0.84	1.44	0.72
6.1.1.1: Evidence to suggest that existing services and programs have been designed based upon student and stakeholder requirements	1.3	0.48	1.11	0.33

APPENDIX 1 (*Continued*)

	Round 1 mean	Round 1 s.d.	Round 2 mean	Round 2 s.d.
6.1.1.2: Use of a systematic methodology to translate student and stakeholder requirements into services and program characteristics	1.4	0.69	1.11	0.33
Critical Process 6.1.2: How the library's educational and information delivery offerings are delivered	1.2	0.42	1.22	0.44
6.1.2.1: Use of an established and acceptable model for cause analysis	2.0	0.81	2.11	0.78
6.1.2.2: Procedures exist and are used to verify that corrective measures/actions produce desired results	1.5	0.71	1.33	0.76
Critical Process 6.1.3: How information gathered in designing programs and services are used to achieve better performance	1.5	0.52	1.44	0.52
6.1.3.1: Use of process modeling as a means for identifying opportunities for improvement in processes and resulting operations and services	1.8	0.78	1.66	0.76
6.1.3.2: Use of comparable institutional data or benchmarks as stimuli for identifying opportunities for quality improvement	2.0	0.47	1.88	0.6

APPENDIX 1 (*Continued*)

	Round 1 mean	Round 1 s.d.	Round 2 mean	Round 2 s.d.
Sub-category 2: Library support processes				
Critical Process 6.2.1: How the library designs, implements, manages, and improves support processes	1.3	0.67	1.33	0.71
6.2.1.1: A systematic cause-analysis process is used to diagnose the causes of quality programs and process deviation that occur in support departments	1.4	0.69	1.33	0.71
6.2.1.2: Systems are in place for measuring performance of support functions and feeding data back to the appropriate personnel	1.4	0.69	1.33	0.71
Category 7: Library Performance Results				
Sub-category 1: Student and clientele performance review				
Critical Process 7.1.1: How student performance results are measured and linked to mission-related factors and assessment methods	1.4	0.69	1.22	0.44
7.1.1.1: Evidence that students' performance has improved by access to library resources	1.5	0.71	1.33	0.5
7.1.1.2: Purchasing ratios (e.g. volumes added per faculty or per student) has been improved	3.1	0.73	3.11	0.5

APPENDIX 1 (*Continued*)

	Round 1 mean	Round 1 s.d.	Round 2 mean	Round 2 s.d.
Sub-category 2: Student and stakeholder satisfaction results				
Critical Process 7.2.1: How the library uses student, faculty, and stakeholder satisfaction results to assess effectiveness of programs and services	1.2	0.42	1.0	0
7.2.1.1: Extent to which satisfaction results are used in process improvement	1.1	0.31	1.0	0
Sub-category 3: Faculty and staff results				
Critical Process 7.3.1: How the library uses the results of faculty and staff well-being, development, satisfaction, and performance to improve the library's programs and services	1.5	0.71	1.33	0.71
7.3.1.1: Extent to which satisfaction results of faculty and staff are used to improve the work climate and to improve processes, programs, and services	1.69	0.69	1.66	0.71
Sub-category 4: Library specific results				
Critical Process 7.4.1: What measures are unique to the library that indicate quality, improvement, or effectiveness	1.7	0.82	1.44	0.72

APPENDIX 1 (*Continued*)

	Round 1 mean	Round 1 s.d.	Round 2 mean	Round 2 s.d.
7.4.1.1: Evidence of the specific results that are unique to the library or unit being assessed	1.7	0.82	1.44	0.72
7.4.1.2: Evidence that a specific result that is unique to the library or unit being assessed has improved from past performance or can be compared to benchmark institutions	1.8	1.03	1.55	1.01
7.4.1.3: Evidence of increased usage of library gateway information	1.33	0.71	1.16	0.40

APPENDIX 2
LIST OF PREDICTIONS WITH MEANS AND STANDARD DEVIATIONS OF QUESTIONNAIRE RESPONSES

Data on Prediction 1	Invisible access gateways: users will be unaware of whether the library has played a role in giving them access to desired information; library as "place" will be minimal in 1–15 years.

	Round mean of occurrence	Round s.d. of occurrence
Round 1	2.11	0.92
Round 2	1.83	0.98

	Round mean of importance	Round s.d. of importance
Round 1	2.0	0.86
Round 2	1.83	0.98

APPENDIX 2 (*Continued*)

Data on Predication 2	Changing nature of scholarly communication and its impact on the role of libraries; changes in pedagogy; distance education and use of technology; changes in the way we work due to the introduction of new technologies

	Round mean of occurrence	Round s.d. of occurrence
Round 1	1.22	0.44
Round 2	1.0	0

	Round mean of importance	Round s.d. of importance
Round 1	1.11	0.33
Round 2	1.0	0

Data on Prediction 3	Internet: already changing the breadth and scope of use and "institution." Major changes will occur in five years

	Round mean of occurrence	Round s.d. of occurrence
Round 1	1.33	0.5
Round 2	1.16	0.4

	Round mean of importance	Round s.d. of importance
Round 1	1.22	0.44
Round 2	1.0	0

Data on Prediction 4	The nature of learning programs and the scholarly communication process will change. We must be prepared to be partners not intermediaries in both. We must help design courses and become publishers and packagers of information. We must be able to identify the outcome/impact of the work (the value we add) and demonstrate we manage our resources effectively.

	Round mean of occurrence	Round s.d. of occurrence
Round 1	1.77	1.0
Round 2	1.33	0.81

	Round mean of importance	Round s.d. of importance
Round 1	1.44	0.88
Round 2	1.33	0.81

APPENDIX 2 (*Continued*)

Data on Prediction 5	Twenty years is far too long for any credible prediction. Technology, however, will drive all significant change.	
	Round mean of occurrence	Round s.d. of occurrence
Round 1	1.77	0.83
Round 2	2.0	0.89
	Round mean of importance	Round s.d. of importance
Round 1	1.77	0.83
Round 2	2.16	0.75

Data on Prediction 6	The proportion of new "acquisitions" will shift more heavily to the area of electronic resources	
	Round mean of occurrence	Round s.d. of occurrence
Round 1	1.33	0.5
Round 2	1.0	0
	Round mean of importance	Round s.d. of importance
Round 1	1.55	0.52
Round 2	1.33	0.51

Data on Prediction 7	Expectation that information resources in digital format will be available whenever needed, to whomever needs them, wherever they need them. What was traditionally the domain of physical library collections will move out such that "libraries" and "collections" as we have defined them will disappear	
	Round mean of occurrence	Round s.d. of occurrence
Round 1	1.77	0.66
Round 2	1.5	0.54
	Round mean of importance	Round s.d. of importance
Round 1	1.77	0.83
Round 2	1.16	0.4

Data on Prediction 8	Commercialization of information and privatization of knowledge	
	Round mean of occurrence	Round s.d. of occurrence
Round 1	1.88	0.78
Round 2	2.16	0.98

APPENDIX 2 (*Continued*)

	Round mean of importance	Round s.d. of importance
Round 1	1.33	0.5
Round 2	1.16	0.4

Data on Prediction 9	Customization and personalization of resources and services for a diverse and dispersed clientele	
	Round mean of occurrence	Round s.d. of occurrence
Round 1	1.66	0.71
Round 2	1.0	0
	Round mean of importance	Round s.d. of importance
Round 1	1.33	0.5
Round 2	1.16	0.4

Data on Prediction 10	Close involvement of library staff in curriculum development and instructional design/delivery	
	Round mean of occurrence	Round s.d. of occurrence
Round 1	2.22	0.97
Round 2	1.83	0.75
	Round mean of importance	Round s.d. of importance
Round 1	1.77	0.83
Round 2	1.5	0.83

Data on Prediction 11	Increased marketing and promotion of library services to meet increased competition from commercial and independent sources	
	Round mean of occurrence	Round s.d. of occurrence
Round 1	2.11	1.11
Round 2	2.16	0.4
	Round mean of importance	Round s.d. of importance
Round 1	1.44	0.72
Round 2	1.16	0.4

APPENDIX 2 (*Continued*)

Data on Prediction 12	The Internet's explosion into the lives of the academy: teachers and students alike	
	Round mean of occurrence	Round s.d. of occurrence
Round 1	1.11	0.33
Round 2	1.0	0
	Round mean of importance	Round s.d. of importance
Round 1	1.44	0.72
Round 2	1.5	0.83

ABOUT THE AUTHORS

Gail Bader is Assistant Professor, Department of Anthropology, Ball State University, Muncie, Indiana. A cultural anthropologist, Bader's research interests include educational anthropology, the cultural construction of work, computing and technology, and U.S. and Japanese culture.

John M. Budd is Professor and Associate Director of the School of Information Science and Learning Technologies at the University of Missouri – Columbia. He is the author of numerous journal articles and books, including *The Academic Library* and *Knowledge and Knowing in Library and Information Science.*

Bambi Burgard has served as Assistant Dean for Academic Affairs/Student Achievement at the Kansas City Art Institute since May 2002. Upon completion of her undergraduate education, she began doctoral study in counseling psychology at the University of Missouri-Kansas City where she earned her Ph.D. in 1999. She completed her predoctoral and postdoctoral internships at the University of Missouri-Kansas City counseling center.

Harvey R. Gover is on the library faculty of Washington State University (WSU) Libraries and is the Assistant Campus Librarian for WSU Tri-Cities. Formerly, he was Public Services Librarian, Tarleton State University, a branch campus of Texas A&M. He was a principal author of the 2000 edition of *ACRL Guidelines for Distance Learning Library Services.*

William Graves III is Associate Professor of Humanities at Bryant College in Smithfield, Rhode Island. A linguistic anthropologist, Graves is interested in the diverse roles that language and communication play in social and cultural change. He has conducted fieldwork on issues of social and cultural change among Native Americans, in diverse organizational settings in the U.S., in enterprises undergoing privatization in Russia and, most recently, among small-scale entrepreneurs in Belarus.

José-Marie Griffiths served as the Chief Information Officer at the University of Michigan and Vice Chancellor for Information Infrastructure at the University of Tennessee. She was responsible for strategic IT planning; the development and implementation of academic and administrative computing, telecommunications and networking activities; and IT alliances with external organizations. She is the recipient of numerous awards for her contributions to information science, the development of the IT industry, and support for women in computing. She currently holds an endowed chair and professorship in the School of Information Sciences at the University of Pittsburgh and is Director of the University's Sara Fine Institute for Interpersonal Behavior and Technology.

John B. Harer has been a school and academic librarian for over twenty-seven years. As an academic librarian, he has held various positions in access services, reference, and personnel administration. He is currently the Director of the Library at Catawba College in Salisbury, NC.

Donna Meyer's career has included management of computer labs, teaching computer skills, designing curricula that integrated information skills into core subject areas, creating web sites, and managing library collections. She currently works as Director of Library Resources at Northcentral University in Prescott, Arizona, providing quality online graduate research services.

Rush Miller has been Hillman University Librarian and Director of the University Library system at the University of Pittsburgh for eight years. He serves as co-chair for the Association of Research Libraries e-Metrics Project. Miller is active in the profession and writes regularly on library management, international librarianship, diversity, digital library content and e-Metrics.

James M. Nyce, a cultural anthropologist, is interested in how information technologies are used in and can change workplaces and organizations, particularly in medicine and higher education. A docent at Linköping University, Nyce's research interests include the historical, social aspects of library and information science, the design and evaluation of information systems, and information use in science and medicine. Nyce is Associate Professor at the School of Library and Information Management, Emporia State University, Emporia, Kansas, and Visiting Associate Professor at the Indiana University School of Medicine, Indianapolis.

Charles Oppenheim is Professor of Information Science at Loughborough University, Loughborough, UK. His main professional interest is where the law interacts with information services. He is also interested in knowledge management, measuring the value and impact of information, citation studies, bibliometrics, national and company information policy, the electronic information and publishing industries, ethical issues, chemical information handling, patents information and policy issues related to digital libraries and the Internet.

Roswitha Poll is chief librarian of the University and Regional Library Münster. From 1991 to 1993 chair of the German Association of Academic Librarians, since 1997 chair of the German Standards Committee for Information and Documentation. She chaired the IFLA group for the handbook on performance measurement in libraries and is now convener of the ISO working group for the International Standard of Library Statistics and member of the ISO group for performance measurement. She is working in national and international groups on collection preservation, quality management, statistics and cost analysis in libraries.

Mary Jane Rootes is a Public Services librarian at Abraham Baldwin Agricultural College in Tifton, Georgia. She worked previously at the Pitts Library of Andrew College in Cuthbert, Georgia.

Sherrie Schmidt is the Dean of University Libraries at Arizona State University. She began her tenure at ASU as Associate Dean of Library Services in 1990 and was named Dean in 1991. Prior to that, she worked at Texas A&M University, the University of Texas at Austin, the FAXON Company, the University of Texas at Dallas, AMIGOS, the University of Florida, and Ohio State University. Most of her professional activities relate to the use of technology in libraries.

Joan Stenson is a Research Associate in the Department of Information Science at Loughborough University, Loughborough, UK, where she is currently undertaking a doctorate.

Richard Wilson is Professor of Business Administration and Financial Management at Loughborough University, Loughborough, UK. He has inter-disciplinary interests in the valuation of information assets. His publications reflect his research interests in management control, financial control, marketing control and strategic control.

SUBJECT INDEX